REFERENCE ONLY

THE ENCYCLOPEDIA OF DEAFNESS AND HEARING DISORDERS

Diagram of the ear.

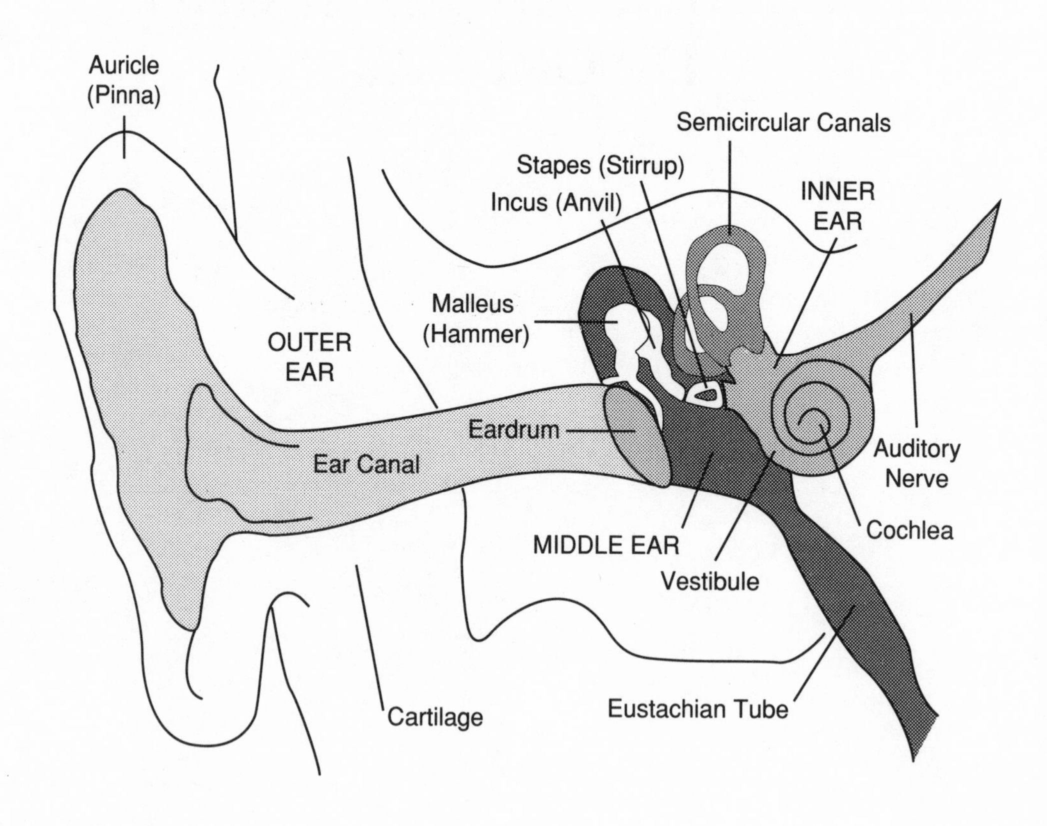

THE ENCYCLOPEDIA OF DEAFNESS AND HEARING DISORDERS

REFERENCE ONLY

Carol Turkington and
Allen E. Sussman, Ph.D.

ST. THOMAS AQUINAS COLLEGE
LOUGHEED LIBRARY
SPARKILL, NEW YORK 10976

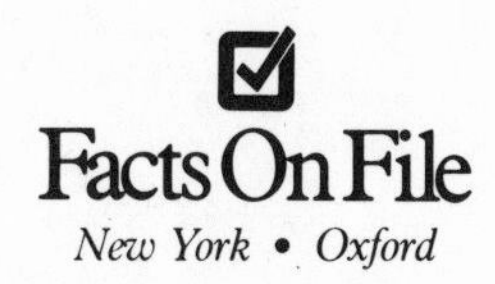

Facts On File
New York • Oxford

THE ENCYCLOPEDIA OF DEAFNESS AND HEARING DISORDERS

Copyright © 1992 by Carol Turkington and Allen E. Sussman, Ph.D.

All rights reserved. No part of this book may be reproduced or utilized in any form or by any means, electronic or mechanical, including photocopying, recording, or by any information storage or retrieval systems, without permission in writing from the publisher. For information contact:

Facts On File, Inc.
460 Park Avenue South
New York NY 10016
USA

Facts On File Limited
Collins Street
Oxford OX4 1XJ
United Kingdom

Library of Congress Cataloging-in-Publication data
Turkington, Carol.
The encyclopedia of deafness and hearing disorders / Carol Turkington and Allen E. Sussman.
p. cm.
Includes bibliographical references and index.
ISBN (invalid) 0-8260-2267-4
1. Deafness—Encyclopedias. 2. Ear—Diseases—Encyclopedias. I. Sussman, Allen. II. Title.
[DLM: 1. Audiology—encyclopedias. 2. Deafness—encyclopedias. 3. Hearing Disorders—encyclopedias. WV 13 T939e]
RF290.T93 1991
617.8'003—dc20
DNLM/DLC
for Library of Congress 91-16451

British data available on request from Facts On File.

Facts On File books are available at special discounts when purchased in bulk quantitites for businesses, associations, institutions or sales promotions. Please contact the Special Sales Department of our New York office at 212/683-2244 (dial 800/322-8755 except in NY, AK or HI).

Composition by the Maple-Vail Book Manufacturing Group
Manufactured by Hamilton Printing Company
Printed in the United States of America

10 9 8 7 6 5 4 3 2 1

This book is printed on acid-free paper.

CONTENTS

ACKNOWLEDGMENTS

The authors would like to thank the staff members at Gallaudet University who so generously offered their time during this project. In particular, we wish to thank the staffs at the university's library, public relations office, university press, information center and law center.

In addition, we appreciate the efforts of countless people from national organizations, services and government agencies concerned with deaf and hard-of-hearing people who offered a great deal of helpful information, statistics and support.

Thanks also to Elca Swigart, Ph.D., director of the Speech and Hearing Center at Reading Hospital and Medical Center, and audiologist Robert Gance for their valuable technical assistance and review; and to staffers at the National Library of Medicine and the medical libraries of Hershey Medical Center, the University of Pennsylvania Medical Center and Reading Medical Center. Hats off as well to public relations personnel at the National Institute of Mental Health and the National Institutes of Health.

We would also like to thank our editors at Facts On File—Kate Kelly, Nick Bakalar and Gary M. Krebs—for their thoughtful suggestions and editorial guidance. We are also grateful to Bert Holtje of James Peter Associates for his valuable support.

Finally, thanks to friends and family for their patience and understanding. And a very special thank you to Michael and Kara.

PREFACE

One out of 10 Americans has some degree of hearing loss, and one out of every 400 is profoundly deaf. Yet many hard-of-hearing and deaf people in this country do not consider themselves handicapped, at a disadvantage or lacking in any way. They do not believe their hearing loss makes them less—just different—and they look upon the deaf community as a separate culture, as rich and diverse as that of the hearing world.

The Encyclopedia of Deafness and Hearing Disorders reflects the continuing struggle within the deaf community to maintain its integrity following years of segregation and misunderstanding. Although educators, linguists, experts in the field of deafness, and deaf and hard-of-hearing people have come a long way toward replacing antagonism with cooperation, there still remain areas of controversy.

Where there are conflicting philosophies on a particular point, we have tried to identify and explain all sides. An extensive bibliography at the end of the book will assist anyone who wishes to explore any specific topic in further depth.

In addition, we made a great effort to include comprehensive appendixes that reflect the diverse range of organizations and support services available to deaf and hard-of-hearing people. We have tried to list as many of these special groups and services as we could find, together with current addresses and phone/TDD numbers.

Entries include all facets of deafness and hearing disorders: physiology of the ear, experts in education, science, linguistics and communication, famous deaf individuals, organizations and groups for deaf people, brief outlines of deaf culture in foreign countries, and more. All entries are cross-referenced to related subjects.

Although information presented in this book comes from the most recent sources available, readers should keep in mind that changes can occur very rapidly in medicine and technology. The very latest technical information on hearing aids and on assistive and telecommunications devices should be obtained from specialists. The authors would also like to stress that information in any medical entry should not be substituted for prompt medical attention.

Carol Turkington
Morgantown, PA

Allen E. Sussman, Ph.D.
Washington, DC

A

acoupedic method See AUDITORY-ORAL METHOD.

Acoustical Society of America Founded in 1929, this group is interested in learning more about ACOUSTICS and the promotion of its practical applications. In addition to regular meetings to discuss research, the society publishes the *Journal of the Acoustical Society of America*. The society holds two meetings a year to discuss current research.

acoustic impedance Some sounds that enter the ear canal and reach the eardrum are reflected, while others are absorbed and eventually reach the inner ear. The tendency of the ear to oppose (reflect) the passage of sound is called its acoustic impedance.

How great the acoustic impedance will be depends on the size and stiffness of the eardrum membrane and the ossicles.

Testing a person's acoustic impedance gives important information about the health of the middle ear. This is because a person may have an ear disease with very little hearing loss. Unlike more routine hearing tests, impedance tests can detect both the presence and characteristics of middle-ear diseases. (See ACOUSTIC IMMITANCE; AUDIOMETRY.)

acoustic immitance The measure of acoustic immitance can be defined as either acoustic admittance or ACOUSTIC IMPEDANCE. ''Admittance'' refers to how easily energy flows through a system, while ''impedance'' represents the opposition to the flow of energy. A system with high acoustic impedance to the flow of sound will have low acoustic admittance.

Acoustic immitance tests are used as an adjunct to hearing tests, since a patient may have a significant ear disease with little hearing loss. While most hearing tests can uncover type and degree of hearing loss, they may not reveal specific ear diseases.

Unlike most hearing tests, acoustic immitance can reveal middle ear disorders without requiring any active participation by the patient. This is particularly helpful in the testing of young children. (See also AUDIOMETRY.)

acoustic nerve See AUDITORY NERVE.

acoustic neuroma A rare benign tumor (also called an auditory nerve tumor or Schwannoma) arising from the Schwann cell sheath of cranial or spinal nerve roots most commonly involving the auditory (eighth cranial, or hearing) nerve. This type of tumor can cause HEARING LOSS on the affected side and is usually slow-growing. About 5% to 7% of brain tumors fall into this type, which occur more often in women between ages 40 and 60.

Almost all are located within the internal auditory canal and originate from the vestibular division of the AUDITORY NERVE, although occasionally these tumors arise from the cochlear division of the nerve.

Symptoms begin with TINNITUS in one ear with a progressive high-frequency hearing loss. There is often a loss of speech discrimination out of proportion with the hearing loss, probably due to the lessened ability of the cochlear nerve to conduct sound because of the tumor's pressure. Compression of the blood vessels within the internal auditory canal may also cause hearing loss because of the reduced blood flow to and from the COCHLEA. As it enlarges, it may press on the brainstem and cerebellum, causing lack of coordination, and eventually may press on the fifth cranial nerve (causing pain in the face) or the sixth cranial nerve (causing double vision). As the vestibular nerve cells within the internal auditory canal degenerate, unsteadiness or VERTIGO can result.

When occurring in both ears, it represents an inherited form of acoustic neuroma diagnostic of central neurofibromatosis (elephant man's disease).

Diagnosis is confirmed by hearing and balance tests, AUDITORY BRAINSTEM RESPONSE TEST, and by brain scans. (Most acoustic neuromas affect the size and shape of the internal auditory canal by eroding the bone, which can be detected through scanning.)

While these tumors rarely become malignant, early detection while hearing loss is still minor is imperative, since hearing may be spared with early intervention. (See also AUDITORY NERVE TUMORS.)

acoustic reflex A reflex contraction of a small muscle in the middle ear that stiffens the chain of ossicles (hammer, anvil, stirrup) to protect the inner ear.

acoustics The science concerning the properties, production, control, transmission, reception and effects of sound. Acoustics, a subdivision of physics, has two major branches: architectural acoustics and environmental acoustics.

Architectural acoustics includes the study of how sound waves operate in closed spaces and how to create the best acoustical conditions for a variety of purposes (such as sound transmission in concert halls and theaters). Environmental acoustics focuses on noise pollution and its control, including improved insulation, room partitions and so forth.

Other branches of acoustics include musical acoustics (the operation and design of musical instruments and the study of how musical sounds affect listeners), engineering acoustics (development of high-fidelity sound recording and reproduction), ultrasonics (acoustical phenomena with vibration rates above the audible range of 20,000 hertz), underwater sound, mechanical vibration and shock and speech communication.

acoustic spectrum The distribution of the intensity levels of various frequency components of a sound.

acoustic trauma Ear damage resulting from a sudden, intense noise (such as a gunshot) including an immediate sense of fullness, TINNITUS and HEARING LOSS. If the noise is loud enough, it can rupture the EARDRUM and disrupt the ossicular chain (hammer, anvil, stirrup), causing a conductive hearing loss without much accompanying nerve damage because the middle ear defect now protects the inner ear.

Generally, the tinnitus and feeling of fullness subside after the injury, and hearing improves—although there may be a degree of permanent hearing loss. The amount of the loss depends on the intensity and duration of the noise and the sensitivity of the ear. In milder cases, the hearing loss is only in the ear closest to the noise.

Hearing loss from damage to the middle ear can sometimes be corrected; a ruptured eardrum can heal by itself in time, and the small bones of the ear may be repaired or replaced.

Normally, permanent loss is mild (a high tone dip between 3,000 to 6,000 hertz), although the loss may be greater if the ear is very sensitive or the noise was quite loud. Because there is almost always some amount of temporary hearing loss following acoustic trauma, some time must pass before the amount of permanent damage can be measured.

In addition, the body may sustain other types of damage from excess noise: Since the body's equilibrium is partly controlled by inner structures, intense sound can cause motion sickness, dizziness and disorientation. (See also NOISE; OCCUPATIONAL HEARING LOSS.)

acupuncture Although acupuncture has been used to treat deafness in the People's Republic of China, there has been no scientific evidence of its usefulness for SENSORINEURAL HEARING LOSS.

adenoidectomy The surgical removal of the ADENOIDS, the twin lymph nodes at the back of the nose above the tonsils. This operation is usually performed on a child with abnormally large adenoids that are causing recurrent middle ear or sinus infections which could lead to hearing loss. Often, an adenoidectomy is performed at the same time as a tonsillectomy.

There are few aftereffects of the operation, and the patient can usually begin to eat normal meals one day afterward.

adenoids The two lymph nodes above the tonsils at the back of the nose that are partly responsible for protecting the body's upper respiratory tract against infection. Although they tend to enlarge during childhood when these types of infections are common, adenoids usually shrink after about age five and disappear by adolescence.

However, they sometimes continue to grow, obstructing the eustachian tube and causing hearing problems. In addition, if secretions behind the nose are obstructed by oversized adenoids, this can lead to infections of the nose (rhinitis) that can spread to the middle ear.

Occasional infections can be treated with antibiotics, but surgery to remove the adenoids (ADENOIDECTOMY) may be needed if infections become chronic.

adhesive otitis media A chronic middle ear infection that scars the eardrum. The eardrum collapses and adheres to the ossicles (hammer, anvil, stirrup) and middle-ear promontory, causing hearing loss. A chronic infection such as this can also cause new bone to form in the middle ear lining. Treatment involves drainage and the use of antibiotics. (See also OTITIS MEDIA.)

adventitious deafness Also called acquired deafness, this is a hearing loss that occurs later in life. (See also HEARING LOSS.)

aero-otitis media Also called barotrauma, this is a temporary yet painful condition that can interfere with hearing. It is caused by unequal external air pressure and pressure in the middle ear and is usually caused by rapid descent in a poorly-pressurized airplane when a head cold does not allow normal equalization of air pressure in the ear. The symptoms may include severe pain, inflammation, bleeding and rupture of the eardrum membrane. Underwater divers and airplane pilots are also susceptible to this problem.

The middle ear (located behind the eardrum) is connected to the nasal cavity by a thin tube called the EUSTACHIAN TUBE. Normally, when the external air pressure rises or falls, air from the nose goes through the eustachian tube and equalizes pressure in the middle ear cavity. Air pressure can also be equalized by periodically opening the eustachian tube by swallowing or yawning. But fluids from head colds, tumors or enlarged tonsils, can block the eustachian tube and interfere with the equalization process.

In a descending airplane, the external air pressure increases and in order to equalize pressure in the middle ear, air must pass from the eustachian tubes to the middle ear. In an ascending airplane, air in the middle ear expands as external air pressure falls; if the eustachian tube is blocked, the expanding air in the middle ear has nowhere to go and presses against the eardrum, bulging it outward.

It is usually harder to equalize pressure when descending rather than ascending in a plane, as the increasing external pressure creates a vacuum in the middle ear that seals the eustachian tubes.

As pressure in the ear equalizes, the pain subsides unless the eardrum has already been damaged. Although the eardrum membrane can rupture because of the difference in pressure on its two sides, most often the pain continues until the middle ear fills with fluid.

Rupture of an eardrum membrane relieves the pain and pressure, but it can cause dizziness, partial hearing loss and middle ear infections. Usually, pain and hearing loss produced during a flight under these conditions is temporary and disappears by itself. If there are no complications, a ruptured eardrum heals itself in about a month.

Deep sea divers encounter the same problem: Every 10 to 15 feet as they descend in the water, they must equalize the pressure in their ears to the external pressure of the sea.

age-related hearing loss See AGING AND HEARING LOSS.

aging and hearing loss About 12 million Americans experience some form of hearing loss as they age—and about half of those over age 75 experience some hearing loss. These late-deafened adults make up the vast majority of the elderly with hearing problems. They are usually not profoundly deaf and are not likely to know sign language or consider themselves a part of the deaf community.

Hearing loss among the elderly is much more prevalent among men than women, among whites than blacks, among people earning less than $7,000 per year and among people who didn't graduate from high school. One explanation for these characteristics could be that those in lower economic brackets are likely to become ill more often, and chronic health conditions can lead to or exacerbate hearing problems.

If ignored and left untreated, the hearing problems among this country's elderly interfere with communication, curtailing social activities and unnecessarily limiting an older person's circle of friends.

Hearing loss among the elderly can be caused by a variety of things, including infections of the outer, middle or inner ear; blood clots; loud noises; hereditary conditions; bony growths in the middle ear; and adverse reactions to drugs or medication.

However, the most common cause of deafness in the elderly is PRESBYCUSIS—a progressive deterioration of the hearing organ leading to an intolerance for loud noises but not total deafness. Although presbycusis is usually blamed on old age, not every senior citizen is affected. The loss of hearing sensitivity may be caused by chemical and mechanical changes in the inner ear and breakdown of these structures or by complex degenerative changes along the nerve pathways leading to the brain. These changes slow the signals traveling from the ear to the brain. Although these breakdowns also happen in the outer and middle ear, the most significant changes occur in the inner ear.

Researchers do not definitely know what causes presbycusis, but there are several things that may contribute to it: prolonged exposure to loud noise, reduced blood flow to the inner ear and atherosclerosis.

Damage to the outer or middle ear causes CONDUCTIVE HEARING LOSS, which involves the blocking or impairment of movement in the outer or middle ear so that sound waves can't travel through it. With this type of hearing loss, sounds are perceived as soft and muted. Talking louder often helps a person with this type of loss, and HEARING AIDS may help people with this problem. Conductive loss is usually caused by IMPACTED EARWAX, extra fluid, abnormal bone growth in the ear or infection.

Central deafness is quite rare among the elderly, although it can occur. It is caused by damage to the hearing nerve centers inside the brain and affects not the perception of sound but the understanding of language. Causes range from an extended illness with high fever, to head injuries, circulation problems or tumors.

Damage to the inner ear or auditory nerve causes a SENSORINEURAL HEARING LOSS in which perception of pitch and loudness may be affected. People with this type of loss can often hear sounds but cannot understand words (for example, ''hem'' for ''hen,'' ''pin'' for ''tin.'') Hearing aids may help, but they will not eliminate the distortions associated with sensorineural hearing loss.

Many older people experience hearing loss, but they don't all experience loss in the same way; the kind of hearing loss depends on where the damage in the ear has occurred and the severity may range from mild to profound. For example, some older persons have high frequency losses, which means they have trouble hearing high-pitched sounds. Thus, the higher-pitched voices of women and children may be more difficult for them to understand.

Warning Signs and Management of Hearing Loss Warning signs that a person's hearing is beginning to fail may be suspected if there is a history of ear infections and the person experiences TINNITUS (ringing in the ear) and starts talking loudly, increasing the TV or radio volume, complaining that others are mumbling and confusing words that have similar sounds. The person may also be unable to hear soft or high-pitched sounds.

The early signs of hearing loss may be very slight, but the earlier it is diagnosed, the better chance there is of successful management. The important first step is a correct diagnosis by a physician who specializes in the ear and evaluation by an AUDIOLOGIST to identify the degree and type of hearing loss. Audiologists can also design a rehabilitation program and offer hearing aid evaluation and orientation together with training in lipreading techniques and speech.

Services for Senior Citizens Senior citizens who begin to experience hearing loss may find particular help from SELF HELP FOR HARD OF HEARING PEOPLE (SHHH), which is primarily designed for the needs of late-deafened people. Founded in the early 1980s by a former senior officer in the Central Intelligence Agency, the group stresses self-assertiveness and advocacy.

Other special services for senior citizens with hearing problems include the GALLAUDET UNIVERSITY summer program "Elderhostel" designed for late-deafened adults and a special section for late-deafened adults as part of the ALEXANDER GRAHAM BELL ASSOCIATION FOR THE DEAF.

AIDS.Net A special computer bulletin board established by DEAFTEK.USA. AIDS.Net is an information-sharing network about AIDS established after a conference on AIDS and deafness held in 1988 in Toronto.

Information for the bulletin is provided by the National Information Clearinghouse on AIDS, together with agencies and professionals serving deaf people. Currently, members in the United States, Canada and England are participating in AIDS.Net. Subscribers are also free to ask questions of experts provided by the bulletin board. CONTACT: International Communications Ltd., PO Box 81, Fayville, MA 01745; telephone 508-620-1777 (voice/TDD).

AIDS and hearing loss Infection with human immunodeficiency virus (HIV) can result in acquired immune deficiency syndrome (AIDS) or AIDS-related complex (ARC). Both AIDS and ARC are associated with neurological complications that include hearing loss: An estimated 75% of adult AIDS patients and 50% of all ARC patients have auditory system abnormalities.

Why this happens is unknown, although direct infection of the nervous system by HIV is well documented. Hearing disorders in AIDS could be caused directly by HIV infection of the cochlea or the central auditory system.

On the other hand, many AIDS complications are the result of opportunistic infections rather than HIV itself—the most prevalent infection, CYTOMEGALOVIRUS (CMV), is known to damage the auditory system in congenital infections. More than 90% of AIDS patients have CMV.

air bone gap The difference between air- and bone-conduction thresholds. (See also AUDIOMETRY.)

air conduction Transmission of sound to the inner ear via the ear canal and middle ear.

air conduction audiometry A subjective method of estimating hearing sensitivity by evoking responses of the patient to air conducted pure tones. (See also AUDIOMETRY.)

air conduction test, pure tone See AUDIOMETRY.

alarms, sound sensitive See ALERTING DEVICES; WAKE-UP ALARMS.

alarms, visual See ALERTING DEVICES; WAKE-UP ALARMS.

Alberti, Salomon (1540–1600) This 16th century German physician and professor at the University of Wittenborg was the first to call attention to people hard of hearing—those who can hear loud sounds and are not deaf—and attributed deafness to "some lack" in the development of the fetus. He claims to have discovered the cochlea, and knew about the modiolus.

alerting devices A compensatory device that alerts deaf and hard-of-hearing persons to a sound (doorbell, crying baby, telephone, timer) by activating a visual light signal.

These visual alarms often feature one or more flashing lights, (one lamp or all the lights in the house). The lights are turned on either through direct wiring or by using a signal transmitted through the building's wiring system. Some systems can even alert to different sounds by using different light patterns for each sound. (See Appendix 3.) for the addresses of companies that sell these. (See also WAKE-UP ALARMS.)

Alexander Graham Bell Association for the Deaf A private, nonprofit organization serving as an information center, publisher and advocate of effective ways of teaching deaf and hard-of-hearing persons to communicate orally.

Since its inception in 1890 as the American Association to Promote the Teaching of Speech to the Deaf, the association has had one primary purpose: to promote the use of speech, SPEECHREADING and residual hearing by hard-of-hearing people.

Most of the first members of the group were articulation teachers who used the VISIBLE SPEECH method, a system of written symbols representing the anatomical formation of speech sounds, invented by Alexander Melville Bell (Alexander Graham's father). Since then, the association has grown into an international organization serving 4,500 members in 38 countries. Its members fall into four categories: professionals in the deafness field, parents of hard-of-hearing children, deaf adults who can speak and speechread and others who believe in the importance of oral communication.

Although it began as an active proponent of speech for deaf people, the organization has gradually expanded its interests to include research, family support and financial assistance to help deaf students attend classes with hearing peers. It also sponsors workshops and biennial conventions and publishes the *Volta Review,* a professional journal published six times a year; *Newsounds,* a newsletter published 10 times a year; and *Our Kids Magazine.* In addition, the association sells books of interest to members through mail-order catalogs and presents books on various oral topics for teachers, parents and deaf and hard-of-hearing adults.

Three distinct sections within the organization focus on the needs of three specific groups: deaf adults (Oral Deaf Adults Section), parents (International Parents Organization) and teachers (International Organization for the Education of the Hearing Impaired).

Oral Deaf Adults Section This voluntary, nonprofit service section was formed in 1964 to help improve the education, employment and social opportunities of deaf people. Members receive a newsletter, a membership directory and scholarship support and have access to programs designed to help parents of children with hearing problems.

International Parents Organization This section provides special help to families of children with hearing problems who are interested in promoting aural/oral education. Membership is open to any member of the association and includes a magazine, *Our Kids Magazine,* family workshops, educational scholarships and a family support network throughout the United States and Canada.

International Organization for the Education of the Hearing Impaired This special section, formed in 1967, promotes excellence in aural/oral education for deaf children and adults. The aims of this group include the development of effective oral education and communication programs, research into oral communication and an information exchange among educators. (See also BELL, ALEXANDER GRAHAM; VOLTA BUREAU.)

Contact: Alexander Graham Bell Association for the Deaf, 3417 Volta Place NW, Washington, DC 20007; telephone (voice and TDD): 202-337-5220.

Alport's disease A genetic disease that causes kidney inflammation in childhood, followed by a sensorineural hearing impairment in young adulthood and eye problems later in life. It is more common among men than women.

There is no clear relationship between the extent of kidney disease and onset of deafness.

Treatment is supportive, since glucocorticoids and cytotoxic agents are ineffective. The disease is not known to recur following transplantation.

alternate binaural loudness balance test The ABLB test measures RECRUITMENT (the abnormal rapid increase in loudness above the THRESHOLD level) with a device that allows the client to set controls so that the loudness of a tone heard by the defective ear matches the tone heard in the normal ear.

By repeating this comparison at several intensity levels, the presence or absence of recruitment can be identified. This test is used to diagnose a SENSORINEURAL HEARING LOSS affecting primarily one ear.

alternative listening systems

AM Systems With this method, a person with a hearing problem can listen via an individual AM receiver headset or a portable radio to sounds transmitted on an AM radiowave. The AM transmitter can also be connected to a public address system. Unfortunately, this system is open to the same interference that disrupts regular AM radio broadcasts.

FM Systems The frequency modulation system includes both a transmitter and receiver; it picks up sound and transmits it over a specific FM frequency for a distance up to 300 feet to a person wearing a special receiver. The Federal Communications Commission has set aside the FM frequencies between 72 and 76 megahertz for such use by both public and private services.

The transmitter can be connected directly to the source of the sound, such as a television set or a microphone; the sound is carried on a specific FM radio frequency through the air until it reaches an FM receiver turned to the same frequency. The receiver changes the signal, and the electrical energy is sent to the ear either through a headset or a hearing aid. If a hearing aid with a telecoil is used, it can connect to a necklace loop attached to the receiver. Alternatively, a hearing aid with direct audio input capability can be linked to the FM systems with a special attachment called a boot, which fits on the bottom of a behind-the-ear hearing aid and connects to the receiver by a wire. With characteristically good sound quality, FM systems can be very helpful for people with severe or profound hearing problems.

Infrared Systems Some large group rooms and public places are equipped with a public address system that is plugged into an infrared light emitter that transmits sound via invisible lightwaves. An infrared transmitter may be connected directly to a sound source or a microphone; the transmitter then uses harmless infrared light rays to transmit sound to portable infrared receivers (available with headphones or "stethoscopes") which then change the signal into electrical energy and back into sound.

Although a person without a serious hearing loss may use the headphones without a hearing aid, someone with a greater hearing loss may connect a hearing aid directly to an infrared receiver or use the aid's TELECOIL capability together with a neckloop or silhouette inductor. With a neck loop, the infrared receiver sends the electrical signal to the loop, where it creates an electromagnetic signal picked up by the hearing aid. This signal is converted into electrical energy and then converted into sound at the aid's receiver.

Unlike FM transmissions, lightwaves do not pass through walls and are not affected by neighboring radio frequency signals. However, infrared transmission may be affected by intense sunlight.

Infrared devices are most helpful for those who have a mild to moderately severe hearing loss.

Audio Loop Systems This system, also called an induction loop system, features a loop of wire placed around an entire room that is connected to a microphone and an amplifier. The system's microphone picks up sound and changes it into electrical energy that is then amplified and sent through the coil of a wire (also called an induction loop) strung around the room.

The electrical energy flowing through the wire coil creates a magnetic field that can be picked up by a hearing aid containing a very small coil of wire called a TELECOIL or "T-coil." (See also ASSISTIVE LISTENING DEVICES.)

Ambrosi, Gustinus (1893–1975) Born in Eisenstadt, Austria, this talented musician and sculptor was best known for his classic sculptures in bronze and marble.

A child prodigy on the violin, he lost his hearing at the age of six after a bout of meningitis and smashed his treasured instrument when he realized he could no longer hear. However, as Ambrosi grew to adulthood he began to consider his deafness a blessing in disguise.

Finding he was no longer able to continue in music, Ambrosi studied woodcarving at the age of eight and became an apprentice at 14 with a sculpting firm in Prague. Within five years he had won two major art prizes, and in 1908 Emperor Fran Joseph gave him lifetime use of an atelier.

Considered a Renaissance man, Ambrosi was a gifted poet, graphic artist and philosopher, although he was known primarily for his lifelike busts.

When old age began to interfere with his ability to sculpt, Ambrosi committed suicide on July 1, 1975, in Vienna.

American Academy of Otolaryngology-Head and Neck Surgery The largest professional organization in this field, representing physicians who specialize in the treatment and surgery of the ear, nose and throat and related structures of the head and neck. It provides continuing medical education and various professional publications and also presents the interests of otolaryngologists to legislators. Its annual convention includes an intensive continuing education program offering a wide range of courses in the latest research and advanced techniques in cosmetic facial reconstruction, cancer surgery, patient management and treatment of allergic, sinus, laryngeal, thyroid and esophageal disorders.

The association publishes leaflets related to ear problems and a monthly journal, *Oto-*

laryngology-Head and Neck Surgery and also provides physician referrals. (See also OTOLARYNGOLOGIST.) Contact: American Academy of Otolaryngology-Head and Neck Surgery, One Prince St., Alexandria, VA 22316; telephone: 703-836-4444.

American Annals of the Deaf The oldest professional educational journal in the United States, *American Annals of the Deaf* is published jointly five times a year by the Convention of American Instructors of the Deaf (CAID) and the Conference of Educational Administrators Serving the Deaf (CEASD).

The journal, which was first published in 1847 by the faculty of the American School for the Deaf in Hartford, Connecticut, has passed through many different editorial hands. Its primary focus is to publish information of broad interest to those concerned with the education of deaf people. This information includes statistics on deafness, research into the psychology and sociology of deafness, conference reports and philosophical discussions. In addition, the publication includes an annual directory of services for the deaf. Contact: *American Annals of the Deaf,* Gallaudet University, 800 Florida Ave. NE, Washington, DC 20002.

American Association for the Promotion of the Teaching of Speech to the Deaf The original name of the ALEXANDER GRAHAM BELL ASSOCIATION FOR THE DEAF, this group—founded in 1890—first changed its name to the Volta Speech Association for the Deaf in 1948 and then changed to its present name in 1953.

American Athletic Association of the Deaf (AAAD) Founded in 1945, this group was established to encourage athletic graduates of deaf schools to continue in sports competition. It promotes intramural competition among deaf athletic clubs, supervises regional tournaments and, since 1957, gives financial support to deaf athletes wishing to participate in the WORLD GAMES FOR THE DEAF.

From the early 1900s, deaf athletes discussed the possibility of having a national basketball tournament for deaf people. In 1945 the first competition for the National Champion of the Deaf was held in Akron, Ohio, pitting top players from teams in Akron, Buffalo, Philadelphia, Kansas City and Los Angeles. (Buffalo won the tournament.) At the same time, members from deaf clubs all over the country voted to make the tournament an annual event and formed the American Athletic Union of the Deaf to oversee its organization. The AAUD later changed its name to the American Athletic Association of the Deaf to avoid its being confused with the Amateur Athletic Union of the United States.

After the AAAD became affiliated with the Comité International des Sports des Sourds, sponsor of the World Games of the Deaf, the AAAD was able to hold three World Games for the Deaf in the United States: summer games in Washington, D.C. (1965) and in Los Angeles (1985) and winter games in Lake Placid, NY (1975).

The AAAD, which administers more than 150 clubs in eight regions, sponsors annual basketball and softball tournaments, names an annual Athlete of the Year and hosts an AAAD Hall of Fame to honor outstanding deaf athletes, coaches and sports figures. In addition, AAAD is affiliated with four national athletic organizations (skating, ice hockey, tennis and volleyball), the U.S. Olympic Committee's Handicap in Sports Committee and the Amateur Softball Association. Contact: American Athletic Association of the Deaf, Inc., 1052 Darling St., Ogden, UT 84403.

American Coalition of Citizens with Disabilities This national nonprofit group, founded in 1974 by the directors of about 150 disabilities groups, was the only one of its kind directed by disabled people. Although no longer in existence, at one time it promoted the human and civil rights of America's 30 million disabled people on local, state and national levels, encouraged research and training and provided information and referral programs.

The coalition also published the *ACCD NewsNet,* which covered disability-related issues and books related to disabilities.

American Deafness and Rehabilitation Association (ADARA) A nonprofit, interdisciplinary group that promotes efforts to improve and expand rehabilitation services for deaf people, encourage research in deafness and promote the recruitment and training of professionals to work and communicate with deaf individuals.

Formerly called the Professional Rehabilitation Workers with the Adult Deaf (PRWAD), the organization was founded at a national conference of the Rehabilitation Services Administration in 1966. At that time, there was no national group serving those who worked with deaf people (the Convention of American Instructors of the Deaf was only interested in education and teachers, and the National Rehabilitation Association had no section for those who worked with deaf clients). The PRWAD welcomed rehabilitation counselors, psychologists, social workers and other professionals whose clientele were mostly deaf people.

After several years of debate, the name was changed to its present form during the group's 1978 convention, placing ''deafness'' before ''rehabilitation.''

Today, ADARA works closely with other organizations to develop legislation serving the needs of deaf people and publishes the quarterly *Journal of American Deafness and Rehabilitation Association* as well as various monographs sold as separate publications. The association also organizes national and regional conferences, workshops, training seminars and continuing education programs.

Although ADARA does not conduct research itself, its conferences and publications provide scientists with information and bibliographical support. The biennial conference provides a forum for professionals to learn about developments in the field, special problem areas and new treatments and advances. Several states have chapters that continue the work of the national group at the local level.

ADARA has grown from a group of about 300 in 1967 to more than 2,000 members in 1991. Separate sections within the organization address DEAF-BLINDNESS, mental health counseling, social work, and vocational and psychological assessment. (See also JOURNALS IN THE FIELD OF DEAFNESS.) Contact: American Deafness and Rehabilitation Association, P.O. Box 55369, Little Rock, AR 72225; telephone (voice and TDD): 501-663-7074.

American Hearing Research Foundation A nonprofit agency that promotes and finances medical research into the causes and treatments of deafness, hearing problems and balance disorders, encourages collaboration between clinical and laboratory research and works to broaden teaching and professional aims. Contact: American Hearing Research Foundation, 55 E. Washington St. Suite 2022, Chicago, IL 60602; telephone: 312-726-9670.

American Humane Association A national federation of local, state and regional animal care and control agencies. It started the first formal hearing ear dog training program in 1976 and helped create other training programs across the country.

Today, American Humane's Center for Hearing Dog Information assists local hearing dog training programs through publications and training aids and helps deaf individuals obtain dogs of their own. (See also CENTER FOR HEARING EAR DOGS; HEARING EAR DOGS.) Contact: American Humane Association, P.O. Box 1266, Denver, CO 80201; telephone: 303-695-0811 (voice); 303-695-4531 (TDD).

American manual alphabet See FINGERSPELLING.

American Ministries to the Deaf An evangelical organization whose aim is to proclaim the gospel of Jesus Christ among deaf people around the world. Contact: American Ministries to the Deaf, 7564 Brown's Mill Road, Kaufman Station, Chambersburg, PA 17201; telephone (voice and TDD): 717-375-2610.

American School for the Deaf The oldest school for deaf students in the United States. It offers a wide range of programs guided by the TOTAL COMMUNICATION philosophy—a philosophy implying acceptance of all methods of communication (speech, speechreading, aural, oral, American Sign Language and other manual communication systems).

The school began as a joint collaboration between THOMAS HOPKINS GALLAUDET, a young Andover, Massachusetts divinity student, and Dr. MASON FITCH COGSWELL, a surgeon and professor at Yale Medical School. When Dr. Cogswell saw Gallaudet's success at teaching Cogswell's young deaf daughter, he was inspired with the idea of reaching other hard-of-hearing students around the country. Gallaudet was sent to Europe by Cogswell and the Hartford, Connecticut city fathers to study both the French and English methods of teaching deaf students.

However, when Gallaudet arrived in England, he discovered that the founder of the English method demanded payment in turn for sharing his knowledge of deaf education. Unable to pay, Gallaudet continued on to France.

In Paris, Gallaudet worked closely with ABBÉ ROCH AMBROISE CUCURRON SICARD, director of the French Institute for the Deaf (now the Institut National des Jeunes Sourds) and his two assistants, JEAN MASSIEU and LAURENT CLERC. Eventually, Gallaudet returned to the United States with Clerc to set up a school for deaf students in Hartford.

The American School for the Deaf (originally known as the American Asylum for the Education and Instruction of Deaf and Dumb Persons) opened its doors April 15, 1817, with a class of seven students.

Immediately successful, it became the first recipient of state aid to elementary and secondary education in the United States when the state government awarded the school a legislative grant in 1819.

Since then, almost 5,000 students have graduated from this school, which has evolved from a small educational institution for deaf children to a multifaceted organization offering more than 75 different programs and services to the deaf community and the general public, including:

- Parent-Child Counseling Program—a home-based early intervention program serving families of hard-of-hearing infants and children through school age.
- PACES program—comprehensive and highly structured psychoeducational and dormitory life for emotionally and behaviorally disordered hard-of-hearing children and adolescents.
- Adult Vocational Services—New England's center for vocational rehabilitation services for hard-of-hearing individuals seeking job training and skills necessary for employment. The comprehensive resource center serves deaf people who need help preparing for, finding and keeping jobs.
- Community Audiological Services—a comprehensive hearing health care service including hearing tests; hearing aid evaluations, dispensing, fitting and repair; earmold impressions; and electroacoustical analysis of hearing aids and amplifications equipment.
- Camp Isola Bella—a recreational residential summer camp for deaf children between ages 6 and 18, located in the southern Berkshire hills of Salisbury, Connecticut.

Other services at the American School for the Deaf include preschool and kindergarten programs; academic and vocational instruction; residential opportunities; extracurricular, cultural and social activities (scouting, athletics, Junior Achievement, student body government); professional consultation and training; and summer recreation and education programs. Contact: American School for the Deaf, 139 N. Main St., West Hartford, CT 06107; telephone (voice and TDD): 203-727-1300.

American Sign Language (ASL) A visual-gestural language used as a primary means of communication by a very large portion of the deaf population in the United States (estimates suggest between 100,000 to 500,000 people). Often called the language of deaf people, ASL has a unique grammar and syntax and is unrelated to English, although it reflects English influences. It also includes FINGERSPELLING (the manual alphabet) to spell out words, including proper names and technical phrases. Some deaf individuals use sign exclusively, others use ASL in combination with SIGNED ENGLISH.

For many years, ASL was not considered a language at all. Critics claimed it lacked grammatical structure and warned that it relegated deaf people to an isolated subculture. Because ASL was considered "grammatically incorrect" by many educators, its usage was forbidden in schools and educational programs for deaf children. Thus, for years ASL was considered a suppressed language, despite its wide use by deaf children and adults from one generation to the next.

However, on the basis of new research, linguists today believe ASL is indeed a language—a visual language that requires many nonmanual features, including facial expressions and body language. It is passed on from parents to children, and children whose parents are deaf and fluent signers learn ASL as a first language.

Many linguists believe that it is only when sign language differs completely from English that it may properly be called AMERICAN SIGN LANGUAGE, although some use ASL as a catch-all term to describe a whole range of manual communication.

At one extreme of the sign language continuum is FINGERSPELLING, in which handshapes are used to spell out each word of the English language while speaking or moving lips. This method (also called the Rochester method or visible English) is occasionally used in a few schools, but it is an unpopular method of communication and can be tiring to use and interpret.

Farther along on the continuum are MANUALLY CODED ENGLISH systems, which use fingerspelling but also include signs and markers. The most common forms of this system are SIGNED ENGLISH and SIGNING EXACT ENGLISH, which base their signs on ASL but include other aspects of the English language.

They often use the first letter of the word (also called initialization) with the basic movement of the sign to give hints to the intended word. These systems also include markers for prefixes, suffixes, plural endings and tenses, together with signs for articles, infinitives and all forms of the verb "to be." Although this system is often used in schools, it is not used by deaf adults except for some initial signs and endings that have found their way into popular usage.

In the middle of the sign language continuum is a system called PIDGIN SIGN ENGLISH (PSE), the system used most often by hearing people learning to communicate with deaf people.

PSE combines the English language with the vocabulary and nonmanual features of ASL and is the preferred method of communication by many deaf people. Signs for definite and indefinite articles are omitted, and only one sign is used for the verb "to be" unlike the manually coded English systems.

Finally, American Sign Language, when used in its true sense to mean the patterns used by deaf persons when they communicate in sign in a non-English style, is at the other end of the sign language continuum.

Studies have shown that signs used this way are indeed a recognizable language with its own grammatical pattern, and nonmanual behaviors are an important part of this system. Neither articles nor speech are used, although fingerspelling is used for proper names.

In the United States, variations in ASL can often be traced to different residential schools and educational programs for different deaf communities. For example, the segregation of black deaf students in the South resulted in a variation of ASL used by the majority of the white population. It featured different words and even some different grammatical structures.

The acceptance and resultant surge in the use of ASL by both deaf and hearing people is reflected in the increase of ASL classes, videos and instructional books. Today, ASL has been incorporated with Signed English, speech, speechreading and other modes of communication in many educational programs for deaf students from elementary to postsecondary levels.

Still, there is some resistance to the use of ASL, especially in education where many school officials acknowledge the language but do not officially recognize it as a teaching tool. Despite research to the contrary, these school administrators believe teaching in ASL will interfere with the development of English skills.

In fact, there is still disagreement among deaf people themselves about ASL. Some find a source of pride and an example of cultural identity in the language, but others feel more ambivalent about its use in the wider hearing society. (See also SIGN LANGUAGE; SIGN LANGUAGE INTERPRETERS; SIMULTANEOUS COMMUNICATION; TOTAL COMMUNICATION.)

American Society for Deaf Children (ASDC) An organization providing advocacy, information and support to more than 20,000 parents, professionals and families with deaf or hard-of-hearing children. The organization was founded in 1967 by members of the CONVENTION OF AMERICAN INSTRUCTORS OF THE DEAF and promotes TOTAL COMMUNICATION as a way of life for deaf children and their families.

ASDC is the only national, independent, nonprofit organization whose sole purpose is to provide support, encouragement and information about deafness to families of deaf and hard-of-hearing children. The fundamental goal of ASDC is to improve education for deaf and hard-of-hearing students and to involve parents in the decision-making process.

Its "Two Years of Love" program includes a range of personalized services presented to a family with a deaf child—ASDC membership and a monthly shipment of books, toys, letters and journals.

In addition, the group provides a speakers' bureau, sponsors task forces, holds regional meetings and a biennial convention, and publishes various brochures, position papers and a quarterly newsletter, *The Endeavor*.

Parent groups can become affiliate members of ASDC, and organizations, agencies and educational institutions can become organization-affiliate members. Contact: American Society for Deaf Children, 814 Thayer Ave., Silver Spring MD 20910; telephone (voice and TDD): 301-585-5400 or 800-942-ASDC.

American Speech-Language-Hearing Association (ASHA) The national professional and scientific organization founded in 1925 for speech language pathologists and audiologists concerned with communication disorders. The group provides information and a toll-free helpline number (800-897-8682) for individuals with questions about speech, language or hearing problems.

With more than 40,000 members, ASHA maintains high standards of professional competence, develops good clinical service programs, stimulates research and offers continuing communication about speech and hearing.

New members must hold a graduate degree (or equivalent) in speech-language pathology, speech and hearing science, audiology or allied disciplines. Members in independent clinical practice must meet specific requirements in order to receive the Certificate of Clinical Competence.

Publications include three quarterly publications, *Journal of Speech and Hearing Disorders, Journal of Speech and Hearing Research* and *Language, Speech and Hearing Service in Schools* in addition to monographs, reports and directories. (See also JOURNALS IN THE FIELD OF DEAFNESS.) Contact: American Speech-Language-Hearing Association, 10801 Rockville Pike, Rockville, MD 20852; telephone (voice and TDD): 301-897-5700.

Americans with Disabilities Act This law signed in 1990 guarantees a number of rights to all handicapped Americans in four important areas: employment, transportation, public services and telecommunications.

Specifically, the law applies to deaf people as follows:

- A job can't be denied a deaf person if that person is qualified for the job. Businesses must make ''reasonable accommodation'' for deaf employees—including TDD (TELECOMMUNICATIONS DEVICE FOR THE DEAF) availability and interpreters.
- Medium- and large-sized hospitals, libraries, museums, hotels, restaurants, stores, parks and zoos must make interpreters and TDDs accessible for deaf patrons.
- By 1993, the United States must have developed a TDD relay system for all its deaf citizens, which will allow deaf people to call anyone anywhere at anytime.

A TDD relay system takes telephone calls in voice and transfers them to a TDD and vice versa. This new national relay system will give deaf people equal access via telephone to libraries, doctor's offices and so forth. In addition, the law provides that all emergency services must have TDD access.

American Tinnitus Association This nonprofit group founded in 1971 provides education and information about TINNITUS to patients and professionals in addition to raising money for research.

Founded by Dr. Charles Unice, who suffers with severe tinnitus himself, the organization offers a wide range of services, including information and a resource center, referral to a worldwide network of tinnitus clinics, local self-help groups and activities, professional workshops and seminars, counseling and guidelines for organizing tinnitus self-help groups and publishes a newsletter about tinnitus. Contact: American Tinnitus Association, P.O. Box 5, Portland, OR 97207; telephone: 503-248-9985.

Ameslan See AMERICAN SIGN LANGUAGE.

amoxicillin This broad-spectrum penicillin is one of a group developed to treat bacteria and is frequently prescribed for the treatment of ear infections. Amoxicillin is also useful in treating infections caused by certain types of bacteria leading to cystitis, bronchitis, etc., and is sensitive to penicillinase, an enzyme that makes penicillin ineffective. (See also OTITIS MEDIA.)

amplification See HEARING AIDS.

amplified hearing aid See HEARING AIDS.

amplified telephone See ASSISTIVE LISTENING DEVICES.

amplitude One of three measurements detecting the vibration of a sound wave (the other two are wavelength and frequency).

Amplitude is the vertical vibration that reflects the intensity of sound.

ampulla The expanded end of the semicircular duct contained in each SEMICIRCULAR CANAL of the inner ear.

anacusia Term meaning total deafness. Also spelled "anakusis" or "anacusis."

anacusis See ANACUSIA.

anoxia The complete loss of oxygen within a body tissue that can kill cells unless corrected very quickly. Anoxia is very rare, as opposed to hypoxia (reduced oxygen supply), which is a more common disorder.

Anoxia and hypoxia are the most frequent causes of damage to the organ of Corti, the body's hearing organ, during birth, since any disturbance of the infant's breathing or circulation can cause the loss of oxygen in the blood.

Anoxia can result from long labor, heavy sedation of the mother, obstruction of the baby's respiratory passages with mucus, poor lung development or congenital circulatory or heart defects. The only treatment for anoxia is prevention of these conditions.

antibiotics and deafness Studies have shown that aminoglycoside antibiotics have ototoxic effects when treatment is continued for more than 10 days.

These antibiotics include amikacin, gentamicin, kanamycin, neomycin and streptomycin. Neomycin is considered the most toxic of all drugs to the cochlea, and damage may result in hearing loss that continues irreversibly after treatment is stopped. Warning signs may include tinnitus or impaired balance, but these symptoms do not always occur.

Other types of antibiotics, including erythromycin and viomycin, can also cause hearing loss. All known cases of erythromycin ototoxicity (hearing loss and tinnitus) have been reversed once the drug is discontinued. Only large doses (more than four grams per day) have been associated with erythromycin toxicity. Viomycin, on the other hand, can cause permanent hearing loss. (See also OTOTOXIC DRUGS.)

antitragus A bump on the pinna (outer ear) opposite the tragus (located in front of the ear canal). The antitragus projects cartilage in the pinna near the opening of the ear canal.

anvil The middle of the three bones in the MIDDLE EAR that transmit sound vibrations, also known as the incus. The body of the incus is tightly bound to the head of the malleus (hammer); as the eardrum membrane moves, these two OSSICLES move in and out as a unit. With moderate sound, the third bone of the ossicles (the stapes or stirrup) moves with them, and all three then vibrate as a single mass, transmitting the vibration across the middle ear to the fluid-filled inner ear, the ORGAN OF CORTI, through the neural pathway and on to the central nervous system and the brain.

aphasia A disturbance in the ability to speak, write and/or comprehend and read, aphasia is caused by damage to the brain rather than by a problem with hearing or sight. Most often, head injury or a stroke in the dominant cerebral hemisphere—especially the Wernicke's and Broca's areas important for language—causes the brain damage that results in aphasia.

Some recovery can be expected following head injury or stroke with speech therapy. In general, the more severe the aphasia, the less chance for recovery.

Architectural and Transportation Barriers Compliance Board This independent federal agency is responsible for enforcing the ARCHITECTURAL BARRIERS ACT of 1968, which prohibits architectural barriers to the handicapped in federally-funded buildings and public transportation systems.

(These buildings cannot have barriers to people in wheelchairs or using crutches or who are blind or deaf. Buildings and transportation systems covered by this act must meet the minimum standards for accessibility established by the American National Standards Institute.)

Any person who believes there has been a violation of the act in a building built with federal funds can file a written complaint with the board describing the problem and giving the name and address of the building.

The board, which investigates every complaint it receives, first seeks voluntary compliance in a friendly, informal way if a violation is found. If no informal resolution is possible, the board's executive director may begin legal action by filing a citation before an administrative law judge, who then calls a hearing. (The person bringing the complaint does not need to appear at the hearing and will remain anonymous unless specific permission to reveal the name is given in writing.)

After the hearing the judge makes the final decision. If the judge's decision supports the board's findings, the judge may issue an order requiring correction of the problem within a specific amount of time.

The board also has a range of other responsibilities, including the development of advisory standards and provision of technical assistance to groups covered in the civil rights section of the Rehabilitation Act of 1973. (See also LEGAL RIGHTS.)

Architectural Barriers Act Also known as Public Law 90-480, this 1968 law requires federally-funded buildings and public transportation systems to be accessible to handicapped persons. This law applies to those with vision and hearing problems in addition to those in wheelchairs or with other physical handicaps.

The act also sets minimum standards for the design and construction of buildings under the supervision of the General Services Administration, the Department of Housing and Urban Development, the Defense Department and the U.S. Postal Service. These four agencies issued joint standards (the Uniform Federal Accessibility Standards) that include specifications for visual warning alarms, a permanently installed or portable listening system for hard-of-hearing people and at least one volume control on public telephones.

In order to enforce the act, Congress created the ARCHITECTURAL AND TRANSPORTATION BARRIERS COMPLIANCE BOARD in its Rehabilitation Act of 1973 (section 502), giving the board power to conduct investigations and issue orders of compliance. Those who don't comply can face withholding of federal funds. (See also LEGAL RIGHTS.)

Aristotle (384 BC–324 BC) Ancient Greek philosopher who coined the term "deaf and dumb." "Men that are deaf are in all cases also dumb," he wrote, "that is, they can make vocal sounds, but they cannot speak." Although Aristotle's use of the term "dumb" meant speechless, it came to take on other, more negative connotations (such as stupid or unable to comprehend). The negative connotations of this word have deeply influenced the rights of deaf people from Aristotle's time up to this day.

ASCII The language of most personal computers in the United States today. This data code standard (the American Standard Code for Information Interchange) was adopted in 1968 by the federal government in response to the rapid growth of computers.

The code is composed of 128 characters, including the upper and lower case alphabet, numerals and many special characters. It is used by more than 20 million personal computers in the United States and is the accepted language for most data communications.

Although it is not the language of the TDD (TELECOMMUNICATIONS DEVICE FOR THE DEAF), some of the newest TDD machines offer a combination of ASCII and the traditional BAUDOT CODE, allowing TDD users to communicate with personal computers over the telephone lines.

aspirin and deafness High doses of salicylates (aspirin) can cause TINNITUS and a hearing loss of up to 40 decibels—both directly related to the amount of the drug in the blood.

Although many drugs can be toxic to the delicate sensory tissue of the ear and can cause permanent hearing loss, aspirin is unusual in that the inner ear hearing loss it causes is reversible. Both hearing loss and tinnitus will disappear within one to three days after drug treatment is stopped. Normally, more than 12 aspirin tablets per day must be taken before there is a danger of hearing loss, although each person's sensitivity to the drug varies.

Patients with nerve deafness may also notice that aspirin will have a greater effect on hearing at lower frequencies.

Drugs containing quinine may also cause a similar, reversible hearing loss. (See also OTOTOXIC DRUGS.)

assistive listening devices Personal devices that can be used by hard-of-hearing people to assist their hearing and comprehension under a wide variety of circumstances.

There are many types of these devices, including those that offer input to the ear, extension microphones and telephone and television devices.

Input to the Ear There are several ways that listening devices can provide sound directly to the ear.

Induction A magnetic field capable of transmitting sound can be generated by a coil connected to the sound source, transmitting sound to a specifically-equipped hearing aid. This coil can be a loop of wire strung around a room, worn around the neck, embedded in a small, flat plastic device hooked over the ear or placed in the receiver of a compatible telephone. A second coil that picks up this magnetic signal is built into many HEARING AIDS. Called a TELECOIL, it is activated by use of the "T-switch" on hearing aids.

One advantage of the T-mode is that the microphone in the hearing aid is usually turned off, so background noise does not interfere with the sound from the induction system. For hearing aids without a T-switch, special receivers are available that have a telecoil that picks up and amplifies the induced sound.

Direct Audio Input Direct audio input (DAI) makes it possible to transfer sound directly to the hearing aid, taking advantage of the hearing aid's amplification and eliminating through-the-air noise. With some aids, the DAI signal can be heard while in the T-mode, turning off the microphone and further eliminating background noise. The hearing aid must be equipped to accept a DAI attachment.

Earphone Earphones are generally used by people not yet fitted with a hearing aid or whose aid has neither a T-switch nor DAI capability.

Speaker For people with a mild hearing loss, a loudspeaker close to the ear is enough to improve comprehension.

Extension Microphones The purpose of extension microphones is to extend the microphone closer to the sound source rather than rely solely on the microphone built into the hearing aid. Because microphone sensitivity drops rapidly with distance, an extension makes the signal stronger and tends to minimize background noise.

There are several types of extension microphones, including hard-wired, amplified and wireless.

Hard-wired This type of extension microphone consists solely of an additional microphone connected via cable and coupled to the hearing aid either by earphones, induction (neck loop or ear hook) or DAI. Most devices need an amplifier worn in the pocket, on the belt or held in the hand, but there are palm-sized models combining microphone with amplifier. Recent "super-directional" models have become available that make it possible to accurately pick up a voice 6 to 10 feet away if there is not too much background noise.

Amplified For people who need less amplification and don't wear a hearing aid, there are amplified microphones attached to a battery powered pocket/belt amplifier. The amplifier can be connected to the ear by an earphone or a built-in speaker held close to the ear. As with the hard-wired microphone, the amplified microphone cable can be as long as needed.

Wireless (Personal FM system) Considered the ultimate in extension microphones, this transmitter can broadcast 150 to 300 feet without connecting cables and can provide for another microphone in addition to the one built in. Receivers can use earphones, induction couplers or DAI but have no built-in speaker. Each unit is about the size of a cigarette package and can be useful in public auditoriums if the receiver frequency matches the one being broadcast.

Telephone Devices The telephone is often one of the biggest obstacles in communication for a deaf person because the sound is frequently distorted and visual cues are impossible.

The hearing aid telecoil was developed in America to take advantage of a defect in telephone design—the fact that the magnetic signal leaks and that leak can be picked up by a hearing aid equipped with a T-switch. In the United States, all telephones sold must be labeled "Hearing Aid Compatible," and all public phones, by law, must meet these requirements.

Minimizing feedback There are telephone attachments that minimize the feedback that occurs when the telephone receiver is held against a hearing aid. For a less expensive approach, a plastic-foam filled cap designed for telephone comfort can be slipped over the receiver instead. Using a T-switch on the hearing aid with a compatible phone will also eliminate feedback.

Amplifying handset An amplifying handset is available that features an amplifier built into the receiver, with a wheel for adjusting volume. Some models have another push button that gives additional volume as well. There is also a modular portable amplified handset that may be substituted for unamplified handsets of similar modular units when away from home.

Attachable portable amplifier There are two types of attachable portable amplifiers. One increases the audio signal from either a model that slips over the handset receiver or a small box-shaped model that plugs into the modular fitting at the base of the phone and amplifies the signal there. The second type slips over the receiver and converts the audio signal into a strong magnetic signal that is picked up by the T-switch of a hearing aid. There is also an attachable amplifier that combines both types.

TDD A TELECOMMUNICATIONS DEVICE FOR THE DEAF (TDD) is a visual typewriter connected to the telephone line by a modular plug or acoustic modem with the conversation appearing on a moving screen above the keyboard.

Television Devices There are several ways to improve sound for the hard-of-hearing TV watcher.

Hard-wired If a listening jack is provided in the TV set, a hard-of-hearing person can simply plug in earphones.

Amplified A cable can be connected from the listening jack of the TV to the microphone jack of a portable amplifier, or an extension microphone can be mounted near the TV speaker if there is no listening jack available on the TV.

TV band radio A small portable radio that receives both UHF and VHF audio broadcasts of the TV, with usually better sound quality, can be placed nearby, the radio's speaker or its earphone can be used.

Audio induction loop For people with a T-switch-equipped hearing aid, this method will eliminate background noise. An amplifier that converts the TV audio signal to an induction signal is needed, and either a neckloop or a loop system around the wall or under the viewer's chair can be used. Loop and/or wire can be permanently installed, avoiding a cable stretched across the room.

Infrared light This method picks up the TV sound with a microphone and then transmits it by invisible infrared light (the same technique used for TV remote control units). A viewer wears a stethoscope or a clip-on receiver; sound is transmitted to the ear via either earphone, neckloop or DAI. (See also ASSISTIVE LISTENING SYSTEMS.)

assistive listening systems In a large room, a person with a hearing problem may have trouble understanding speech even when using the most powerful hearing aid. Background noise and vibration can compound hearing problems and interfere with a hearing aid's ability to pick up specific sound.

Because of this, large public meeting rooms, concert halls, auditoriums and churches are sometimes equipped with one of a number of different alternative listening device systems that help hard-of-hearing people. These include AM systems, FM systems, infrared systems and AUDIO LOOP SYSTEMS.

Association of Late-Deafened Adults This group serves as a resource and information center for late-deafened people and works to increase public awareness of the special needs of ADVENTITIOUS DEAFNESS. If offers a publication, *ALDA NEWS*. Contact: Association of Late-deafened Adults, 1027 Oakton, Evanston, IL 60202.

atresia The absence or closing of a body's orifice. Atresia of the ear usually occurs during development of the fetal PINNA (external ear), external ear canal or middle ear and usually affects only one ear. It is an uncommon birth defect (one out of every 30,000 live births). In addition, atresia of the external ear can follow burns, tumors, accidents and infections.

Surgery can repair the ear's appearance and restore hearing by creating a passage for sound to reach the inner ear. Complete external and middle ear atresia in one ear only usually causes a 60 decibel (dB) hearing loss for speech. Hearing loss after surgery depends on the severity of the ear's malformation, but 50 percent of the time there is generally at least a 20 dB improvement.

audiogram A graph produced as part of certain hearing tests, and used to represent at what level of loudness an individual can hear sounds of different frequencies.

The audiogram form is arranged so that octave and half-octave frequencies range across the top with the frequency increasing from left to right. The hearing level scale on the left side of an audiogram shows the strength of the test sound in decibels. (See also AUDIOMETER; AUDIOLOGIST; AUDIOMETRY.)

audiologist A licensed and/or certified professional trained to identify and measure hearing loss and rehabilitate those with hearing and speech problems.

Audiologists are trained to determine where hearing loss occurs. They also assess the effect of the hearing loss on the ability to communicate and offer hearing aid evaluation and orientation, auditory training, training in speechreading techniques and speech conservation and counseling. Audiologists are not physicians and thus cannot treat infections or other ear diseases.

Services Audiologists work in a wide variety of settings, including universities, hospitals, schools, medical offices and private practice.

When employed by a university, audiologists may teach, supervise clinical practice and direct clinical services.

At medical centers, hospitals and rehabilitation agencies, audiologists test hearing, including the pre- and postoperative evaluation of otologic surgical patients. Referrals come from a wide variety of professionals, including OTOLARYNGOLOGISTS, neurologists, neurosurgeons, pediatricians, geriatricians, family doctors and internists. In hospitals with acute care pediatric nurseries, audiologists direct hearing screening programs for infants at risk for hearing problems. In addition, hospital audiologists often dispense hearing aids and, in veterans' hospitals, test and rehabilitate veterans with hearing problems.

Since most school districts require some type of hearing screening tests for students, audiologists serve as directors of these programs and work with teachers to help with special educational needs of students with hearing problems. In schools with special classes for students with hearing problems, audiologists equip and maintain classroom amplification systems.

Audiologists are also employed by private practice physicians (especially otolaryngologists) to test hearing, evaluate vestibular function and dispense hearing aids.

Recently, audiologists have begun branching out into private practice themselves, primarily to dispense hearing aids directly to clients with hearing problems. What separates them from traditional hearing aid commercial dealers is the in-depth professional rehabilitation program they can offer their customers.

Audiologists in private practice also work with industry to protect the hearing of employees in noisy environments, as required by the Occupational Safety and Health Act and the Workman's Compensation program.

Finally, community hearing and speech centers employ audiologists to work with adults and children as rehabilitation specialists to test hearing, select hearing aids and help improve speech and reading skills.

Tests Audiologists use both formal and informal tests to determine a person's ability to hear and understand. Although these tests usually measure hearing abilities, the audiologist may also test skills at interpreting gestures and facial expressions.

The audiologist routinely tests three aspects of hearing: the degree of hearing ability, the kind of hearing loss (if any) and the ability to understand speech under different conditions. (See also AUDIOMETRY.)

Employment Settings of ASHA Audiologists

Employment	Number	Percentage
College/university	660	12.1
School	525	9.7
Health service	1,401	25.8
Government health service	252	4.6
Private practice	478	8.8
Other	602	11.1
Unknown	1,513	27.9
Total	5,431	100.0

Source: J. Punch, "Characteristics of ASHA Members," *ASHA*, 25 (1983): 10.

Training An audiologist needs a bachelor's degree in speech-language pathology or a related field, a master's degree in audiology and a certificate of clinical competence in order to practice independently. Some states also require a license.

The certificate of clinical competence is widely acknowledged as evidence that the person is able to give independent audiologic services to children and adults with hearing problems. This standards program was set up by the American Speech-Language-Hearing Association (ASHA) in 1952, and certification standards are set by the Council on Professional Standards in Speech-Language Pathology and Audiology.

In order to take the certification exam, audiologists must have completed a master's degree and a minimum number of credits covering both the normal and disordered processes of hearing, speech and language. In addition, an applicant must have completed at least 300 hours of supervised clinical experience within the academic program, at least half of which is at the graduate level, followed by nine months of full-time professional experience under the supervision of a certified audiologist.

In order to attain certification, the applicant must then pass the National Examination in Audiology, a written test covering basic auditory sciences and clinical issues. Audiologists are not required to be active members in ASHA in order to be certified.

audiology The study of the entire field of hearing, including the nature and conservation of hearing, identification and assessment of hearing loss and the rehabilitation of all those with hearing impairments.

Within the field, there are specialities of diagnostic work, rehabilitation, research and teaching. (See also AUDIOLOGIST; AUDIOMETRY.)

audio loop A loop of cable (also called an induction coil) through which electricity passes, creating an electromagnetic field that can be converted into audible sounds by someone wearing a hearing aid equipped with a special device called a TELECOIL or T-coil. The loop can be worn around the neck or—as in part of an AUDIO LOOP SYSTEM—placed around the room, under the carpet and so forth. (See also ASSISTIVE LISTENING DEVICES; ALTERNATIVE LISTENING SYSTEMS.)

audio loop system In a large room, a person with a hearing problem may have trouble hearing even with the most powerful hearing aid. Background noise can compound hearing problems and interfere with a hearing aid's ability to pick up sound. To alleviate this problem, large public meeting rooms can be equipped with an audio loop system that utilizes a loop of wire placed around an entire room, a microphone and an amplifier. The electric current flowing through the loop creates an electromagnetic field that can be picked up by anyone wearing a special hearing aid sitting near or within the loop. Portable receivers are available for people without the special hearing aids.

The system's microphone picks up sound and changes it into electrical energy that is then amplified and sent through the coil of a wire (known as an induction loop) strung around a room. The electrical energy flowing through the wire coil creates a magnetic field that can be picked up by a hearing aid containing a very small coil of wire called a TELECOIL or T-coil.

The telecoil is activated by the T-switch and acts as an antenna that picks up the electromagnetic energy and delivers it to the hearing aid's receiver, where the energy is converted to sound.

An induction loop may be connected to a microphone or plugged directly into a TV or stereo jack. It can be coiled around a room, desk or chair or can be worn around the neck or in the ear (as a silhouette inductor). But a hearing aid cannot be used with a loop system unless it also contains an electromagnetic device (the telecoil). (See also ASSISTIVE LISTENING DEVICES; ALTERNATIVE LISTENING SYSTEMS.)

audiometer An electronic device used to test hearing that produces simplified PURE TONES or speech of a defined intensity and frequency. The audiometer includes a signal generator, an amplifier, an attenuator (which controls and specifies the intensity of sounds) and an earphone.

The hearing in one ear is measured over the full range of normally audible sounds, usually ranging up to 100 DECIBELS (dB) in steps of five. The 0 dB level represents normal hearing for young adults in favorable laboratory conditions.

There are several types and classes of electric audiometers, divided into two main types: pure tone and speech. A single instrument may be designed to serve both functions.

Pure Tone Audiometers These devices provide pure tones of selected frequencies and of calibrated sound-pressure levels, including wide range (which cover most of the human auditory range in frequency and sound pressure level) and must include the means for AIR CONDUCTION and BONE CONDUCTION tests and masking. A limited-range pure tone audiometer offers a more restricted range of frequency or sound pressure level, and may only allow air conduction tests. A narrow-range audiometer offers limited range of frequency and sound pressure levels. Audiometers vary in scope from limited to wide range.

Speech Audiometers A speech audiometer provides spoken syllables, words or sentences at known sound-pressure levels. It can be a separate unit but more often is a function included on diagnostic audiometers.

Automatic Audiometers These units provide both interrupted and continuous stimuli and may be operated by the client. The Békésy audiometer is a classic example of an automatic audiometer. They have largely been replaced by electrophysiologic testing.

Immitance Equipment Tests with this device include tympanometry, static measurements, acoustic reflex threshold determination and acoustic reflex decay. (See also AUDIOMETRY.)

audiometric zero The zero reference setting for the tone-intensity control at each selected frequency on a pure-tone audiometer. The tone intensity at zero is assumed to represent the average normal hearing threshold at each frequency used for testing. (See also AUDIOGRAM; AUDIOMETER; AUDIOMETRY.)

audiometrist A person without a degree in AUDIOLOGY who has been given informal training in the administration of hearing tests. An audiometrist must work under the supervision of an audiologist or a physician, and can neither diagnose hearing disorders nor interpret AUDIOGRAMS. (See also AUDIOMETRY.)

audiometry Measurement of a person's ability to hear through the use of hearing tests that provide accurate and quantitative results. Tests can determine if a HEARING LOSS exists, the amount and nature of the hearing loss and can yield some indication of the benefits that are possible through available treatment.

Basically, hearing tests measure sensitivity (the level at which a person can first detect sound) and DISCRIMINATION. A person's hearing loss is measured in DECIBELS (dB); however, two people with the same decibel loss may actually perceive speech quite differently, depending on the amount of structural damage to the ear and the age at onset of hearing loss.

Many methods have been used in the past to measure hearing, including monochords, whispered voice, watch ticks and whistles. Today, there are five basic types of hearing tests: screening or identification audiometry, routine diagnostic audiometry, acoustic-immitance audiometry, special audiometric tests and electrophysiologic tests.

Screening or Identification Audiometry Used to measure hearing of large groups, such as schools or industry, the audiologist can use a screening test to rapidly sift through the majority of hearing clients to identify the few with hearing loss. These tests are for detection of loss, not for description nor quantification. The most common is the pure tone sweep check tests.

Every child should have a hearing test as part of a school screening during the first two years of school and routinely throughout the school years, according to the Better Hearing Institute. The institute also recommends that every adult who is regularly exposed to high noise levels should have a hearing test at least once a year.

Routine Diagnostic Audiometry includes both air and bone conduction tests.

Pure Tone Air Conduction Air conduction refers to the process by which stimuli travels through air to the ear's conductive mechanism, which stimulates sensory endings of the eighth cranial nerve. This test evaluates how softly a client can hear across the spectrum of frequencies and measures the threshold of sound detection—the lowest hearing level at which the client responds correctly to pure tones 50% of the time.

Pure Tone Bone Conduction Bone conduction is the process by which sound vibrates the skull and thus the cochlear mechanism, bypassing the conductive apparatus of the ear. This test is designed to bypass the air conduction pathway and stimulate the cochlea. It also provides data on sensorineural mechanisms and the cochlear system.

The air bone gap (the difference between the thresholds measured by air and bone conduction) are attributed to pathological states in the outer or middle ears. Patients whose bone conduction results are normal or near normal and who have significant hearing loss by air conduction tests may be candidates for surgical or medical treatment.

Pure tone bone and air conduction tests measure hearing through the use of pure tones (a single frequency) by sending a tone through earphones to one ear at a time. The decibel loudness when these sounds can first be heard is the pure tone hearing threshold (or hearing level) for that frequency. People with normal hearing will usually hear each pure tone frequency at the zero point or close to it; people with a hearing loss will only hear pure tones much louder than zero.

Pure tones are usually in octave or half-octave steps, and cover the frequencies between 250 and 8,000 hertz (Hz). Because speech falls within this range, it is possible (in a limited fashion) to measure a person's ability to hear a conversation by testing with pure tones. The disadvantage of testing hearing with pure tones is that the sounds heard every day are not pure tones, but complex ones.

With the electronic AUDIOMETER, it is possible to measure a person's threshold of hearing for a series of pure tones at 11 different frequency points, starting at 125 cycles per second and ending at 8,000. This includes the three octaves between 500 and 4,000 Hz that are most important for speech. Audiograms test hearing at most of these 11 points.

When there is a large difference between the hearing thresholds of two ears, the AUDIOLOGIST will mask the better ear to prevent it from responding and giving a false reading while the poorer ear is tested. The better ear is masked by presenting a band of noise through the earphone at about the same frequency as the one being tested.

In addition to air and bone conduction tests, there are a number of special audiometric measures.

Speech Audiometry Pure tone thresholds tell the nature and extent of the hearing loss, but don't reveal the extent of communication problems. In addition to pure tone tests, a hearing evaluation often includes some measurement of a person's sensitivity to speech (or the lowest level at which speech is heard). In speech audiometry, the clinician gives verbal messages (live or taped) through earphones or loudspeakers to determine the lowest level the client can hear two-syllable words (spondees) well enough to repeat them (the speech reception threshold) and how clearly the client can discriminate one-syllable words while listening at a comfortable level (speech discrimination, or word recognition). The speech discrimination test determines the person's ability to understand important sounds (primarily consonants) and measures how well a person can discriminate speech at intensities 30 to 40 decibels (dB) above the speech reception threshold. (See chart on interpretation of discrimination scores, page 25).

Speech audiometry results are important because patients with hearing loss in one ear with poor discrimination at high loudness levels may require additional audiometric or X-ray studies to rule out possibility of a tumor on the hearing nerve. Secondly, speech discrimination results may be beneficial in predicting the extent to which a person with sensorineural hearing loss will benefit from a hearing aid.

Acoustic-Immitance Tests Immitance tests measure the response of the eardrum, ossicles and small muscles attached to the ossicles. Immitance is a measure of how easy it is to transfer sound energy from the external ear through the middle ear to the COCHLEA.

The measure of ACOUSTIC IMMITANCE can be defined as either acoustic admittance or acoustic impedance. "Admittance" refers to how easily energy flows through a system, while "impedance" represents the opposition to the flow of energy. A system with high acoustic impedance to the flow of sound will have low acoustic admittance, and vice versa. The most common acoustic-immitance test is the tympanogram, a measure of eardrum stiffness as a function of air pressure change. It can determine with a good degree of accuracy whether there is fluid behind the eardrum or whether air pressure condition in the middle ear is abnormal.

Another acoustic-immitance test is the acoustic reflex test, which is helpful in testing young children. This tests measures the reflex contraction of muscle in the middle ear.

Acoustic immitance tests are used as an adjunct to hearing tests, since a patient may have a significant ear disease with little hearing loss. While most hearing tests can uncover type and degree of hearing loss, they may not reveal specific ear diseases. Unlike most hearing tests, acoustic-immitance can reveal middle ear disorders without requiring any active participation by the patient. This is particularly helpful in the testing of young children.

Special Audiometric Tests These determine whether a sensorineural loss is located in nerve endings in the inner ear or hearing nerve. They include tone decay tests, the short increment sensitivity index (SISI), loudness balance tests, and Békésy audiometry. These have largely been replaced by electrophysiologic tests.

Electrophysical Tests Other tests that do not require the client to give a conscious response include electrophysical tests: electroencephalic (EEG) audiometry and evoked response audiometry. For the very young, hearing thresholds for pure tones can be deciphered from these electrophysical methods.

The electroencephalogram is a graphed representation of the electrical activity of the brain but is not widely used. With this method, a click causes a small variation in the electrical potentials recorded by the EEG. Through the aid of a computer and repeated presentation of clicks, the child's auditory threshold can be determined. Although very closely matching findings from conventional audiometry, the EEG readings cannot pinpoint the site of any hearing problem.

As nerve impulses pass through the lower levels of the brain from the auditory nerve on their way to higher brain centers, they make connections in the brainstem near the base of the skull. The most widely used electrophysiologic test is the AUDITORY BRAINSTEM RESPONSE TEST (ABR), which measures this electrical activity in the brainstem to see how well certain portions of the auditory system in the brain respond to a presented stimulus.

This noninvasive test is useful for the detection of hearing loss in newborns and infants, for the medical diagnosis of auditory disorders (including tumors) and for confirming nonorganic hearing loss. The ABR can be performed on individuals of any age—even the youngest infant.

In the test, clicks or tone pips are fed into the ear and a computer analyzes the results to see if the brain activity changes. Rather than a true test of the entire process of hearing, the ABR determines whether auditory signals are reaching the brain. Development of new stimulus delivery systems and recording electrodes now permit the use of ABR for intraoperative monitoring and monitoring patients with head injuries.

Another type of electrophysical test is the ELECTROCOCHLEOGRAM, which measures impulses in the cochlear nerve by inserting a thin electrode through the eardrum into the promontory of the basal turn. This indicates how well the cochlea is functioning.

Interpretation of Discrimination Scores

Discrimination Score	Interpretation
90–100%	Excellent understanding of speech
80–88%	Good understanding of speech
70–78%	Fair understanding of speech
60–68%	Poor understanding of speech
0–58%	Marked reduced understanding of speech

Who Tests Hearing? Although general practitioners or pediatricians may test hearing in the office, these simple tests can give only crude, unreliable results. Much better results can be expected from two kinds of experts on hearing who cooperate on diagnoses and treatment: the AUDIOLOGIST and the OTOLOGIST.

The audiologist is a nonmedical professional with a master's or doctorate in audiology who is trained to evaluate hearing and knowledgeable about types of hearing loss and their management.

The otologist is a surgeon specializing in the diagnosis and treatment of diseases of the ear. Otologists may make their own audiograms or rely on an audiologist's findings. While speech pathologists may also have qualifications in audiology and may be very helpful with deaf children's speech, not all are experts in deafness.

In addition, a nonaudiometric test is sometimes used as a very basic way to test hearing. The most common of these are the tuning fork tests (WEBER, SCHWABACH and RINNE).

auditory adaptation A perceived decline in loudness of a sustained acoustic signal commonly found in people with lesions of the cochlea or auditory (eighth cranial) nerve. People with normal hearing, when presented with the same sustained signal, experience no "tone decay" or decrease in loudness over time.

It is also possible to differentiate between lesions of the cochlea and the auditory nerve, since auditory nerve lesions cause a more rapid and extensive tone decay.

Auditory adaptation is measured by Békésy AUDIOMETRY or conventional tone-decay tests.

auditory agnosia A defect, loss or failure in development of the ability to comprehend spoken words caused by disease, injury or malformation of the hearing centers of the brain. A person with auditory agnosia may or may not respond to an audiometric test or may give very different results at different times.

auditory analgesia The control of pain by listening to music or WHITE NOISE through earphones, with the volume under control by the patient.

Because most subjects become less sensitive or insensitive to certain kinds of pain when listening to very loud noise or music, auditory analgesia is sometimes used in dental and obstetrical situations.

auditory aphasia See AUDITORY AGNOSIA.

auditory brainstem response test (ABR) As nerve impulses pass through the lower levels of the brain from the auditory nerve on their way to higher brain centers, they make connections in the brainstem near the base of the skull. The ABR measures this electrical activity in the brainstem and can determine how well certain portions of the auditory system in the brain respond to a presented stimulus.

This noninvasive test is useful for the detection of hearing loss in newborns and infants, for the medical diagnosis of auditory disorders and for confirming nonorganic hearing loss. The ABR can be performed on individuals of any age, even the youngest infant.

In the test, a brief tone causes a small variation in the electrical potentials that can be recorded from the scalp. Clicks or tone pips are fed into the ear, and a computer analyzes the results to see if the brain activity changes. Rather than a true test of the entire process of hearing, the ABR determines whether auditory signals are reaching the brain.

By repeating the stimulus up to 100 times and averaging the response by computer, the responses can be enhanced while eliminating random background electrical activity. This way, auditory thresholds can be established that are quite close to those that can be obtained in conventional AUDIOMETRY.

Development of new stimulus delivery systems and recording electrodes now permit the use of ABR for intraoperative monitoring and monitoring patients with head injuries.

auditory discrimination The ability to discriminate one speech sound from another.

auditory evoked potentials Slight electrical signals in the brain that have a characteristic pattern and occur in response to repetitions of identical sounds. The characteristic pattern, or wave form, indicates that the brain has responded to the test sound and, therefore, the sound must have been heard by the client. Tests of auditory evoked potentials are useful in those who cannot participate in hearing tests, such as the very young or the retarded. (See also AUDIOMETRY; AUDITORY BRAINSTEM RESPONSE TEST).

auditory feedback The ability to hear one's own speech, in which the output is fed back to the ear, producing a self-monitoring regulation of speech.

auditory-global method See AUDITORY-ORAL METHOD.

auditory nerve The part of the vestibulocochlear nerve (the eighth cranial nerve) concerned with the sense of hearing; also called the acoustic nerve or hearing nerve.

auditory nerve tumor This type of tumor, located along the eighth cranial nerve, can cause hearing loss on the affected side and is usually slow-growing and benign. Although several types of tumors can grow on the auditory nerve, the most common is an acoustic neuroma (also called a neurinoma or schwannoma). The cause of these tumors is unknown, except for the few that are associated with neurofibromatosis, a hereditary neurologic disorder.

Untreated, the acoustic nerve tumor first distorts the eighth cranial nerve and then, as it grows larger, presses on the seventh cranial nerve next to it. Eventually it can grow so large it protrudes from the canal into the brain behind the mastoid bone and, if untreated, can eventually cause death.

There are no typical symptoms, but people who have inner ear problems should be evaluated to eliminate the possibility of an acoustic neuroma. Most people with these tumors have hearing problems in one ear together with ear noise or tinnitus and sometimes have balance problems as well. Auditory, balance and hearing tests (including a brainstem auditory evoked response test and a CAT [computerized axial tomography] scan) can be used to diagnose the acoustic tumor.

Although the surgical removal of these tumors is complex and delicate, few patients die from the surgery because of modern technology and early detection. Still, long-term eye problems affect at least half of those who have had an acoustic neuroma removed, in addition to possible taste disturbances, problems with voice or swallowing and—if the facial nerve has been injured or removed during surgery—some degree of facial paralysis.

With small tumors, it may be possible to save what is left of the patient's hearing, but medium or large tumors have usually destroyed hearing, and this cannot be restored through surgery. The particular hearing problems common to people who have had acoustic neuromas include locating the direction of sound, hearing a person speaking softly and understanding speech in a noisy environment.

auditory neuritis Neuritis (inflammation) of the auditory nerve can follow infections such as scarlet fever or typhoid fever or other infections with high fevers. Hearing loss may be noted immediately, although deafness usually progresses over several days or weeks.

The insidious development of neuritis can cause sensorineural deafness very similar to PRESBYCUSIS but it occurs much earlier in life and is usually attributed to ANOXIA (absence of oxygen), anemia, nonspecific viruses and LABYRINTHITIS (inflammation of the fluid-filled chambers of the inner ear).

auditory-oral method A method of teaching speech to deaf and hard-of-hearing children. Proponents believe that using residual hearing in the most efficient way to develop speech. Therefore, children are encouraged to perceive speech of others through audition alone. This method is also referred to as acoupedic, aural-oral, auditory approach, unisensory-auditory and auditory-global. (See also MULTISENSORY TEACHING APPROACH; SPEECH TRAINING.)

auditory perception The mental awareness of sound.

auditory rehabilitation A variety of modern techniques are available to help people with HEARING LOSS. These include specialized programs for deaf children; customized personal HEARING AIDS; help for specific situations through the use of ASSISTIVE LISTENING DEVICES for telephone communication, television and group listening; COCHLEAR IMPLANTS; tinnitus maskers; tactile aids and alerting devices, and counseling (when necessary. (See also AUDITORY TRAINING.)

auditory training The process of teaching a person with a hearing loss to take full advantage of any sound cues that can still be heard. Like SPEECHREADING, auditory training can help people with hearing losses become aware of cues they might not notice otherwise. The form of auditory training used depends on when the person lost hearing and the type of hearing loss.

Auditory training helps children born deaf learn how to understand the weak or distorted sounds they can still hear; it can also help people with acquired hearing loss learn to pay attention to the act of listening and to separate background noise from speech. It also helps those with HEARING AIDS adjust to the task of using the device.

A person's need for auditory training depends on the ability to understand speech with or without a hearing aid. Often, auditory training is combined with speechreading training in a total AUDITORY REHABILITATION program.

aural Pertaining to the sensation of hearing or to the ear itself.

aural-oral method See AUDITORY-ORAL METHOD.

auricle See OUTER EAR.

Australia As many as 750,000 Australians, 5% of the population, have problems with hearing. Of those, 168,000 have trouble understanding speech even with a hearing aid.

Most of these deaf or hard-of-hearing Australians are elderly and began to lose their hearing after finishing school. Only about 40,000 were born with hearing problems or lost hearing early in life. In addition, conductive hearing loss is particularly high among the aborigines, since most native Australian children have chronic suppurative OTITIS MEDIA. Australia has the lowest prevalence rate of deafness among those developed countries for which statistics were available (35 per 100,000).

Education Because the educational system in Australia is administered at the state level, most families with children who cannot hear have access to some guidance and counseling during the child's early years. All states have a kindergarten/preschool service for children with hearing problems, generally with large centers in cities and satellite programs in rural areas. The preschools are usually special schools for deaf students, but children may also attend regular preschools if they wish.

As deaf children enter elementary school, services become more fragmented from state to state, although most states do have elementary day schools for deaf students. (When deaf education began in Australia at the end of the 19th century, there were large state residential schools, but by the end of World War II their enrollment dropped; today most deaf students commute to special schools.)

At the high school level, deaf students are generally taught academic subjects by elementary teachers; secondary teachers trained in deafness generally teach vocational studies. Because of the differing pattern of services among states, the educational level of deaf students in Australia ranges from superior to below normal.

There are no specialist higher-education services for Australians. Although deaf high school graduates have the ability to go on to universities, very few do so.

Communication Because most deaf people in Australia lose their hearing late in life, they rely on HEARING AIDS and SPEECHREADING to communicate. Most schools and services supplement their oral-aural curriculum with a manual system, which is usually a mixture of signs, FINGERSPELLING and SIGNED ENGLISH. Occasionally, cued speech is used.

AUSTRALIAN SIGN LANGUAGE is a direct descendent of BRITISH SIGN LANGUAGE, introduced by the founders of two large state schools for deaf students. Although Catholic schools for deaf students at first used Irish Sign Language, today these Catholic schools rely on the oral method and use cued speech. There are few people left in Australia who use Irish-Australian Sign Language.

Because Australian Sign Language, like all sign languages, has a grammar alien to English, Australian educators believed it was less useful in schools and have tried to employ Signed English by adding various fingerspelled markers for grammar (tense, plurals and so forth) to Australian Sign Language. Australian aborigines developed an extended communication sign system of their own, and this is now used with deaf aboriginal children.

The National Acoustic Laboratories provide free hearing aids to all military personnel, senior citizens and Australians under age 21 (which allows most school-age children with hearing problems to be properly fitted with hearing aids). The labs are the second-largest provider of hearing aids in the world, and were founded in 1948 to produce hearing aids for the deafened veterans of World War II and children deafened by the rubella outbreaks in the early 1940s.

Organizations for the deaf include the Australian Association of Teachers of the Deaf, the Association of Welfare Workers with the Deaf and the Federation of Australian Deaf Societies.

Australian Sign Language The sign language used by most deaf Australians incorporates the British two-handed system together with some use of the Irish and American one-handed alphabets.

The British two-handed system was brought to Australia in 1860 when the first two schools for deaf students were established; subsequent Irish Catholic schools introduced IRISH SIGN LANGUAGE.

A *Dictionary of Australasian Signs* was published in 1982 and includes the signs used in Australian schools in English word order.

Although there are no accurate census figures, estimates suggest that about 9,000 deaf Australians use Australian Sign Language.

autocuer This assistive device is a speech processor that breaks units of speech down into cues. These cues are activated by tiny light-emitting diodes, which show up in digital form on special eyeglasses worn by the deaf person. As with CUED SPEECH, that person will have to read the lips of the speaker as well as the cues on the eyeglasses in order to get the whole message. Cues and lips can be lined up and read at the same time by moving the head. The equipment consists of the eyeglasses and a small box-like speech processing microcomputer.

The autocuer was invented by Dr. Orin Cornett (the inventor of Cued Speech) and was developed by Dr. Cornett, Dr. Robert Beadles and a team of researchers in the North Carolina Research Triangle Institute's Center for Biomedical Engineering.

automatic audiometry Hearing tests in which the audiometers are operated by the patient. (See also BÉKÉSY AUDIOMETER).

B

bacterial labyrinthitis See LABYRINTHITIS.

bacterial meningitis See MENINGITIS; POSTNATAL CAUSES OF HEARING LOSS.

barotitis See AERO-OTITIS MEDIA.

barotrauma See AERO-OTITIS MEDIA.

barry five slate system A printed system to help deaf children learn to speak, read and write syntactically correct sentences.

Devised in 1899 by Katherine Barry, this system is similar to the five sentence parts system of ABBE ROCH AMBROISE CUCURRON SICARD. Barry's method utilized five large slates, each with one column, to help children categorize the parts of speech in sentences. Each slate contained one part of speech: subject, verb, object of the verb, preposition and object of the preposition.

basilar membrane A flexible membrane that is attached to the bony shelf and divides the coil of the COCHLEA lengthwise into two compartments. On one side of the membrane is the PERILYMPH fluid of the SCALA TYMPANI; on the other side is the ORGAN OF CORTI. As sound vibrations disturb the perilymph fluid, they are transferred through the basilar membrane to the organ of Corti and on to the hair cells inside.

battery hearing aid See HEARING AIDS.

Baudot code A code invented by Emile Baudot in 1874 that recognizes 32 characters—the capital letters of the alphabet and six other characters. The Baudot code was chosen in the early 1900s as the language of the teletype (TTY) machines by inventor ROBERT H. WEITBRECHT, and the TDD (TELECOMMUNICATIONS DEVICE FOR THE DEAF) network is based on the language of the Baudot code.

A person with a TDD that uses Baudot code cannot communicate over the phone lines with a personal computer (which uses ASCII) since the TDD and the computer "speak" different languages.

However, it is now possible to buy a TDD with both Baudot and ASCII capability. A TDD user transmitting or sending over the ASCII code can process information about five times faster than when using the Baudot code; this speedier ASCII rate is called 300 Baud.

The ASCII capability feature on a TDD also allows the user to have access to many personal computer bulletin boards. While the number of these bulletin boards are constantly changing, estimates range from 1,500 to 5,000 (See also ELECTRONIC MAIL.)

Beethoven, Ludwig van (1770–1827) A German musical genius widely regarded as one of the greatest composers who ever lived, Beethoven's life was marked by a heroic struggle against encroaching deafness. Some of his most important works were composed during the last 10 years of his life, when he was completely unable to hear.

During the first part of his life, his art stayed within the bounds of 18th-century technique. However, he experienced a change in direction as he gradually realized he was becoming deaf. The first symptoms appeared in 1800 before he was 30, and by 1802, when he could no longer deny that his hearing disorder was both permanent and progressive, he considered suicide. "But only Art held back," he wrote, "for it seemed unthinkable for me to leave the world forever before I had produced all that I felt called upon to produce."

As his hearing became worse, his piano playing degenerated, although he continued to appear in public from time to time. By 1819 he was totally deaf, and friends communicated to him using "conversation books" in which they wrote down questions and he replied orally.

By 1824, Beethoven finished his last large-scale work—the Ninth Symphony—with the aid of a type of audiophone. Holding a "sound stick" in his teeth with one end touching the piano, Beethoven would feel sound vibrations traveling through the stick to his teeth, the bones of his skull and into his inner ear.

At the end of the premiere of the Ninth Symphony, Beethoven, as conductor, stood alone in front of his orchestra. Totally deafened, he was unable to hear the thunderous applause and stood unaware until one of the soloists made him turn to face the audience.

behind-the-ear hearing aids These devices include a microphone, amplifier and receiver inside a small curved case worn behind the ear and connected to the EARMOLD by a short plastic tube. It can help all but the most severe hearing loss. Batteries are located in the base of the aid.

Some models have a tone control, volume control and telephone pickup device (T-switch), although all types of aids will amplify speech from the phone if the phone receiver is brought close enough to the hearing aid's microphone. (See also HEARING AIDS; TELECOIL.)

Békésy audiometer An instrument developed by GEORG VON BÉKÉSY in 1947 to provide automatic AUDIOMETRY. This device automatically tracks auditory thresholds for tones on a moving chart.

With the Békésy audiometer, the client makes his own audiogram tracing by pressing a button as long as he can hear a pure tone given during a hearing test. As the button is pushed (threshold response), the tone automatically decreases in intensity. When the button is released, the sound gradually increases again until the patient taps the button to indicate that he can again hear it. As the frequency is slowly increased, a graphic recording is made that produces a complete AUDIOGRAM in less than 10 minutes.

Auditory thresholds for pulsed and sustained tones are recorded, and the audiograms are evaluated on the basis of the separation between threshold tracings for pulsed and sustained tones. This procedure is basically a test for auditory adaptation for the sustained tone since most people, both deaf and with normal hearing, show adaptation for pulsed tones.

In a sweep-frequency Békésy audiometer, thresholds can be charted as a function of frequency; a fixed-frequency Békésy audiometer charts thresholds as a function time at a given frequency. (See also BÉKÉSY AUDIOMETRIC TEST.)

Békésy audiometric test A special hearing test that is given to older children and that can sometimes detect certain types of hearing problems of the inner ear and of the hearing nerve beyond the inner ear.

With the Békésy automatic recording audiometer, the patient controls the level of the tone by pressing a button as long as he can hear the tone. As the button is pushed, the tone automatically decreases in intensity. When the button is released, the sound gradually increases again until the patient taps the button to indicate that he can again hear it.

As the frequency is slowly increased, a graphic recording is made that provides a complete AUDIOGRAM in less than 10 minutes. (See also AUDIOMETRY; BÉKÉSY, GEORG VON; BÉKÉSY AUDIOMETER.)

Békésy, Georg von (1899–1972) The inventor of the modern theory of BASILAR MEMBRANE resonance, this Hungarian-born communications engineer wanted to understand the difference between the quality of the human ear and the telephone system. While director of the Hungarian Telephone System Research Laboratory, he studied long-distance communication problems and became interested in the human hearing mechanism.

He studied the inner ear by building mechanical models of the COCHLEA. From this work, he developed his traveling-wave theory, which describes how a sound impulse sends a wave sweeping along the basilar membrane, increasing its amplitude until it reaches a maximum when it falls off sharply until the wave dies out. The point of greatest amplitude is the point at which the frequency of the sound is detected by the ear. He developed highly sensitive instruments that made it possible to understand the hearing process, differentiate between types of deafness and choose proper treatment.

Von Békésy also found that high-frequency tones were perceived near the base (or entrance) of the cochlea and lower frequencies toward its end. He also discovered that location of nerve receptors are most important in determining pitch and loudness. For this theory, Békésy received the Nobel Prize in physiology and medicine in 1961. (See also BÉKÉSY AUDIOMETER.)

Belgian Sign Language (BSL) The sign language of Belgium includes many regional dialects. Although the country has two official languages (Dutch in the north and French in the south), sign languages in these two areas are quite similar, possibly because the deaf schools in Brussels have included students from both sections of the country.

Belgian Sign Language began in schools for deaf students and was based on signs from the old French Sign Language. Although this country has been traditionally oralist, support for BSL and both the manual codes of Signed Dutch/Signed French (used in communicating between deaf and hearing people) has been growing.

Belgium The deaf population in Belgium reflects the deep communication divisions between the Flemish and French-speaking natives. The provision of services for deaf Belgians, therefore, depends on the difference between the two groups.

The total number of deaf students in the country is unknown, but there are about 1,500 pupils in special schools for deaf children. Because early diagnosis is stressed in Belgium, most deaf children are diagnosed by the age of one. It is one of the few countries in which deafness rates are declining, reporting 60 per 100,000 for 1950 and 51 per 100,000 in 1974. The differences may reflect a sampling error, however.

Education/Communication For many years, as in most of Europe, Belgian teachers stressed the oral method of education. Manual communication, although not repressed, was not encouraged. Gradually, Belgian educators have decided that an exclusively oral education does not benefit all students; now many promote a combination of oral and manual communication in order to acquire a command of spoken language.

Cued speech is very popular, as is a Belgian invention called AKA (alphabet of assisted kinemes, or lip movements), which is used to complement spoken language in order to make speechreading easier. In addition, the total communication method using Signed French together with speech is used as an alternative to cued speech or in combination with it. Signed French is based on signs of BELGIAN SIGN LANGUAGE.

Mainstreamed students must learn through speechreading, hearing aids or written material, since there are no sign language, cued speech-interpreters or deaf teachers to help deaf students in schools for hearing students.

Services Special education is free in Belgium, and the national health service helps pay for hearing aids. All Belgian families receive allowances for children, which are doubled for deaf children.

Little has been done to make television or telephone accessible to deaf consumers, although the national French-speaking television network provides sign interpretation five days a week. There is no systematic captioning system.

Bell, Alexander Graham (1847–1922) This Scottish-born American inventor dedicated his life to improving methods of communication for deaf students, and was instrumental in instituting the oral method of deaf instruction at almost every school in the United States.

Born in Edinburgh, the son of Melville and Eliza Bell, Alec (as he was then known) was a brilliant child whose interest in inventions would preoccupy him for the rest of his life. With his father, he was also interested in speech disorders and elocution, in part because his mother had severe hearing problems since her childhood. However, she could speak well, used an EAR TRUMPET (a mechanical device to improve hearing), and played the piano.

Bell's father was a pioneer of the "VISIBLE SPEECH" system, in which he tried to develop a universal language for mankind. This system described oral sounds through written symbols and was created in order to improve elocution. Although the system was not originally designed to be used in teaching deaf students, a British teacher recognized its potential and began working with young Alec Bell. With the success of his first experience in teaching deaf students with visible speech, Bell accepted an invitation to teach the method at the Boston School for Deaf Mutes in 1870.

Three years later, Bell was hired as a private teacher for 15-year-old Mabel Hubbard; in 1877 the two were married, forming a union that lasted for 45 years. This remarkable woman was one of the strongest influences on Bell and helped shape his theories of education for deaf children.

In New England, Bell taught instructors at leading schools of deaf students the visible speech system but discovered that, in the long run, the symbols were too abstract for the teacher to apply, and the system fell into disuse.

During this time in New England, Bell began to promote his belief in day schools, instead of the residential facilities then common for deaf students. His first day school was started in 1878 in Scotland with three pupils. Back in the United States, Bell opened a day school in Washington, D.C. in the same building as a kindergarten class for hearing students; his hope was that the two groups would mix.

Bell was an ardent supporter of the ORAL APPROACH, and as he grew older, he focused his efforts on promoting oralism and founding schools to teach deaf students to speak. He was considered the champion of oral education in America and believed it was an educator's job to help deaf students speak English and read lips. He objected strongly to SIGN LANGUAGE because he believed it would prevent students from achieving integration into the hearing world.

Although some proponents of the MANUAL APPROCH argued that sign was the natural language of deaf people, Bell disagreed. He agreed that sign language was of great benefit in developing the intellect, but integration into society was far more important to him than developing the mind. Bell strongly believed that all deaf children could be taught to speak and read lips.

Because of his strong opinions against sign language—he considered a signing deaf adult a "failure"—many deaf adults hated him. They saw his attempts to eliminate sign language as an attack on their culture and identity.

Bell was also a supporter of eugenics, the science of improving hereditary characteristics through controlled mating, and opposed marriages between deaf people because he believed it would eventually create a race of deaf people. After studying statistics of deaf families, he concluded that deafness was often inherited and that those who inherited deafness should only marry hearing people. He wanted to have marriages between people with inherited deafness outlawed but gave up this idea when he decided that such legislation was unrealistic. He advocated that deaf students should not be segregated in schools, that deaf teachers should no longer be hired to teach deaf students and, of course, that sign language should be abolished.

It is not surprising that most of these ideas made him even more unpopular among the deaf population, at least among those who had adjusted to their inability to hear and considered themselves normal. But Bell, dreaming of a utopian society and brought up in a family that prized oral communication, saw deafness as a problem for society, not as an individual condition.

Bell also gave financial support to the cause of oral education. On May 8, 1893, young HELEN KELLER attended groundbreaking ceremonies for Bell's VOLTA BUREAU, an international information center promoting the oral education of deaf people. In 1890 he used his share of royalties from the invention of the Graphophone (a type of tape recorder) to finance the American Association to Promote the Teaching of Speech to the Deaf (ASPTSD) (now called the ALEXANDER GRAHAM BELL ASSOCIATION FOR THE DEAF). Today this association is a leader in the support of oral education, organizing meetings and conventions, lobbying and publishing a journal, the *Volta Review,* in its efforts.

Bell had an extraordinary impact on the educational methods used to teach deaf students in this country. When Bell formed the ASPTSD, only about 40% of deaf students were taught to speak. At the time of his death 30 years later, that number had risen to more than 80%.

Berthier, Jean-Ferdinand (1803–1886) A political leader of the French deaf "nation," Berthier was born in Louhans, France, and became the most outstanding advocate for deaf people in 19-century France.

A firm believer in promoting public understanding of deafness, he also supported "natural sign language" and thought it helped students learn written French.

Berthier attended the famous Institut National de Jeunes Sourds in Paris and was the first deaf man to receive the Legion of Honor medal. He spent his life fighting negative attitudes toward deaf people, testifying before parliament to revamp laws dealing with (and ignoring) deaf people, and researching the history and heritage of deaf people. (See also INSTITUT NATIONAL DES JEUNES SOURDS.)

Better Hearing Institute A nonprofit educational organization that offers general information about hearing loss and help available through medicine, surgery, amplification and rehabilitation. It also distributes films, technical information, news and human-interest features.

Founded in 1973, the organization is supported entirely by private donations. Contact: Better Hearing Institute, P.O. Box 1840, Washington, D.C.; telephone: 703-642-0580 or 800-EAR-WELL.

BI-CROS hearing aid BI-CROS (bilateral contralateral routing of signal), aids, usually of the eyeglass type, used for those with an unequal hearing loss in both ears, one of which cannot be helped by amplification.

Unlike the CROS HEARING AID, which utilizes only one microphone, the BI-CROS system uses two microphones (one above each ear) sending signals to a single amplifier. Sound is picked up by microphones in both ears, transmitted to a single receiver and transferred to the better ear via a conventional earmold. (See also HEARING AIDS.)

Bilingual, Hearing- and Speech-Impaired Court Interpreter Act This law, enacted by Congress in 1979, amends the 1978 Court Interpreters Act and requires the court to appoint a qualified interpreter for deaf, speech-impaired or non-English speakers in any criminal or civil action initiated by the federal government.

The director of the administrative office of the U.S. Courts determines the qualifications required of court-appointed interpreters. Each district court must maintain a list of certified oral and manual interpreters for deaf people, obtained in consultation with the NATIONAL ASSOCIATION OF THE DEAF and the REGISTRY OF INTERPRETERS FOR THE DEAF.

However, an interpreter is *not* provided for a deaf person who initiates a lawsuit. Although many states will provide an interpreter for a deaf defendant in a criminal trial, few offer one at the time of arrest or in a civil case.

binaural Pertaining to both ears.

binaural hearing aids Two complete HEARING AIDS, one in each ear. Any type of hearing aid may be worn in both ears, if the listener can tolerate two aids and can benefit from amplifying residual hearing in both ears.

Some wearers find that the binaural system increases directional sense and helps separate desired sound from unwanted background noise. Although it is sometimes assumed that using an aid in each ear should improve hearing, tests of people wearing these aids do not always support this theory.

bionic ear A popularized misnomer for the COCHLEAR IMPLANT.

body hearing aid Also known as ''on-the-body'' aids, these devices feature a microphone and amplifier that are larger than in other HEARING AIDS and are carried inside a pocket or attached to clothing in a case about the size of a cigarette case. The external receiver attaches directly to the EARMOLD, and its power comes through a flexible wire from the amplifier.

The devices always include a volume control and an on/off switch and may also offer tone control and a microphone/telephone selection switch (T-switch) that disconnects the microphone and allows the electromagnetic pickup of telephone conversations without background noise.

On-the-body hearing aids are more powerful and easier to adjust than smaller devices. However, their size and body location and the problem of noise from clothing make this aid an unpopular choice. These aids are still in use by people who need larger controls and for infants who are not old enough to wear ear-level hearing aids. (See also TELECOIL.)

bone conduction Sound transmitted from the source through the skull bones directly to the COCHLEA, which is partly how we hear our own voice. The resulting sound is indistinguishable from air conduction signals. Bone conduction sounds reach the cochlea by several routes, unlike air conduction. Vibrations are sent through the skull wherever contact is made, reaching both ears almost at the same time.

With higher frequencies, the skull vibrates in segments, and these vibrations are transferred to the cochlear fluids by directly compressing the otic capsule (the bony enclosure surrounding the inner ear). The resulting movements of the basilar membrane can stimulate the ORGAN OF CORTI. This form of conduction is known as compression bone conduction.

With frequencies below 1500 hertz, the skull moves as one rigid piece. Because the OSSICLES are only loosely attached to the skull, they are less affected than the cochlea and the OVAL WINDOW and move less freely. As a result, the oval window moves with the footplate of the stapes in a type of bone conduction known as inertial.

Because the ear disease otosclerosis hardens the stapes, this disease interferes with inertial bone conduction but does not affect compressional bone conduction.

bone conduction test See AUDIOMETRY.

bone conduction vibrator An instrument placed on the mastoid bone behind the external ear as a way to present pure tones as part of bone conduction audiometry.

bone conductor hearing aids Bone conduction aids are mostly for people with conductive hearing loss that has not been effectively treated by surgery. This type of hearing aid, which allows sound to be heard through the bone behind the ear, is used when the ear canal is closed or drainage from the ear is poor. (See also HEARING AIDS.)

bone hearing level A measurement, determined through part of a hearing test, that indicates how well pure tones are heard through the bone behind the ear. (See also AUDIOMETRY.)

Bonet, Juan Pablo (1579–1623) The author of the first published book of oral teaching methods for deaf people. Bonet was born on July 1, 1579, in a little town in Spain, Torres de Berrellen. After serving in the army and learning Italian and French, he was hired as secretary by the Duke of Frias. The duke's second son, Luis, was deaf, and Manuel Ramirez de Carrion was employed to teach Luis, using the methods developed by PEDRO PONCE DE LEON. Bonet spent some time watching Ramirez and took over the education of Luis when Ramirez left.

After about three years, Bonet published *Simplification of the Alphabet and the Art of Teaching Mutes to Speak,* in which he explained the Ramirez-de Leon technique. The text was not his own method, but by writing down the system, Bonet was able to interest a wide variety of European teachers in the possibility of oral education for deaf children.

Bonet believed in teaching reading and spelling, speech instruction and fingerspelling. However, he did not support the teaching of speechreading.

bony labyrinth See LABYRINTH, INNER EAR.

Bove, Linda (b. 1945) One of the most influential deaf women in the performing arts, this totally deaf actress may be best known for the character she plays in public television's *Sesame Street.*

In addition, Bove is a founding member of both the NATIONAL THEATRE OF THE DEAF and the Little Theatre of the Deaf, and remains the national theatre's ambassador-at-large.

Bove was born congenitally deaf in Garfield, New Jersey to deaf parents and graduated from Gallaudet University, where she had been active in drama. She toured internationally with the National Theatre of the Deaf, and in 1973 she played ''Melissa Hayley,'' a deaf character on the television soap opera *Search for Tomorrow;* other TV appearances include *The Dick Cavett Show, Happy Days* and *A Child's Christmas in Wales.* She first appeared in public television's *Sesame Street* in 1971; by 1976 she was a permanent member of the cast, portraying a deaf member of the neighborhood.

Bragg, Bernard (b. 1928) A cofounder of the NATIONAL THEATRE OF THE DEAF, Bernard Bragg is an actor, mime, director and lecturer known for his development of "sign-mime," a variation of sign language that features graceful, poetic body movement and motion to highlight dialogue.

Born deaf to deaf parents in Brooklyn, Bragg graduated as class valedictorian from the New York School for the Deaf and went on to Gallaudet University where he excelled in dramatics as an actor and director, and received the Teegarden Award for poetry upon graduation.

Bragg taught for 15 years at a California school for deaf students, where he also performed for Marcel Marceau. The celebrated French mime then invited Bragg to study with him in Paris; after Bragg's return to California, he began performing in small clubs in San Francisco and was named one of the best small club performers by *Life* magazine.

Internationally, Bragg has served as artist-in-residence with the Moscow Theatre of Sign Language and Mime and served on the U.S. Intelligence Agency's Overseas Speaker's Program in 1977, traveling all over the world conducting workshops in sign for both deaf and hearing audiences.

He currently serves as artist-in-residence at Gallaudet University.

Braidwood, Thomas (1715–1806) A pioneer Scottish educator of deaf people best known for his refusal to pass on his methods in oral instruction to anyone outside his own family. This reticence was responsible for the early emphasis on manual education of deaf students in the United States.

Thomas Braidwood taught his first deaf pupil in 1760 and was so pleased with his success in helping the boy speak and understand language that he decided to concentrate on teaching deaf students.

His first school, the Academy For the Deaf and Dumb, opened in Edinburgh in the early 1760's. By 1779, the academy had 20 pupils who were taught to speak, read and write. Although his exact methods were not divulged, it was known that he based his method on the articulation theories of educator Thomas Wallis. This was an oral method, but the use of natural signs and the manual alphabet was not forbidden.

In response to an offer from King George III to set up a school for deaf students in London, Braidwood opened Grove House in 1792 and then a separate school for needy deaf children, where Braidwood's nephew Joseph Watson was headmaster.

Braidwood's schools were successful, but the oath of secrecy kept by the Braidwood family had important consequences for the future of deaf education in the United States. THOMAS HOPKINS GALLAUDET, who had studied the manual communication system in France developed by ABBÉ ROCH AMBROISE CUCURRON SICARD, came to Britain to learn the oral method from Braidwood.

When he got to London, he found that the three English schools for deaf students were all controlled by the Braidwood family, who were unwilling to share their methods freely, as was the custom at the time.

Consequently, Gallaudet returned to Paris to study the French manual system, which he subsequently introduced into the United States. This method became the basis of deaf education and communication in U.S. schools for deaf children.

brainstem audiometry See AUDITORY BRAINSTEM RESPONSE TEST.

brainstem auditory evoked potential See AUDITORY BRAINSTEM RESPONSE TEST.

brainstem evoked potential See AUDITORY BRAINSTEM RESPONSE TEST.

brainstem testing See AUDITORY BRAINSTEM RESPONSE TEST.

Brazil Deaf citizens in Brazil receive limited funds from the state and federal government for diagnosis, treatment, education and rehabilitation. Free diagnosis of simple cases of deafness and routine prescription of hearing aids are provided by the government through its own otolaryngologists and through agreements with private clinics. The state mandates minimal educational and treatment provisions and helps finance the training of teachers for deaf students. Numerous private charitable groups also serve deaf Brazilians. Many large cities maintain good private clinics and professionals, but the treatment cost is often beyond the reach of many Brazilians.

Although there are no exact figures, estimates suggest that there are up to a half million profoundly deaf Brazilians out of a total population of 120 million people. More than half of the deaf students who receive assistance attend school in special classes, one-fourth are in integrated classes, and one-fifth attend special schools.

The predominant philosophy in the schools and programs for deaf citizens throughout the country is to integrate deaf people into the hearing world by developing speech and speechreading skills and utilizing residual hearing. The use of sign language was discouraged between 1950 and 1970, but today its use is spreading slowly across the country.

Brazilian Sign Language A number of dialects make up Brazilian Sign Language, but communication among people is surprisingly easy for so large a country.

Although Brazilian schools for deaf students became completely oral after the Milan Congress in 1880, there has been more interest in Brazilian Sign Language since the 1970s, and at least one school has adopted the educational philosophy of TOTAL COMMUNICATION.

Brazilian Sign Language is similar to both American and European sign languages, and its one-handed manual alphabet is quite similar to the French system. In Brazilian Sign Language, fingerspelling is used for proper names, fingerspelled signs, technical terms and negative emphasis. The system utilizes hand and body movements, facial expressions, eye gaze, pauses and changes in the rhythm of signing to indicate grammatical and structural meanings, and the space around the body provides an important frame of reference, indicating spatial agreement between verbs and subjects/objects, reference for directional verbs, and so forth.

Breunig, H. Latham (b. 1910) A chemist, statistician and leading proponent of oral education, Breunig founded the Oral Deaf Adults Section of the ALEXANDER GRAHAM BELL ASSOCIATION FOR THE DEAF. Along with two others, he set up Teletypewriters for the Deaf, Inc., to acquire and recondition surplus teletypewriters donated by American Telephone and Telegraph.

Born in Indianapolis, he lost part of his hearing when he was three years old, a condition exacerbated by an attack of scarlet fever at age five. Two years after that, a skull fracture left him with a 115 dB loss. He attended the Clarke School for the Deaf in Northampton, Massachusetts where he met his future wife, and then attended a public school, where he worked on the school newspaper, became an Eagle Scout and was accepted into the National Honor Society.

He received a degree in chemistry from Wabash College in Indiana and completed his Ph.D. at Johns Hopkins University. While a full-time researcher with the pharmaceutical firm of Eli Lilly, Breunig was active in national organizations for deaf people and was director of the Indianapolis Speech and Hearing Center for 21 years. Committed to the idea that deaf people need to be able to communicate with the hearing world in order to take advantage of opportunities, he attributed his own success in business and as a professional chemist to his ability to speak and speechread.

Brewster, John Jr. (1766–1854) Considered one of New England's most accomplished folk artists, he was also one of the most successful traveling artists of his day.

Brewster was born deaf to hearing parents, Dr. John and Mary Brewster, in Hampton, Connecticut. Able to communicate in sign language and adept at an early age in art, he obtained several commissions for portraits of family and friends despite a lack of formal training.

Brewster faced great difficulties as an independent artist forced to communicate constantly with strangers in inns or homes. He traveled by horseback in Massachusetts and Maine and was gifted at capturing a model's personality in his portraits.

When the Connecticut Asylum for the Education and Instruction of Deaf and Dumb Persons opened in Hartford (now the American School for the Deaf), Brewster, at the age of 54, was one of its first six pupils. During the three years he lived at the school, he was able to support himself through painting. He left the school in 1820 to continue painting. His paintings hang today in museums in Maine, Massachusetts and New York.

Bridgman, Laura Dewey (1829–1889) The first deaf and blind person to be educated in the United States, Laura Bridgman was born in Hanover, New Hampshire to a successful farm family. Always a delicate child, at age two she contracted scarlet fever, which destroyed her sight and hearing and left her ill for two years. During this time, she forgot the few words she had learned to speak before her illness, and she retreated into silence.

Bridgman was introduced in 1837 to Samuel Gridley Howe, the founder of the Perkins Institution for the Blind in Boston. Although Laura could barely communicate with her family (she understood shoves and pats on the head), Howe was convinced she was extremely bright and would benefit from instruction.

Her parents brought her to Perkins in 1837, where Howe constantly worked with her to establish a form of communication using labels with raised letters pasted on common objects. When she finally learned that the labels actually represented objects, the greatest obstacle to meaningful communication had been crossed. At Perkins, she studied a variety of subjects, such as fingerspelling, handsewing and how to use a sewing machine.

Although she never learned to talk, she could make about 50 sounds, which she used as names for people she knew. At the age of 23, she was sent home where it was assumed she would be happy with household chores. But the sudden loss of noise and activity affected her poorly; she became bedridden and near death until she was returned to Perkins, where she remained for the rest of her life.

British Sign Language This highly complex system is the language of the deaf community throughout Great Britain and Northern Ireland, although there are regional dialects. As in many natural sign languages, BSL has a topic-comment structure: for example, "Drink—you want more?" instead of "Do you want another drink?" It includes an inflection system, with which it is possible to show person or number by the way signs move.

As in AMERICAN SIGN LANGUAGE, BSL and English are quite different, although the two-handed BSL manual alphabet is based on the English alphabet.

There are no exact figures on the number of people who use BSL, but estimates suggest that as many as 30,000 profoundly deaf people in the United Kingdom use BSL and were educated through its use. It includes a two-handed fingerspelling system that was first published in 1680.

Although the use of BSL was widespread by the mid-19th century in combination with English, it fell out of favor as oralism reached popularity in Britain. Today, BSL is becoming increasingly well accepted and is a topic of research and study by linguists.

Bulwer, John This 17th-century English physician was very interested in manual communication as an orator but later became involved in its uses as a tool to educate deaf students.

Bulwer believed it was possible for deaf-mutes to learn speechreading and speech, although he believed that sign language and manual alphabets were more practical. His *Philocophus, or the Deafe and Dumbe Man's Friend,* published in 1648, was the first major English book on deafness. In it, he discussed the anatomy and physiology of speech and the etiology of deafness. He also explored the elements of phonetics, describing specific movements for each speech sound and insisting that speech is *movement* rather than *position*.

However, Bulwer was not a teacher of the deaf and never applied any of his theories. Although he hoped to establish a school for the deaf to teach communication methods to hard-of-hearing students, he never accomplished his goal.

C

Canada As in the United States, about one in ten Canadian citizens have some type of hearing problem. Nearly 4,000 children with hearing problems are in special programs, almost half of these students are profoundly deaf. These numbers, however, are estimates since there has been no national deaf census and the figures do not include native Canadians in the far north, among whom hearing loss is reportedly endemic. According to 1941 statistics, Canada's prevalence rate of deafness is 63 per 100,000 (an average rate), although much lower than the United States' rate of 100).

The result is a small and widely scattered minority population served only by a small number of professionals, in a country with a decentralized method of administering social services. This decentralization, in which the provinces fiercely maintain sole right to administer social services for its people, virtually guarantees a crazy-quilt pattern of services for deaf people across the country. Most important, education for Canada's deaf students has no uniform, comprehensive standards or administration.

Although deaf Canadians have made strides in civil rights, including the rights to legal interpreter services and to become adoptive parents, they have not been as successful in effecting improvements in postsecondary education, audiological service delivery and research.

Canada's history has been closely linked to England and France, but the country has allied itself with the United States in its development of educational services for its deaf citizens.

The first school for deaf Canadians was opened in 1831 in Champlain, Quebec by Ronald McDonald, who had spent a year at the American School for the Deaf at Hartford training under Thomas Gallaudet and Laurent Clerc. All schools gradually evolved from reliance on a manual to an oral educational philosophy.

American signs and AMERICAN SIGN LANGUAGE (ASL) have remained the preferred method of communication, although the small French deaf community within the country uses French-Canadian Sign Language. Across the country, there are regional differences in sign.

A bilingual dictionary of the basic vocabulary of sign language used in Canada is being compiled by the Canadian Coordinating Council on Deafness and will include the signs used in French Canada.

Because most Canadians prefer sign language, many disagree with the school-based English sign systems used as part of Total Communication in many educational programs. Many Canadians support a bilingual approach to learning language, with ASL as the first language and English signs as an added benefit to a student's curriculum.

Approximately 80% of Canadians have access to a telecommunication device for the deaf (TDD), and message relay centers operate in large cities.

Captioned television became available with the development in 1982 of the Canadian Captioning Development Agency, which captions a wide variety of Canadian programs in English and French. For a time, the agency also captioned French language telecasts around the world since there was no closed captioning system available to the French.

The Canadian Coordinating Council on Deafness and the Canadian Association of the Deaf are major national organizations with affiliated groups throughout the provinces. Contact: Alberta Association of the Deaf, 10004-105 St., Alberta, Canada T5J 1C4.

Canadian Sign Language Just as the culture of Canada has evolved along two lines, French and English, so has the language of the deaf community. Canada's deaf community speaks two completely different sign languages: Canadian Sign Language (CSL)—used primarily by deaf people in the English Canadian community—and Langue des Signes Quebecoise (LSQ)—used primarily by deaf French Canadians.

As in many sign languages around the world, much investigation is still being done into the structural properties of the communication methods. It appears, however, that CSL may share certain properties with British Sign Language, and LSQ may be similar to the sign language used in France (Langue des Signes Francaise [LSF], also called French Sign Language). There is also some evidence that CSL shares some structural similarities with American Sign Language. Still, research also suggests that both CSL and LSQ have different structures from English and French.

Although the Canadian constitution stipulates that English and French are equal official languages, it is extremely rare for a deaf student to be taught both CSL and LSQ.

As with many other sign languages, CSL and LSQ depend on systematic changes in movement, space and facial expression as linguistic devices to change meaning.

canal hearing aid Designed for mild to moderate hearing loss, this tiny device is even smaller than the in-the-ear devices and fits almost completely into the ear canal. It does not normally have a T-switch capability. Further, the ear canal must be of the right shape and size in order to use this type of hearing aid. Successful wearers are able to place the tiny unit into the ear, and utilize its even tinier controls. Cosmetically, it is the most appealing of all HEARING AIDS. (See also TELECOIL.)

cancer of the outer ear Cancer of the outer ear usually appears as a small, painless ulcer covered by a dry scab that slowly deepens in areas exposed for years to the sun. Treatment involves complete removal of the cancerous area and radiation therapy.

More serious—and more rare—is cancer that begins in the ear canal, where it may spread to the bone before being discovered and can therefore be more difficult to cure. (See also ACOUSTIC NEUROMA, CHOLESTEATOMA, CHORISTOMA.)

Caption Center This nonprofit service of Boston's WGBH Educational Foundation was the world's first television captioning agency.

The center began offering open captioning (captions visible on all TV sets) on programs in the early 1970s to stations affiliated with the Public Broadcasting Service (PBS). Usually, the first showing of a program had no captions, and rebroadcasts carried open captions.

Today, the center produces captions for every segment of the entertainment and advertising industries and offers an array of services, including real-time captions (live captions created as a program is broadcast) and open captions. Its development of software programs has enabled agencies and schools to caption their own programs and events.

In 1991 the center received a $6 million three-year grant from the U.S. Department of Education to provide real-time captioning services for national news and public affairs programs on commercial and public television. This grant doubles the total number of captioned hours available. The three major TV networks (ABC, NBC and CBS) will assume up to one-third the cost for their network news. The share for the "MacNeil/Lehrer Newshour" public TV show will be contributed by The John D. and Catherine T. MacArthur Foundation. (See also CLOSED CAPTIONS; NATIONAL CAPTIONING INSTITUTE; TELECAPTION DECODER.) Contact: The Caption Center, 125 Western Ave., Boston, MA 02134; telephone (voice and TDD): 617-492-9225.

Captioned Films/Videos for the Deaf A loan service of theatrical and educational films and videocassettes captioned for deaf viewers. Established in 1958, the project is funded by the captioning and adaptations branch of the U.S. Department of Education to promote the education and welfare of deaf people through the media. This branch also provides funds for several closed-captioned TV programs, including the live-captioned news on the ABC, NBC and CBS networks.

Captioned Films/Videos for the Deaf grew out of a private, nonprofit corporation established by the Junior League of Hartford and the CONVENTION OF AMERICAN INSTRUCTORS OF THE DEAF that was designed to caption films for deaf people. Because the expense and size of the job soon became too much for the small company, Congress passed Public Law 85-905, which established Captioned Films for the Deaf as a government service.

In 1965, Congress changed the name to Media Services and Captioned Films/Videos for the Deaf in order to broaden its services to include other people; however, subsequent Congresses did not appropriate money for this larger purpose. (See also CLOSED CAPTIONS; NATIONAL CAPTIONING INSTITUTE; TELECAPTION DECODER) Contact: Captioned Films/Videos for the Deaf, 5000 Park St. N, St. Petersburg, FL 33709; telephone (voice and TDD): 800-237-6213.

carhart notch A loss in bone conduction hearing acuity at 500, 1,000, 2,000 and 4,000 Hz first discovered by audiologist Raymond Carhart in patients with OTOSCLEROSIS. The loss is not attributed to impairment of the COCHLEA but to blockage of cochlear fluid movement by the STAPES which have become fixed in place.

CASE See CONCEPTUALLY ACCURATE SIGNED ENGLISH.

catarrhal deafness Hearing loss caused by inflammation of the mucous membrane of the air passages in the head and throat together with a blocked EUSTACHIAN TUBE. Since this is an early stage of an acute ear infection, antibiotic drug treatment is generally prescribed, together with decongestants to alleviate symptoms.

catarrhal otitis media See SEROUS OTITIS MEDIA.

cauliflower ear A deformity of the shape of the outer ear (pinna) caused by blows or friction that are sharp enough to start bleeding within the soft cartilage of the ear itself. It is most commonly found in boxers and can be prevented by using a protective helmet.

After a severe blow to the ear, swelling can be reduced by applying an ice pack, and blood can be drained from the ear with a needle and syringe. Repeated injuries to the ear, however, will distort its shape in a way that can only be repaired through plastic surgery.

CC Acronym used to denote closed captioning on TV programs, videocassettes and so forth. (See CLOSED CAPTIONS.)

Center for Bicultural Studies, Inc. This group promotes public education about the interaction between deaf and hearing cultures and fosters public acceptance, understanding and use of AMERICAN SIGN LANGUAGE and other natural signed languages. It disseminates information on deaf culture and American Sign Language, sponsors forums, public discussions and video projects and publishes the *TBC News*. Contact: Center for Bicultural Studies, Inc., 5506 Kenilworth Ave., Suite 105, Riverdale, MD 20737; telephone: 301-277-3945.

Center for Hearing Dog Information A national advocacy resource and referral center for hearing ear dog programs sponsored by the American Humane Association. The center publishes a Hearing Dog Program Directory, which outlines hearing dog programs and also lists support dog training programs (dogs who assist the physically disabled) and agencies that train dog guides for the blind.

Individuals with a severe to profound hearing loss who can demonstrate a need for such a dog can qualify. Only a few programs place children with dogs because children often cannot maintain the necessary control over an animal. (See also HEARING EAR DOGS.) Contact: Center for Hearing Dog Information, 9725 E. Hampden Ave., Denver, CO 80231; telephone: 303-695-0811 (voice); 303-695-4531 (TDD).

central auditory imperception See AUDITORY AGNOSIA.

central hearing loss A type of hearing loss that results from damage or impairment to the nerves or nuclei of the central nervous system, either in the pathways to the brain or in the brain itself. Central hearing loss may result from congenital brain abnormalities, tumors or lesions of the central nervous system, strokes or from some medications that specifically harm the ear. (See also HEARING LOSS, OTOTOXIC DRUGS.)

cerebral palsy A general term for nonprogressive disorders of movement, posture or speech caused by brain damage during pregnancy, birth or early childhood. About 25% to 30% of people with cerebral palsy have hearing problems.

The degree of physical disability varies widely from slight clumsiness to complete immobility. About two to six infants per 1,000 develop cerebral palsy—90% shortly before or during birth, usually from a lack of oxygen. Sometimes, cerebral palsy can result from a mother's infection that has passed to her unborn baby or from an excess of bilirubin in the blood after birth. After birth, cerebral palsy also can result from a head injury, encephalitis or meningitis.

Although there is no cure for cerebral palsy, it is possible to treat people who have it; physical therapy can help develop muscular control, and speech problems can be treated by speech therapy.

certified hearing aid audiologist An AUDIOLOGIST certified by the AMERICAN SPEECH-LANGUAGE-HEARING ASSOCIATION as qualified to dispense hearing aids. The certified hearing aid audiologist must hold a master's degree in AUDIOLOGY, pass a national certifying examination and hold the certificate of clinical competence.

cerumen See EARWAX.

chickenpox A common and mild childhood infectious disease related to the herpes viruses, which have been known to cause sudden severe deafness in one ear. An attack of chickenpox, which is caused by the varicella-zoster virus, confers lifelong immunity. Afterwards, the virus lies dormant within nerve tissues and may erupt as herpes zoster (shingles) later in life.

The airborne virus is easily spread during the two days before the rash appears and for about a week afterward. Women in the last months of pregnancy are particularly vulnerable and may pass the disease on to their infants, who may have severe cases.

Chickenpox is heralded by a rash on the body, face, upper arms and legs, under the arms, inside the mouth and sometimes in the bronchial tubes. Children usually have only a slight fever, but adults may become quite ill with severe pneumonia and breathing difficulties. Complications include encephalitis (brain inflammation), which can lead to deafness.

Treatment involves rest with acetaminophen to reduce the fever and lotion to relieve the rash, although acyclovir (a drug used to treat other herpes viruses) may also be used in severe cases of chickenpox.

There is no vaccine against chickenpox. (See also VIRUSES AND HEARING LOSS.)

children and deafness The estimates of deafness in the U.S. population vary, but it is particularly difficult to estimate the incidence of deafness among children because it often goes unrecognized or misdiagnosed in the very young. Still, the numbers of hard-of-hearing children are much greater than the numbers of deaf children. Federal government projections have estimated there are about 50,000 deaf and 325,000 hard-of-hearing children in the school-age population. More than 90% of the deaf children and about 20% of the hard-of-hearing children receive special educational services. Data on school children with hearing problems prepared by the Census Bureau in conjunction with the National Center for Health Statistics indicate that in 1982 about 2 out of every 100 people under age 18 had at least some form of hearing problems.

In the book *Deaf Population in the United States,* authors Jerome Schein and Marcus Delk estimate that 1 person in 1,000 is born deaf or is deafened before age three and that 1 in 500 is born deaf or is deafened before the age of 19.

In general, deaf children receive more intensive and comprehensive services while children with a milder hearing loss mainly receive speech-language therapy.

China, People's Republic of There are about three million deaf citizens in China, but services for these people are in woefully short supply. Only about 33,000 of them currently attend schools for deaf students.

The first school for deaf students opened in 1887 at Dengchou, and by 1948 there were 23 such schools, most of which were private. When the People's Republic of China was founded in 1949, the new government mandated major changes in the education of deaf children.

First, the government took control of all schools for deaf students, limited class size to 15 pupils, established a Bureau of the Deaf and Blind to administer education and began research in oral teaching methods. Since then, education for deaf children has grown to more than 30 schools with more than 9,000 staff for 33,000 students.

Students can attend combined schools for deaf and blind children, schools for deaf students only or special classes in regular schools. Still, the school enrollment rate of deaf children is very low, and the system of education is considered poor.

Deaf Chinese citizens are given the same rights as every other member of society and, in cities, receive government-paid medical care and pensions. The government has special rules for its deaf criminals: Since 1980,

Chinese law states that if a deaf person violates a criminal law, he or she can be exempt from punishment or only lightly punished.

Although there were no unified language communication methods for deaf Chinese in the past, research into communication did not begin until the founding of the People's Republic. In 1963 the government adopted the Chinese Fingerspelling Alphabet Scheme, based on the Chinese pronunciation scheme and consisting of 30 separate fingershapes.

The primary association for deaf Chinese is the Chinese Association for the Blind and the Deaf, which is headquartered in Beijing and is a member of the World Federation of the Deaf.

Chinese Sign Language The standard communication mode for the people of mainland China, Chinese Sign Language (CSL) includes 3,000 signs with 41 recurrent handshapes. Although there are three million deaf Chinese, it is unknown how many use CSL.

In general, CSL places the verb last, with the modified followed by the modifier: "Girl sleep not." It has a manual alphabet with 26 letters and four digraphic consonants used to fingerspell words. It is used primarily in schools; deaf Chinese signers rarely use fingerspelling.

Ideograms are still the main type of writing found in China, and 22 of these ideograms are used in CSL. Not surprisingly, given the isolated nature of mainland China, very few of its signs have come from foreign shores.

cholesteatoma This chronic middle ear inflammatory disease is a rare, serious condition in which skin cells and debris collect within the middle ear, usually as a result of a middle ear infection that has caused the eardrum to burst. Cholesteatomas can either be present at birth or appear later in life; the rare congenital variety may appear anywhere in the temporal bone.

Acquired cholesteatoma may be caused by a persistent narrowing of the eustachian tube, eventually pulling the upper part of the eardrum back and forming a sac in the middle ear. The acquired form may also occur because of a tiny hole in the eardrum that allows skin cells of the external ear canal to move into the middle ear.

If the cholesteatoma is not treated, it may grow and damage the small bones in the middle ear and surrounding bone structures, causing a conductive or a mixed hearing loss and serious complications, including secondary infection, LABYRINTHITIS, MENINGITIS or a brain abscess.

The cholesteatoma must be removed either through the eardrum or by MASTOIDECTOMY (removal of the mastoid bone behind the ear together with the cholesteatoma).

Chomsky, Noam (b. 1928) This American linguist is one of the founders of generative grammar, an original system of linguistic analysis. He believes there is a universal pattern in all languages and linguists should study a native speaker's unconscious knowledge of his own language and not the speaker's actual production of language.

Unlike structuralists, who collect samples of language and then classify them, Chomsky developed transformational grammar—a set of rules that can generate structural descriptions for all the grammatical sentences of a language. He then tested results against actual language samples. Transformational grammar has continued to evolve since Chomsky first introduced it in 1957.

Chomsky, whose father was a Hebrew scholar who studied historical LINGUISTICS, teaches modern languages and linguistics at the Massachusetts Institute of Technology.

choristoma A benign tumor in the middle ear that is really a congenital misplacement of the salivary gland and usually occurs with a middle ear malformation. It is treated by complete surgical removal. Although benign, these tumors can cause a conductive hearing disorder by their physical presence—filling the middle ear, destroying OSSICLES and interfering with eardrum movement. (See also TUMORS OF THE MIDDLE EAR.)

classifiers Handshapes that represent or describe certain types of classes of objects or occurrences (for example, upright index fingers brought together to indicate two people meeting).

cleft palate and hearing loss A number of children with cleft palates also have mild to moderate conductive hearing loss because of the cleft condition in the mouth area; this loss is usually medically treatable. A hearing assessment is usually given during speech tests to find out if such a hearing loss is present.

Clerc, Laurent (1785–1869) This leader in education for deaf people was born in LaBalme les Grottes, the son of a family noted in local politics.

Deafened at age one after an infection following a facial burn, Clerc was taken to the famous Royal National Institute for the Deaf in Paris (now the INSTITUT NATIONAL DES JEUNES SOURDS), where he studied with the brilliant deaf instructor JEAN MASSIEU; by the age of 20 he had completed his education and was teaching classes at the institute.

At the school, Clerc met THOMAS HOPKINS GALLAUDET, who had come to learn the manual alphabet developed there. Gallaudet convinced Clerc to return with him to the United States for three years to help establish a school for deaf students.

It was on the ocean voyage to this country that Gallaudet taught Clerc English and Clerc completed Gallaudet's training in manual communication. Once in the United States, Gallaudet and Clerc raised $5,000 at presentations and special programs they conducted throughout New England, an amount that was later matched by the Connecticut general assembly.

With this money, the AMERICAN SCHOOL FOR THE DEAF opened its doors in 1817 in Hartford, Connecticut with seven pupils. The next year, Clerc married one of these, Eliza Boardman, and decided to remain in America. He returned to France to visit only three times.

Although Clerc could not speak, he had great political influence and could write fluently in French and English. With these skills, he was able to convince Americans that deaf children could be educated and that sign language was the best type of communication to use while teaching them. At the age of 73, Clerc retired after 50 years of teaching. He died on July 18, 1869, and was buried beside his wife in Hartford.

closed captions The audio portion of a television program that has been translated into typed dialogue that usually appears across the bottom of the screen. Because viewers who are not deaf could find ordinary subtitles (open captions) distracting, a special TELECAPTION DECODER is needed to see these captions.

Although captioning was at first limited to previously-taped programs, in 1984 the development of computer technology had reached the point where "real time" captioning became available for live broadcasts.

Most captioning is done at the headquarters of the NATIONAL CAPTIONING INSTITUTE (NCI) in Falls Church, Virginia and at WGBH-TV in Boston. When captioning prerecorded programs, an editor records captions on a magnetic disk that is then sent to the TV broadcaster where it is inserted into line 21 of the TV signal. It takes about 30 hours to caption a one-hour program and costs about $2,500.

For live broadcasts, a court stenographer enters phonetic symbols into a computer that then translates the symbols into captions and beams them through the network to viewers about four seconds after words are spoken.

While it works fairly well, captions cannot be edited and mistakes occasionally appear.

Closed captioning was introduced in 1980 and is now used in more than 70% of prime-time programming on networks and cable TV in addition to local and national news, sports and political events. Further, a large number of video movies are now available in closed captioned versions.

A free service of TV and cable networks and home video producers, captioning is funded by corporations, foundations, the government, producers, networks and program sponsors. In addition, people interested

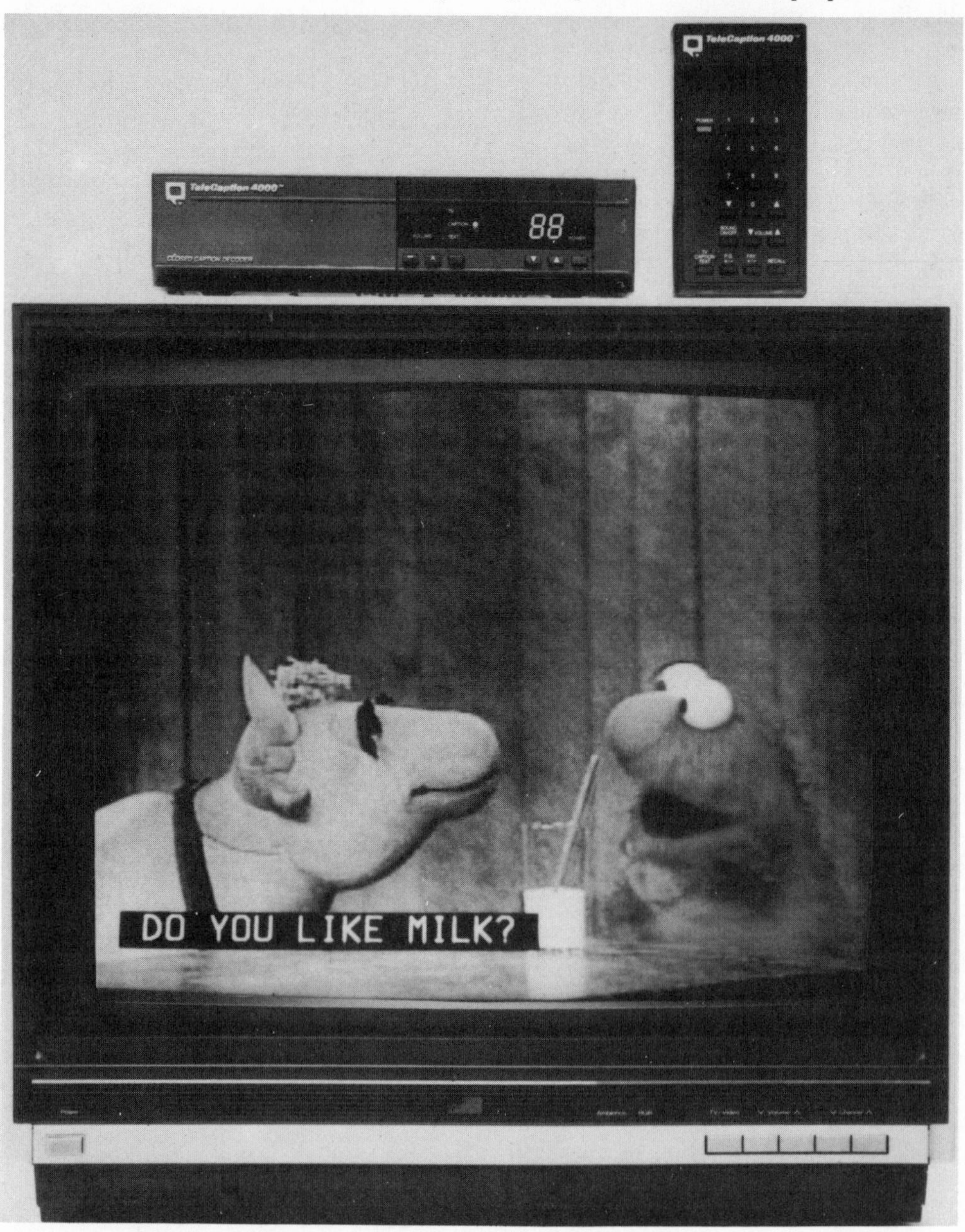

Closed captioning of "Sesame Street"/PBS television show

in closed captioned programs may join NCI's Caption Club, whose membership dues are used to fund captioning of TV programs that reflect viewer's preferences.

Published TV schedules usually mark captioned programs with a "C" or "CC." The TeleCaption decoder itself provides a Program Listing Update Service (PLUS), which is a daily listing of captioned programs and sponsors. TeleCaption decoders are produced by the National Captioning Institute.

There are several different methods of producing closed captions. These include:

Prerecorded Captions Videotaped programs may be broadcast with prerecorded captions, prepared before the airing of the program. In advance, the captioner watches a tape of the program, then writes the captions and types them into a computer together with instructions regarding when and where they should appear on the screen. Then a new tape is made combining the tape of the program and the captions.

Live Display Captions For live TV programs in which there is a script prepared in advance, it is possible to prepare captions before the program airs. The captions are typed into a computer, and when the live program is aired, the captions in the computer are sent to a machine that adds them to the TV signal.

Real-time Captions For live programs with no prepared scripts (such as debates and news conferences), it is possible to create captions as the program is being aired. In this case, a captioner uses a stenotype machine similar to the one used by court reporters, which uses a type of shorthand. As the operator types out the shorthand, the computer converts the symbols into English and organizes them into captions; the captions are then sent to a machine that combines them with the TV signal. They appear on a TV set after a short delay since the operator must hear the word before it can be typed and the computer takes a few additional seconds to perform its functions. These captions are presented in a rolling fashion in order to appear as quickly as possible. There may be mistakes since there is no time to proofread what is typed.

Commentary Captions Some sports shows use this form of closed caption, which does not follow word-for-word what commentators say but simply reports the scoreboard, play-by-play and background information. For the first two types of information, brief descriptions are typed into a computer that types out a more involved caption (the computer might take the brief "out 1" and translate it to "That's the first out for the Red Sox"). Background information is prepared ahead of time in the same way live-display captions are. (See above.)

Combination Some shows may use several types of captioning; for example, a news show with a prerecorded or scripted segment may use live-display together with real-time for those spots that are live with no scripts. (See also CAPTION CENTER.)

cochlea A snail-shaped part of the ear located behind the oval window. The cochlea contains fluid, thousands of microscopic hair cells tuned to various frequencies and more than 20 types of cells. This complex inner ear organ contains the ORGAN OF CORTI, which lies between two fluid channels—the scala vestibuli and the scala tympani.

The sodium-rich PERILYMPH fluid of the scala vestibuli is separated from the potassium-rich ENDOLYMPH fluid of the membranous cochlea by the paper-thin REISSNER'S MEMBRANE. Because these two fluids are separated, they maintain a vital difference in electrical charge imperative for the correct function of the cochlea's sensory cells.

The entire membranous part of the cochlea is surrounded by bone, into which there are two entrances: the round and oval windows.

Sound, traveling through the middle ear, reaches the STAPES (the third bone of the ossicles), which is attached to the oval window by a ligament that allows it to move, transferring sound vibrations to the scala vestibuli. This fluid brushes the tiny hair cells (or sensory cells) where separate pitches are registered, generating an electrical current that telegraphs sound through acoustic nerves to the brain. Once in the brain, the current is then interpreted as sound.

There are two types of hair cells; about 12,000 outer hair cells and about 3,500 inner hair cells lying close to the core of the cochlea. These hair cells are part of the organ of Corti, which lies on the BASILAR MEMBRANE, both part of the membranous cochlea.

When the hair cells of the cochlea die, there is no way to revive or replace them. These cells can die from a variety of causes, including excess noise and the aging process. The hair cells responsible for registering high notes almost always fail first, perhaps because they are located in a more exposed area.

cochlear duct See SCALA MEDIA.

cochlear implant A device that is surgically implanted in the MASTOID BONE to stimulate the hearing nerve and enable a hard-of-hearing person to perceive some sound; the implant does not restore normal hearing.

The implant consists of a magnetic coil surgically placed in the mastoid bone behind the ear. An electrode runs from the magnetic coil and may be placed either within or out side of the COCHLEA (the snail-shaped section of the inner ear containing the hearing-nerve endings). This electrode stimulates the hearing nerve and enables a person to perceive sound.

Cochlear implants have significantly improved the communication skills of some adults who have lost their hearing after they learned to speak. More typically, speechreading ability improves. However, of the 15 million Americans with significant hearing loss, less than 1 percent are potential candidates for an implant.

The simplest version has a single channel, but multichannel implants with more than 20 electrodes (each implanted further along the cochlear duct) have considerably enhanced performance. These electrodes are used with a device that encodes frequencies, providing some pitch discrimination. Implants may transmit only certain features of the speech signal (feature-extraction) or the input signal may be transmitted to the electrodes without extraction specific speech cues (non-feature specific).

Although early expectations were limited to hopes that patients would be able to hear enough sound to increase speechreading abilities, many patients can now understand spoken words without speechreading. Unfortunately, it is not yet possible to predict who will benefit from a cochlear implant to that extent, nor how well one will work for any individual. When tested, people with similar devices score from 0% to 90% on speech comprehension tests.

In addition, there are some risks involved: besides the usual danger inherent in any surgery, it is possible that the implant could damage the inner ear, destroying residual hearing. There is also risk of infection at the site of the skin flap behind the ear, and possible damage to the facial nerve or vestibular system. However, incidence of damage to date has been very slight.

Cochlear implants remain a somewhat controversial choice in the treatment of hearing problems. As yet, it is unclear how much help the implants can provide to hearing or learning spoken or sign language with congenitally deaf children and with those who lost their hearing before acquiring speech or language. Experts stress the implant is not for everyone and research on its value is continuing.

However, new research with implants used in pre- and post-lingually deafened children suggests that they can achieve some awareness of sound with this device. Recently, research suggests some children deaf since birth have obtained some understanding of words with the more advanced multichannel implant system. The long-term changes due to implant-tissue interaction are unknown.

Good candidates for implant surgery include people whose cochlea is completely ineffective but whose hearing nerve endings still respond to direct stimulation. In these cases, sound activating the implanted electrode stimulates the hearing nerve, and the person can hear noise that is usually described as different from the original sound. This difference is because the implant cannot match the normal complex process of the ear as it converts sound into nerve impulses. (See also HOUSE EAR INSTITUTE.) Contact: Cochlear Implant Club International, P.O. Box 464, Buffalo NY 14223; telephone: 716-838-4662 (voice/TDD).

Cochlear Ménière's disease An atypical form of MÉNIÈRE'S DISEASE in which sufferers experience hearing loss, DIZZINESS and TINNITUS—but not the spinning sensation of VERTIGO, as in the classical form of the disorder.

Cogan's syndrome This inflammation of the cornea, which occurs for no known reason, can also damage new bone formation around the ROUND WINDOW and destroy the ORGAN OF CORTI and cochlear nerve cells, resulting in vertigo, tinnitus and severe sensorineural hearing loss. Treatment with steroid drugs is often effective in suppressing disease activity; in some patients drugs may be tapered off and stopped, while others require maintenance level treatment.

Cogswell, Alice (1805–1830) The inspiration behind the establishment of the first permanent school for deaf students in the United States, Alice Cogswell was born in 1805 in Hartford, Connecticut, the third daughter of Dr. MASON FITCH COGSWELL and his wife, Mary.

When Alice was two years old, she contracted cerebrospinal meningitis and lost her hearing before she had completely learned to speak. Whatever speech she had at that point was almost gone by the time she was four, and she could hear very little. Although bright and eager to learn, she fell behind other children her age in spite of the efforts of her family to teach her.

Fortunately for Alice, her neighbors were the THOMAS HOPKINS GALLAUDET family. Alice played with Gallaudet's children and communicated with them using her own code of gestures.

One day, when Gallaudet spelled "hat" for Alice on the ground, using his hat as an illustration, Alice immediately understood that objects had written names and demanded to learn the names of other objects. This was the beginning of real communication between Gallaudet and a deaf child and the start of a lifelong interest for Gallaudet.

When Gallaudet subsequently opened the American Asylum for the Deaf and Dumb in 1817 (now the American School for the Deaf), Alice was first in line to attend, carrying a slate with her to communicate with those who did not know sign language.

Alice, who believed she could not live without her father, died 13 days after he had succumbed to pneumonia in 1830. She was 25 years old.

Cogswell, Mason Fitch (1761–1830) Cofounder of the AMERICAN SCHOOL FOR THE DEAF, this Connecticut surgeon and Yale University professor first became interested in deafness when his daughter Alice became deaf at the age of two from cerebrospinal meningitis, a childhood illness associated with a prolonged high fever.

Cogswell's neighbor was young THOMAS HOPKINS GALLAUDET, who noticed Alice's struggles to communicate with neighbors and began to teach her. Unable to find a school for the deaf in 18th-century America and inspired by Gallaudet's success, Cogswell sent Gallaudet to Europe to learn how to teach deaf children. When Gallaudet returned with a French expert in deaf education, Cogswell—together with Gallaudet and

10 Hartford city fathers—founded the American School for the Deaf in Hartford. (See also CLERC, LAURENT; COGSWELL, ALICE.)

Coiter, Volcher (1534–1600) A Dutch physician who first traced the path of sound waves from the ear canal through the EARDRUM and middle ear bones into the COCHLEA.

A student of anatomy for many years in some of the most celebrated universities of Italy, Coiter also served as personal physician to the mad Prince Ludwig of Bavaria.

He is best known for his book, *De auditus instrumento,* published in 1566 and the first devoted entirely to the ear. The book contained 17 chapters dealing with the various parts of the organ of hearing from anatomical and physiological points of view. His theories were generally accepted by his contemporaries.

Comité International des Sports des Sourds (CISS) This group was organized in 1924 by representatives from six nations (Belgium, Czechoslovakia, France, Great Britain, the Netherlands and Poland) and is similar to the International Olympic Committee in that it regulates olympic-style competition for deaf athletes.

Formerly named the Comité International des Sports Silencieux, CISS is made up of many national sports federations of deaf people and is supervised by an executive committee made up of one deaf person from each of eight different counties. All business at its international meetings and congress is conducted in GESTUNO (international sign language), and no interpreters are used.

It is staffed by volunteers and earns money through dues, fines and competition fees. Officers of CISS are chosen by the executive committee from among federation members. (See also WORLD GAMES FOR THE DEAF.)

compliance The ability of the EARDRUM to accept and transmit sound vibrations from the EXTERNAL EAR CANAL to the MIDDLE EAR. Disorders of the eardrum or the middle ear decrease this ability.

Conceptually Accurate Signed English (CASE) Another term for PIDGIN SIGN ENGLISH or SIGN ENGLISH.

conditioning tests One of several hearing tests designed for infants. In the *visual reinforcement test,* a loud sound is paired with presentation of something visually interesting, such as a flashing light or a puppet. After a number of repetitions, the baby will be conditioned to respond to the sound alone. The sound can then gradually be reduced in intensity and used for testing. Practice sessions may be needed in this test.

In the *conditioned orienting response test,* a sound is sent through one loudspeaker; if the infant turns toward the speaker, a light is flashed. The difference with the conditioned orienting response test from other conditioning tests is that the infant is rewarded for localizing the sound.

In *conditioned play audiometry,* a child is taught to respond to a sound presented through an earphone or loudspeaker by manipulating a toy—for example, putting a peg in a pegboard when a sound is heard. These tests are reliable only if the child is able to respond to the test, usually after the age of two and one half. Adult tests can usually be used after age five.

Sounds used in these tests are either two-syllable sounds, bursts of noise or pure tones. (See also AUDIOMETRY.)

conduction tests See AUDIOMETRY.

conductive hearing loss People with this type of medically treatable hearing loss usually have normal inner ears but specific problems in the outer or middle ear that prevent sound from getting to the inner ear in a normal way. (See also HEARING LOSS.)

Conference of Educational Administrators Serving the Deaf (CEASD) A nonprofit organization committed to improved management in programs for deaf students and educational options for deaf people.

The organization was founded in 1869 as the Conference of Superintendents and Principals of American Schools for the Deaf. The dream of EDWARD MINER GALLAUDET, then president of the Columbia Institution for the Deaf and Dumb (now GALLAUDET UNIVERSITY), was to unite school principals behind his philosophy of communication in the classroom.

Today, the group tries to promote a continuum of educational opportunities for deaf people in North America and to encourage efficient management of schools and programs for deaf people.

The organization holds annual meetings for its members, who must have administrative roles in educational programs for deaf students. In odd-numbered years, its meeting is held at the same time as the CONVENTION OF AMERICAN INSTRUCTORS OF THE DEAF. At these shared meetings, CEASD dedicates one day for its own business, sharing the convention schedule's presentations for the rest of the meeting.

In addition, CEASD (together with the ALEXANDER GRAHAM BELL ASSOCIATION FOR THE DEAF and the Convention of American Instructors of the Deaf) provides certification programs for teachers of deaf students through a confederation called the COUNCIL ON EDUCATION OF THE DEAF.

Conference headquarters are located in Silver Spring, Maryland at Halex House (the building owned by the NATIONAL ASSOCIATION OF THE DEAF). Both CEASD's office and executive director are shared with the Convention of American Instructors of the Deaf. It also shares administrative responsibility with the convention for its journal, AMERICAN ANNALS OF THE DEAF. Contact: President Barry Griffing, P.O. Box 5545, Tucson, AZ 85703; telephone (voice and TDD): 602-628-5261. For journal information contact *American Annals of the Deaf*, Gallaudet University, 800 Florida Ave. NE, Washington DC 20002.

congenital nerve deafness Occurring at or soon after birth, this type of hearing loss may be caused by too little oxygen during a long and difficult delivery. Other causes include kernicterus—a form of jaundice caused by an incompatibility of Rh blood factors between the infant and its mother—and, rarely, an inherited failure of the cochlea to develop properly.

Congenital nerve deafness cannot be cured or improved by surgery, although hearing aids can be helpful to take advantage of whatever residual hearing remains.

Convention of American Instructors of the Deaf Founded in 1850, the convention is one of the oldest American professional organizations interested in education for deaf students.

Its initial meeting in New York, organized by instructors at the New York Institution for the Deaf, marked the first time that a convention for deaf educators was held anywhere in the world. Among other things, conference attendees adopted the *American Annals of the Deaf* as their official publication. Today, the convention and the CONFERENCE OF EDUCATIONAL ADMINISTRATORS SERVING THE DEAF manage the journal as equal partners.

The purpose of the convention is to promote the education of deaf students "along the broadest and most advanced lines." The organization is located in Silver Spring, Maryland in Halex House, owned by the NATIONAL ASSOCIATION OF THE DEAF, and shares its office and executive director with the Conference of Educational Administrators Serving the Deaf. Contact: Convention of American Instructors of the Deaf, P.O. Box 2025, Austin, TX 78768; telephone (voice and TDD): 512-441-2225. (For journal information, see Appendix 9.)

Corti, Alfonso (1822–1888) With the aid of a powerful compound microscope, Corti traced the BASILAR MEMBRANE attached to the lamina and detected thousands of tiny hair cells that rest on the membrane.

Now known collectively as the ORGAN OF CORTI, these cells make up the actual hearing organ and are linked to the brain through the auditory nerve.

cosmetic surgical reconstruction A procedure performed to correct a malformation of the external ear (also called PINNA or auricle). The most common cosmetic reconstruction of the external ear is to treat excessively protruding ears caused by hypertrophic development of the conchal cartilage or insufficient folding of the antehelix ridge. In the worst cases, the ears can extend at a 90 degree angle from the scalp.

If cosmetic surgery is to be performed, it is usually done while the child is young. In the operation, a surgeon cuts the skin behind the ear, excises a portion of the exposed cartilage and moves the antehelix closer to the mastoid bone, holding it in place with stitches.

Cosmetic surgery is also beneficial in the treatment of macrotia (an overdeveloped external ear), which can affect one or both ears.

It is also possible to totally reconstruct the ear. Generally, there is a rudimentary ear already present, which is cut in half horizontally to form the new ear. A piece of tubular skin graft or rib cartilage is placed between the two halves, inserted under the skin over the mastoid bone.

cotton swabs Despite frequent warnings against their use in the ear, these small sticks tipped with cotton are often used to dislodge EARWAX within the ear canal. In actuality, the swabs can push the wax farther into the ear canal, potentially damaging the eardrum. A punctured eardrum with a hole larger than 1.5 mm will produce a conductive hearing loss by interfering with the eardrum's vibration. Larger holes can cause even greater hearing loss; for example, perforation of less than 20% of the eardrum causes a 15 dB hearing loss. Destruction of the entire eardrum can result in a maximum of 45 dB loss. Swabs such as these are particularly dangerous when used to clean the ears of infants, whose uncontrolled movements can force the swab deep into the ear with disastrous results.

An infant's outer ear may be cleaned with a wet washcloth, but nothing should ever be placed into the ear canal. Accumulated earwax in danger of blocking hearing may be removed by a physician; however, most earwax is normal and is a natural way for the ear to protect itself.

Council on Education of the Deaf Founded in 1960, this group, representing more than 10,000 teachers, sets standards for teachers of deaf students, conducts evaluations of teacher training programs and issues certificates for teachers of deaf students. There are about 15,000 teachers serving more than 46,000 deaf and hard-of-hearing students in classes throughout the United States and Canada.

The council coordinates the efforts of three groups involved in deaf education: the CONFERENCE OF EDUCATIONAL ADMINISTRATORS SERVING THE DEAF, the CONVENTION OF AMERICAN INSTRUCTORS OF THE DEAF and the ALEXANDER GRAHAM BELL ASSOCIATION FOR THE DEAF.

The professional certification of teachers of deaf students had first been studied separately by the Alexander Graham Bell Association and the Conference of Educational Administrators Serving the Deaf. The two plans that had been developed by these organizations were administered separately, as a teacher registry (Bell) and as a certification program (CAID) until 1935, when they were joined into a single program.

Council on Professional Standards The primary certification and accreditation board of the AMERICAN-SPEECH-LANGUAGE-HEARING ASSOCIATION (ASHA) located at the association's headquarters in Rockville, MD. Originally established as a certification board in 1959 as the American Board of Examiners in Speech Pathology and Audiology, the group was renamed in 1980 to better describe its larger role as both a certifying and accrediting organization. The council concerns itself not only with the certification of individuals, but with the accreditation of college and university programs and the clinical programs which employ speech-language pathologists and audiologists. Contact: Council on Professional Standards, c/o American Speech-Language-Hearing Association, 10801 Rockville Pike, Rockville, MD 20852; telephone (voice and TDD): 301-897-5700.

Court Interpreter's Act This 1978 act of Congress ensures that people with hearing problems will be given an interpreter if they are involved as the defendant in proceedings brought by the federal government in a district court. It was later amended and broadened by the 1979 BILINGUAL, HEARING-AND-SPEECH-IMPAIRED COURT INTERPRETER ACT. The law requires that either an oral or manual interpreter must be provided at public expense whenever a defendant has a hearing problem that inhibits the ability to communicate or understand testimony.

Before the act was passed, interpreters were allowed but not required, and the decision to have an interpreter was left up to the individual judge. In many occasions, however, judges did not ask for an interpreter, and individuals with hearing problems did not receive communication assistance. Because of this, subsequent appellate court rulings stipulated that without the ability to communicate with lawyers and confront witnesses, hard-of-hearing people are deprived of their constitutional right to due process under the law.

The act requires that the clerk of each U.S. district court maintain a current list of all court-certified interpreters within that court's jurisdiction. The director of the administrative office of U.S. courts is responsible for outlining qualifications for interpreters.

An interpreter may be appointed at the request of the judge, the hard-of-hearing person's attorney or the person himself. Hard-of-hearing people may waive the right to a court-appointed interpreter and use their own interpreters, who will still be paid by the court. The interpreter can interpret simultaneously, consecutively or in summary (although the latter is not recommended).

In court actions outside of federal court, a hard-of-hearing defendant or witness may ask for help from the court clerk in locating an interpreter, but the interpreter may not necessarily be provided at public expense. The presiding judge will determine who should pay for the interpreter.

Further, privileged communications between defendant and attorney through the interpreter are confidential, and the interpreter cannot be required to testify about them. (See also INTERPRETERS AND THE LAW.)

CRIS-CROS hearing aid Because of feedback problems, a person with severe hearing loss in both ears may be unable to wear HEARING AIDS at ear level. (Feedback occurs when the amplifier leaks sound back into the microphone because it is too close to the receiver). In this case, a CRIS-CROS aid uses two CROS HEARING AIDS behind the ear, each unit encompassing the microphone for the other side.

CROS hearing aid Named for "contralateral routing of signals" and also called a "crossover" system, this is a special hearing aid for people with normal hearing in one ear and moderate to severe hearing loss in the other.

This system features a microphone, amplifier and controls beside the poorer ear in a partial mold that feed the amplified signal to the receiver or earphone in the better ear, thereby eliminating "head shadow" (the head blocking sound from the better ear). The amplified sound from the hearing aid on the one side is added to the normal sound entering the healthy ear. The two sides are usually linked by a built-in FM radio signal system, although there are wired models available.

This system may help make speech easier to understand for people with a high frequency loss in both ears. It also allows the listener to understand from which direction sounds are coming.

The benefit of this type of hearing aid system is that it can prevent feedback, which occurs when amplification leaks sound into the microphone located near the receiver. (See also HEARING AIDS.)

Cued Speech This method of communication was developed in 1966 by Dr. ORIN CORNETT as a speechreading support system that, in English, uses eight hand configurations and four hand positions near the mouth to supplement visible speech.

The hand cue signals a visual difference between sounds that look alike on the lips, such as "p" and "b." These cues enable the deaf person to see the phonetic equivalent of what others hear.

Each cue (hand placement or configuration) identifies a special group of two to four speech sounds. The combination of cues and mouth movements makes all the essential speech sounds appear different from each other, so that the spoken message is clarified.

The hand configurations and locations are called cues, not cued speech, which is the combination of the cues with speech (the cues are not readable alone).

Each hand configuration identifies a group of consonants; vowel sounds are shown by position of the hand in one of four ways, all within a few inches of the mouth (the side of the face, throat, chin and corner of the mouth).

Cued Speech can also be used to indicate approximate voice pitch for each syllable uttered, which is important in tonal languages (such as Thai, Cantonese and Mandarin). For example, in Cantonese, the syllable "ma" can mean "mother," "scold," "horse" or "right?" depending on the pitch.

Tone cueing is also helpful in speech therapy. In order to cue tone, a person changes the inclination of the cueing hand to indicate changes in pitch.

Cued Speech has been adapted to many languages, and audiocassette lessons designed for self-instruction by hearing persons are available. (See Appendix 13.) The system is generally the same in all languages.

Cued Speech was developed primarily because some congenitally deaf persons do not become good readers because they don't have an easy way to learn spoken language as young deaf children, according to Dr. Cornett. Proponents believe Cued Speech makes spoken language visually clear and solves the communication problem and also helps youngsters learn a spoken language more easily. It is an easily learned system, taking only about 12 to 20 hours to master. It is most successful when used consistently from early childhood.

Initial research suggests that Cued Speech does help make the spoken language clear, but the long-term effectiveness of the language is not known. One of the recent advances used in conjunction with Cued Speech is the AUTOCUER, a device invented by Dr. Cornett, which contains a miniature computerized speech processor that automatically analyzes speech input and produces cue-equivalents through light signals.

There was a great deal of initial interest in Cued Speech after it was introduced in the 1960s, but it was overshadowed by the spread of TOTAL COMMUNICATION at about the same time. Cued Speech tries to clear up some of the problems with speechreading. However, it has not been widely adopted in schools, and is not widely popular among the deaf population. (See also NATIONAL CUED SPEECH ASSOCIATION.)

cytomegalovirus (CMV) One of the family of herpes viruses, this infection is fairly common in pregnant women; if a woman becomes infected for the first time while she is pregnant, she can pass the infection on to her baby since the virus can cross the placenta. Approximately 80% of adults have CMV antibodies in the blood, indicating prior infection. It usually produces no symptoms.

About 11% of babies born to mothers infected with CMV during pregnancy will have a bilateral, SENSORINEURAL HEARING LOSS of varying severity. Hearing loss in these infants most often is profound, although there are milder losses in some babies.

Some studies suggest CMV has replaced rubella as the most common viral cause of prenatal deafness. This could be because CMV is extremely common—about 80% of adults have antibodies to it in their blood, indicating a previous infection. It is acquired by close personal contact with bodily secretions of someone infected with CMV and is harmless to anyone but a developing fetus. (See also PRENATAL CAUSES OF HEARING LOSS; VIRUSES AND HEARING LOSS.)

D

dactylology A term that generally refers to FINGERSPELLING, although it has been used sometimes to include signs.

DAF See DELAYED AUDITORY FEEDBACK.

Dalgarno, George (1626?–1687) This 17th-century Scottish theoretician's interest in techniques for teaching deaf students grew out of his fascination with the idea of a universal language for all people.

The headmaster of a private grammar school in England, Dalgarno discussed his theories and techniques for teaching deaf students to speak in *The Deaf and Dumb Man's Tutor*, in which he explained that the senses were connected in complex ways. He believed that a person blind from birth could learn quicker than a deaf person. However, with maturity, a deaf person would surpass a blind person in learning because, Dalgarno thought, sight was more essential to education in the long run than hearing. Although he implicitly believed that a deaf person could learn to speak and speechread, he believed that writing and his manual alphabet (a variation of the ROCHESTER METHOD, which he called DACTYLOLOGY) were more practical.

Espousing a natural language approach and early language stimulation, Dalgarno believed that a deaf infant could learn as quickly as a hearing baby if given the proper stimulation.

Danish Mouth-Hand System See MOUTH-HAND SYSTEMS.

Danish Sign Language Considered to be the primary language of deaf people in Denmark, Danish Sign Language has about 6,000 signs and is used together with the INTERNATIONAL HAND ALPHABET introduced by the WORLD FEDERATION OF THE DEAF in 1975. This manual alphabet is now used in Norway, Denmark and Finland. In addition to fingerspelling, a MOUTH-HAND SYSTEM has become an integral part of DSL.

Deaf Danish students were first taught in 1807 using methods based on the French manual method of ABBÉ CHARLES MICHEL DE L'EPÉE. Danish students were using their own signs, but teachers supplemented these with French signs when necessary; this influence by French Sign Language is still noticeable in the Danish sign vocabulary.

Although the oral method of education was introduced in 1881, DSL was never banned from Danish schools. Today, the five deaf schools all emphasize a manual educational method.

In addition, a combination of spoken Danish and sign language is called Signed Danish. It is used, as in many other sign systems around the world, primarily when communicating between deaf and hearing people and in interpreting.

deaf and dumb An archaic term coined by Aristotle meaning that a person can neither hear nor speak. The term is not in favor today because of its negative implication that deaf people are also "dumb" in a literal sense.

Deaf Artists of America This group was organized to bring support and recognition to deaf artists by collecting, publishing and disseminating information about deaf artists. It also provides cultural and educational opportunities and services to members and exhibits and markets deaf artists' works.

The group offers two directories—one of visual artists and one of performing artists. The directory of visual artists (such as painters, sculptors and graphic designers) includes names, addresses, telephone numbers, education, type of artist and availability, along with several photographs of artwork. The directory of performing artists lists information on individual artists and performing arts groups. It includes names, addresses and telephone numbers of actors, dancers, mimes, poets and storytellers with information on their availability, fees and willingness to travel. Contact: Deaf Artists of America, 87 N. Clinton Ave., Suite 408, Rochester, NY 14604; telephone (voice and TDD): 716-325-2400.

deaf-blindness The twin difficulties of the inability to see and hear cause special problems for the individual as well as the person's teachers and rehabilitators. Because deaf-blindness is rare, there has been relatively little help from agencies in this country. The first federal program for deaf-blind people was legislated only in 1968.

This legislation authorized and funded the rehabilitation facility called the National Center for Deaf-Blind Youth and Adults and regional educational programs for deaf-blind students, aimed at helping states educate deaf-blind children.

Although the particular problems of deaf-blind citizens were not widely known, the 1964 rubella epidemic brought the problem to the attention of the U.S. Congress—of the 30,000 infants who suffered visual or auditory systems problems because of this epidemic, about 1,500 were born blind and deaf. In 1966, there were 564 deaf and blind students in this country, but only 177 were enrolled in school. A realization of the impending influx of deaf-blind students prompted Congress to appropriate special funds for their education in 1968.

Deaf-blind people have a loss of two senses in common, but there is wide variation among their other abilities, just as in the hearing and sighted population.

One of the problems faced by deaf-blind people is the definition of deaf-blindness: Different facilities and educational programs define it differently. Further, blindness itself is defined differently across the country. Many groups support this definition: Deaf-blindness involves visual and auditory problems so great that they prevent accommodation in programs for those who are only visually impaired or hard of hearing.

The number of deaf-blind people in the United States is hard to calculate, but a national study commissioned by the Department of Education in 1980 estimated between 42,000 and more than 700,000, depending on how deaf-blindness is defined.

Most people who are deaf-blind are over age 65 because as individuals get older, the risk of impairments increase. More women than men are deaf and blind, which may be related to a woman's longer lifespan. The study also revealed the so-called "rubella bulge" (the excess number of children born blind and deaf during the 1964–65 rubella epidemic), who were from 14 to 16 years old at the time of the study.

In the absence of epidemics, between 250 and 300 deaf-blind children can be expected to be born each year because of genetic problems, accidents and diseases.

Only 1.7% of deaf-blind people are institutionalized, which means that for every person institutionalized, more than 50 are living in the general population.

Despite this national study, many gaps in understanding this population remain. There is no available data on socioeconomic status, education, race, employment or civil status of deaf-blind people, which inhibits efforts to reach this population.

Education Teaching a deaf-blind child is certainly difficult, but it is not impossible. According to the National Needs Assessment of Services for Deaf-Blind Persons, the major obstacle to success is the low opinion of the abilities of deaf-blind people held by parents, teachers and society.

When the Elementary and Secondary Education Act of 1968 was passed, it authorized the establishment of centers for deaf-blind children. But it was not until the passage of the Education for All Handicapped Children Act of 1975 (PL 94-142) that education for all deaf-blind children could be guaranteed, since any local agency could deny education to a student it considered too difficult (or costly) to teach. From 1968 to 1980, enrollment for deaf-blind students increased from 110 to 6,000.

According to research, even children born blind and deaf can be taught to communicate, especially if provided with early intensive intervention soon after birth. Without early efforts to stimulate deaf-blind infants, they develop stereotypical, asocial behavior in an effort to provide the stimulation they don't get from their environment. To counteract this, parents must provide continual, consistent stimulation of taste, feel, smell, movement and temperature together with enhancing whatever residual sight or hearing the child has.

Although deaf-blind children are just as intelligent as sighted and hearing children, their communication problems mean they acquire knowledge more slowly and often show self-stimulatory behavior. This behavior, which appears almost autistic, can include waving fingers, rocking and rubbing their eyes.

History The first deaf-blind student successfully educated was LAURA DEWEY BRIDGMAN, who was taught by 19th-century educator Samuel Gridley Howe, director at the Perkins School for the Blind in Massachusetts. Eight-year-old Laura first learned the names of objects by feeling raised letters that spelled out their names and were pasted on the objects. She later learned the manual alphabet, although she never learned to speak.

Her educational success was followed by Helen Keller's, who was taught by another Perkins school graduate, Anne Sullivan. Keller later attended Perkins and met the elderly Laura Bridgman.

The first school with a formal program for deaf-blind students was Perkins, which established a department for the education of deaf-blind students in 1931. This was followed by seven other schools for deaf-blind students within the next 30 years. (See also KELLER, HELEN.)

D.E.A.F., Inc. The Developmental Evaluation Adjustment Facility, Inc., is a multiservice agency serving deaf people in New England. Acting as a sister organization to GLAD in California, the agency offers independent living services, an evaluation unit, education and training and also sponsors the telephone relay (TDD) service for Massachusetts. In addition, D.E.A.F. sponsors PROJECT ALAS, a service for deaf Latinos and their families. Contact: D.E.A.F., Inc.,

215 Brighton Ave., Allston, MA 02134; telephone (voice and TDD): 617-254-4041.

Deafness and Communicative Disorders Branch This office is part of the Rehabilitation Services Administration in the Office of Special Education and Rehabilitative Services of the federal Department of Education.

Designed to promote better rehabilitation services for deaf, hard-of-hearing, speech-impaired and language-disordered people, the office offers technical assistance to administration staff, public and private agencies and individuals and funds interpreter training programs. Contact: Rehabilitation Services Administration, Department of Education, Mary E. Switzer Bldg., 330 C St. SW, Room 3315, Mail Stop 2312, Washington, DC 20202; telephone: 202-732-1282.

Deafness Research Foundation (DRF) The nation's largest voluntary health organization devoted primarily to furthering research into the causes, treatment and prevention of hearing loss and other ear disorders.

Founded in 1958, this group provides grants for fellowships, symposia and research, provides information and referral services and publishes *The Receiver*.

Second only to the federal government in its research support into hearing loss and ear problems, the DRF also maintains an otologic fellowship program to aid talented third-year medical students interested in research. For example, it awarded more than $1.5 million toward research into age-related hearing loss between 1987 and 1991. Contact: Deafness Research Foundation, 9 E. 38th St., New York, NY 10016; telephone: (voice) 212-684-6556 or 800-535-DEAF, (TDD) 212-684-6559.

Deafness, Speech and Hearing Publications, Inc. (DSHP) A joint venture of the AMERICAN SPEECH-LANGUAGE-HEARING ASSOCIATION and GALLAUDET UNIVERSITY in Washington, D.C., this group was formed to condense information from published sources about the processes and disorders of human speech and hearing. It published a quarterly journal, *dsh Abstracts*.

Formerly called the National Index on Deafness, Speech and Hearing, the DSHP published research abstracts in January, April, July and October. Since 1983, *dsh Abstracts* selected relevant citations from the National Library of Medicine's computerized bibliographic database (MEDLINE), which reviews 3,000 domestic and foreign biomedical journals monthly.

Early in 1985, Gallaudet and ASLHA decided to discontinue subsidizing *dsh Abstracts* and disbanded DSHP; the last issue appeared in October 1985.

DEAFPRIDE A nonprofit, community-based advocacy organization that works for the human rights of all deaf people and their families. DEAFPRIDE helps groups organize and work together for change in the District of Columbia and throughout the country.

DEAFPRIDE also provides interpretative services for residents of the Washington, D.C. metropolitan area, the agencies that employ them and the programs that provide social, health, legal and educational services, including a 24-hour emergency service for medical and legal emergencies.

The organization is working for a changed society where deaf people are understood as persons with their own language and culture and who have equal access to everything society has to offer. The organization has a special focus on deaf people who have the least access to resources and education. Contact: DEAFPRIDE, Inc., 1350 Potomac Ave. SE, Washington, DC 20003; telephone (voice and TDD): 202-675-6700.

DEAFTEK.USA The only international nonprofit organization providing computer ELECTRONIC MAIL service for deaf and hard-of-hearing people. DEAFTEK was established in 1977 by the Deaf Communications

Institute of Framingham, Massachusetts. No longer in operation, the institute was an independent organization that focused on telecommunications services and offered a range of other communications services in addition to DEAFTEK.

The computerized DEAFTEK services include electronic messages, open bulletin boards for sending news of interest to the deaf community, telex, fax, electronic mail for research projects and express mail. Either a computer with modem or a TELECOMMUNICATION DEVICE FOR THE DEAF (TDD) with ASCII must be used to hook up to the service.

An electronic mail network allows a subscriber to communicate with other members of the mail network, using a computer or ASCII-equipped TDD. The system works by transferring a message from one subscriber through a central computer which then transmits the message to the receiver who subscribes to the same system. The message is delivered in seconds to the recipient's "mailbox" (user's name or number), where it remains until that person picks it up by calling the system to retrieve messages. With electronic mail, the same message can be sent to several different mailboxes, saving time and money.

To use DEAFTEK, the caller dials a local phone number to access GTE Telemail (a national electronic mail network) and then types his mailbox name and password to connect to DEAFTEK. A DEAFTEK member can send or receive messages to or from others who belong to DEAFTEK, read "bulletin boards" with news announcements about the deaf community and have access to news items, provided by *USA News Today,* which are updated hourly.

DEAFTEK is available 24 hours a day throughout the world. The service is accessible only by ASCII modems or TDDs with ASCII capability. There is a yearly fee when joining DEAFTEK on GTE Telemail and monthly user fees (like a telephone bill).

In addition, DEAFTEK offers several limited access bulletin boards, spinoff communication networks focused in one area. DEAFTEK's bulletin boards include PSYCH NET (mental health and the deaf community), AIDS.NET (AIDS and the deaf community) and NICD.GALLAUDET, where the NATIONAL INFORMATION CENTER ON DEAFNESS posts messages. Soon to be offered will be a "federal register" for the use of the Department of Education. (See also BAUDOT CODE.) Contact: DEAFTEK.USA, c/o INTERNATIONAL DEAF/TEK, INC., P.O. Box 2431, Framingham, MA 01701; telephone: 508-620-1777 (voice/TDD).

decibel A measure of the intensity of sound. Zero decibel (dB) is the softest intensity of sound or speech that can be heard by a normal person; 100 dB is the most intense sound an audiometer can produce.

degree of hearing loss An indication of how much hearing loss has been sustained. Specific terms are used to define this loss.

Hearing Impairment A hearing loss of any degree in one or both ears.

Mild Loss Loss of some sounds.

Moderate Loss A loss of enough sounds so that a person's ability to understand his surrounding environment is affected, including some speech sounds.

Significant Bilateral Loss Loss of hearing in both ears with the better ear having some difficulty hearing and understanding speech.

Severe Loss Many sounds are not heard, including most speech sounds.

Profound Loss An inability to hear almost all sounds, generally over 90 dB.

Deafness In this sense, the ability to hear is disabled to an extent that precludes the understanding of speech through the ear alone with or without the use of a hearing aid. (This definition was adopted in 1974 by the CONFERENCE OF EDUCATIONAL ADMINISTRATORS SERVING THE DEAF.)

delayed auditory feedback (DAF) Also called delayed side tone, this is a speech signal delayed on the return to the speaker's ears. Research shows that when a person's own speech is delayed to his ears by 200 msec, the delay will cause a change in vocal rate and intensity as the person continues to speak simultaneously with the DAF. This theory can be used in tests to diagnose FUNCTIONAL HEARING LOSS.

diabetes and hearing loss This metabolic disorder results in a decrease or absence of insulin, the hormone responsible for the absorption of glucose into cells, where it is used for energy. Because diabetes tends to degenerate blood vessels and peripheral nerves, compromising blood supply to the ear and the internal auditory canal, it can result in a degeneration of cochlear and vestibular nerves and cause a SENSORINEURAL HEARING LOSS.

Diabetes is diagnosed by testing the urine for a sample of sugar. Treatment is aimed at prolonging life and relieving symptoms while preventing complications. People with insulin-dependent diabetes inject themselves with insulin and follow a restricted diet. With modern treatment and self-monitoring, almost all diabetics can enjoy a normal life.

digital hearing aid A type of aid that allows an external computer to program the hearing aid to match the hearing ability of the wearer. The aid also has the capability to reduce noise and adjust itself and features advanced signal processing techniques and better ways to process speech signals.

The problem with these aids to date is that they consume more power and take up more space than conventional HEARING AIDS. To offset these problems, a hybrid hearing aid has been developed that offers conventional amplifiers and filters that are adjusted automatically by a digital control. These hybrids are small enough to be worn on or in the ear.

diplacusis A condition in which a given frequency produces a different pitch in each ear; this common problem is called binaural diplacusis. The disorder is diagnosed by having the patient adjust the frequency in one ear to equal the pitch to a reference pitch in the other ear.

Although it is normal for a person with normal hearing to have slight differences in pitch between the two ears, people with a cochlear or retrocochlear hearing problem may experience up to an octave difference in pitch.

A related condition, called monaural diplacusis, results in hearing a group of tones when only one tone is actually present.

Often, an individual is unaware of having diplacusis unless he or she is a musician.

direct audio input (DAI) A recent technological advance designed to lessen the problem of hearing aid sound distortion, the DAI features a cord attached to a behind-the-ear aid either by a special outlet or by a connector called a "shoe," which may be added to the hearing aid. This cord is attached to a plug to connect to any type of sound source, such as TV, radios, tape records and FM ASSISTIVE LISTENING DEVICES.

The direct connection eliminates many of the background noises that often disturb the users of HEARING AIDS.

discomfort level The level at which pure tones and/or speech become too loud for comfort to the listener. (See also AUDIOMETRY.)

discrimination The percentage of a word list with or without background noise that is understood by an individual as part of a hearing test. (See also AUDIOMETRY.)

dispensing audiologist An AUDIOLOGIST who sells HEARING AIDS. (See also HEARING AID DEALERS.)

distortion break The level at which sounds become unnatural as HEARING AIDS are turned up.

dizziness This sensation of unsteadiness is a mild form of VERTIGO, which is characterized by a feeling of spinning either of oneself or the surroundings.

Although most attacks of dizziness are harmless, they may occur because of a disorder of the inner ear, hearing nerve or the brain.

In LABYRINTHITIS, a viral infection can inflame the fluid-filled canals within the inner ear, affecting balance; in severe cases, even a sudden movement of the head can cause dizziness and fainting. In the inner ear degenerative syndrome called MENIERE'S DISEASE, dizziness and vertigo are common symptoms.

In more rare cases, a tumor or MENINGITIS affecting the hearing nerve can cause dizziness. Any disorder of the brain stem that connects with the hearing nerve—such as reduced blood supply or tumors—can also result in dizziness.

In cases of dizziness caused by disorders of the inner ear, some physicians may recommend antiemetic or antihistamine drugs.

Doerfler-Stewart test An auditory test used to determine functional or psychogenic hearing loss by testing a patient's ability to respond to spondee words (two long or accented syllables) spoken in the presence of a masking noise presented through earphones. In cases of a functional hearing loss, the patient will be unable to respond consistently to words at varying intensity levels. (See also AUDIOMETRY.)

Down's syndrome A disorder caused by a chromosomal problem and resulting in mental retardation and physical deformities. People born with this syndrome often have irregularities in the middle and inner ears and are susceptible to middle ear infections (OTITIS MEDIA) that can cause conductive hearing loss.

Down's syndrome is caused by an excess chromosome, usually number 21. About one in 650 babies is born with the syndrome, and the incidence of affected babies rises sharply with maternal age, to about one in 40 in mothers over age 40.

In addition to hearing problems, most people with Down's syndrome have a typical facial appearance, including sloping eyes with extra folds of skin, a small face and features and a small oral cavity. The degree of mental retardation varies, although many of these children are educable.

Although medical techniques have improved the prognosis for people with Down's syndrome and have extended their life expectancies, many still do not survive beyond early middle age.

drugs and deafness See OTOTOXIC DRUGS.

dual party relay service See RELAY SERVICE.

Dutch Sign Language Formally known as Sign Language of the Netherlands (SLN), this sign language has five separate dialects, each related to a school for deaf students. There are about 25,000 deaf Dutch people who use sign language.

Dutch Sign Language is based on signs invented in 1827 and later formally taught in a school based on the educational principles of French deaf educator ABBÉ CHARLES MICHEL DE L'EPÉE. However, most other Dutch schools were oral in approach, and these students developed their own signs independent of their schools.

It is only recently that Dutch educators have begun to accept SLN based on new research findings and an awareness of their own rights as compared to deaf Dutch citizens.

dysacusis Meaning "faulty hearing," the term includes any hearing problem not caused primarily by a loss of auditory sensitivity.

From the word "acusis" (or "acousis"), referring to hearing, and "dys," meaning ill or painful, the word is also spelled "dysacusia" and "dysacousia." It is caused by a malfunction or injury of the central nervous system, the auditory nerve or the organ of Corti and is not helped by amplifying speech. Therefore, dysacusis is not measured in decibels.

It must be emphasized that deafness/hearing loss and dysacusis are not necessarily mutually exclusive; for example, a person may have both HEARING LOSS measured in decibels and also a dysacusis in the form of a loss of discrimination.

"Dysacusis" may also be used as a broader term meaning loss of all kinds of hearing—two or three of which may be present in the same person. On the other hand, "hard-of-hearing" implies specifically one kind of problem—loss of sensitivity.

There are several types of dysacusis, including discrimination loss for words, syllables or PHONEMES; reduced intelligibility for sentences; AUDITORY AGNOSIA; phonemic regression; and binaural DIPLACUSIS and monaural diplacusis.

dysphasia Speech or language problem. It is thought that children with dysphasia hear sounds but can't make sense of them, or, if they can make sense, they are unable to put their responses into words. There may be problems with perception, sound discrimination, auditory memory, comprehension, word-finding, reading and writing.

Unlike adults with APHASIA (often following a stroke), there is no loss of previous function; instead, children fail to develop normal language.

Sometimes, deaf children are wrongly labeled aphasic or dysphasic, especially those who don't make progress in oral-only programs. Because there are not any clearcut tests for developmental dysphasia, careful and repeated evaluations are necessary.

E

ear See OUTER EAR. MIDDLE EAR. or INNER EAR.

earache The most common cause of this severe, stabbing pain is an infection of the middle ear (OTITIS MEDIA). Otitis media occurs most often in young children and the stabbing pain is usually accompanied by a fever and a temporary loss of hearing. If the eardrum breaks, the pain and pressure is relieved immediately.

Another common cause of earache is otitis externa (also called SWIMMER'S EAR), which is the inflammation of the outer ear canal, usually caused by an infection. This infection may affect the whole canal or only parts of it and may form an abscess or boil. There may be irritation or itching, discharge and temporary mild deafness as well.

Much more rare is earache resulting from herpes zoster, which causes blisters in the ear canal and can produce pain for weeks or months after the infection has ended.

Earaches that come and go could also occur from a host of problems, including tooth pain, tonsillitis, throat cancer and pain in the lower jaw or neck. In fact, almost any disorder that affects areas near the ear can cause an earache since the same nerves which serve the ear also supply many nearby areas.

Earaches may be treated with painkilling drugs, and antibiotics are often prescribed for infection. Pus in the outer ear may need to be removed or drained via an operation (MYRINGOTOMY) if it is located in the middle ear.

ear canal See EXTERNAL AUDITORY CANAL.

eardrops Eardrops are prescribed for certain conditions in the outer and middle ears but cannot affect the inner ear. Eardrops cannot restore hearing in cases of nerve damage, but they can treat itch, discomfort or ear infection in the outer or middle ears. Eardrops should only be used upon recommendation by a physician.

eardrum An important part of the hearing mechanism, the eardrum (also called the tympanic membrane) separates the OUTER (external) EAR from the MIDDLE EAR and vibrates with sound or speech. The eardrum is thin and slightly transparent; its inner layer consists of mucous membrane, and its outer layer is skin.

Blood vessels supplying the eardrum are extremely tiny, but inflammation can engorge them and can make them so diffuse that the whole membrane becomes reddish and opaque.

eardrum, perforated A hole (perforation) may appear in the EARDRUM as a result of gradual erosion from chronic OTITIS MEDIA (ear infection). Rupture of the eardrum usually is the result of otitis media when pus builds up and—left untreated—bursts the eardrum.

The eardrum may also be perforated by inserting a sharp object into the ear, a blow on the ear, a loud noise, skull fracture, barotrauma (damage from excessive air pressure) or tumor.

The perforation is usually treated with antibiotics to take care of any infection. Except in the case of a chronic otitis media, this is usually the only treatment required. If a perforation does not close within six months, a TYMPANOPLASTY, also called a myringoplasty, may be performed. (See also AERO-OTITIS MEDIA; COTTON SWABS.)

Ear Foundation, The A national, nonprofit organization founded in 1971 and committed to leading the effort for better hearing through public and professional educational programs, support services and applied research. The foundation is particularly interested in problems of ear-related disorders, specifically hearing loss and balance disturbances. From its inception, the foundation has been dedicated to the continuing education of ear specialists and to the development of auditory and vestibular research.

The foundation also administers THE MENIERE'S NETWORK, a national network of patient support groups that provide people with Meniere's disease the opportunity to share experiences and coping strategies. Contact: The Ear Foundation, 2000 Church St., Box 111, Nashville, TN 37326; telephone (voice and TDD): 800-545-HEAR.

ear infection See OTITIS MEDIA.

ear lobe This fleshy hanging lower portion of the outer ear, also called the lobule, is the only part of the external ear that does not contain any cartilage.

ear massage Although it is untrue that pressing on the skull behind the ear or on the neck can improve hearing, gentle massage can restore hearing caused by a problem with the eustachian tube.

However, ear massage can also cause disarticulation of the middle ear bones and is not recommended.

When the eustachian tube doesn't equalize pressure in the MIDDLE EAR cavity (such as during an airplane flight), rubbing the ear gently, yawning, swallowing, chewing and so forth can fill the middle ear with the needed air.

earmold Part of the HEARING AID system, the earmold is a plastic insert that, when fitted into the ear or ear canal, conducts the amplified sound into the ear.

Earmolds come in many shapes, depending on the type of hearing aid and the physical shape of the person's ear. For example, earmolds in canal and in-the-ear aids encase all the hearing aid's components. Earmolds for behind-the-ear and eyeglass hearing aids are placed in the ear and are connected to the hearing aid by a piece of clear plastic tubing. Body type aids have an earmold that allows a button-shaped receiver to snap into a metal ring on its back, with a cord connecting the earmold to the rest of the aid.

When a hearing aid is selected and fitted, the AUDIOLOGIST or dispenser will make an impression of the ear to customize the earmold. Earmolds are made of various types of material, including hard plastic or several varieties of soft, pliant materials. Hypoallergenic earmolds are also available.

An earmold should fit snugly into the ear without pain or a "plugged up" feeling; a loose fit could cause feedback or whistling. Modifications can alleviate problems with earmolds; for example, a hole bored in an earmold can alleviate pressure in the ear canal, and a larger vent can alter the response of the hearing aid so that it is more appropriate in certain types of hearing loss.

ear muffs See EAR PROTECTORS.

earplugs See EAR PROTECTORS.

ear protectors There are two types of ear protecting devices: earplugs, which fit inside the ear canal, and ear muffs, which fit outside the ears. Earplugs and earmuffs worn together provide the most effective protection against noise.

Earplugs Earplugs to be used for protection against noise should not be purchased over the counter, such as the earplugs designed for swimming. In order to be effective in screening out excess noise, earplugs must fit snugly in the ear canal so that no air can get through. In addition, a person's ears may not be the same size, requiring earplugs of two different dimensions.

Custom-fit earplugs are made to fit only one person's ears, usually by an AUDIOLOGIST or hearing aid dispenser. One type of earplug has a valve that allows soft sounds—such as voices or speech—to pass through, but closes for loud sounds.

In fitting the earplugs, the dealer makes an impression of the ear canal and sends the dimensions to a manufacturer, where the soft rubber earplug insert is made. These fitted earplugs should only be used by adults, since the ear canals of children and teenagers change rapidly.

Earplugs must fit properly in order to shut out sound and must be kept clean to avoid infection. Most types give about 30 decibel protection against excess noise.

Earmuffs Earmuffs can provide even more effective sound protection than earplugs and are preferable if there is a draining ear or chronic infection. In addition, some ear canals simply don't accept earplugs without pain.

Earmuffs completely cover the ear; the earpieces are made of sponge material and are held in place by a tension headband. Earmuff protectors generally cost more than earplugs, but they are harder to lose, and some believe they are more comfortable for daily wear than earplugs. Those who wear glasses, however, may find that the glasses interfere with the earmuffs' seal.

Other Protectors Dry cotton is almost useless in preventing excess noise. Some types of disposable ear protectors are made of cotton wax and other specially treated material, and these are somewhat effective.

ear squeeze See AERO-OTITIS MEDIA.

ear structure Ears collect and decipher everything from whispers to screams, and can distinguish not only one musical note from another but even the same note played on different instruments. Superbly crafted to handle our environment, ears contain a sort of gyroscope to help maintain balance, and can protect themselves against noise and selectively tune out unwanted sounds—even during sleep.

The outer and middle ears amplify some sound waves because of the way the ear canal narrows as it proceeds inward, funneling the noise. Once the sound reaches the eardrum, it is transmitted and amplified by the vibrations of the eardrum's skin. Next, the middle ear's three bones (OSSI-

CLES) receive sound through the drum and push it through the oval window into the inner ear.

Once inside the inner ear, the COCHLEA (a small-shaped system of canals located behind the oval window) takes over to interpret pitch. The cochlea contains fluid and about 20,000 tiny hair cells tuned to various pitch frequencies. When the middle ear's stirrup pushes the sound through the oval window, it makes the cochlea vibrate, and the fluid travels to the tiny hair cells where separate pitches are registered. Hair cells responsible for high notes are located near the base of the cochlea, lower-frequency cells are near the apex.

The cochlea generates tiny electrical currents, sending the sound through acoustic nerve connections to the brain, where it is decoded and presented as one of the 350,000 separate sounds a human can recognize. (See also DIAGRAM OF THE EAR; INNER EAR; MIDDLE EAR; OUTER EAR.)

ear trumpet A mechanical hearing aid first created in the 17th century but popularized at the turn of the century, used to increase sound levels by 10 to 15 decibels.

Many of these devices were designed to hide a hearing problem: Men could wear one under beards and sideburns or carry one concealed in the head of a cane. Women could wear an "aurolese phone," a cup-shaped sound collector that was concealed by elaborate hairdos popular at that time.

Ear trumpets were usually cone- or dome-shaped devices and made of metal, rubber, and plastic.

Related to the ear trumpet were the speaking tube and the hearing fan. Speaking tubes were popular in Europe and included a bell-shaped plastic or rubber speaking end connected to a small eartip by two feet of tubing. Hearing fans, which were really a bone-conduction hearing aid, featured a thin rubber fan held between the teeth, kept taut by strings. Sound passed through the fan to the teeth, through bone to the inner ear.

ear tube A small tube that is inserted through the EARDRUM during a surgical incision (MYRINGOTOMY) made in the eardrum to treat a chronic middle-ear effusion in children.

The tube serves to equalize the pressure on both sides of the eardrum, which allows the fluid to drain out of the ear. About six to twelve months after the operation, the tube usually falls out on its own as the eardrum heals.

Water should be kept out of the ear in children with an ear tube, and swimming is usually forbidden. (See also MYRINGOTOMY; SEROUS OTITIS MEDIA.)

earwax A yellow or brown secretion called cerumen, earwax is produced only by glands in the outer ear canal. Any wax deeper inside the canal has been pushed there by a finger or a cotton applicator. The normal function of wax in the ear is to protect the skin of the ear canal by keeping it soft and moist.

Among people who have very narrow or hairy ear canals and among people who work in dirty or dusty environments, wax can build up until it completely blocks the ear canal. When wax is pushed into the ear canal and presses on the EARDRUM, it may sometimes cause ear noises and even dizziness, both of which disappear when the wax is removed.

Earwax is a normal part of the body's function and should not be stopped. Removing earwax with a COTTON SWAB is dangerous; probing can remove protective layers of keratin, opening the way for possible infection of skin cells. There is also a danger that the swab could be pushed through the eardrum, causing problems ranging from severe pain to total deafness. Often cotton swabs push wax farther into the ear canal, which eventually causes impacted earwax. To be kept clean, the ear only needs soap, water and a washcloth.

echolocation The technique of locating objects by emitting bursts of sound and interpreting the echoes; used by sonar and animals such as bats.

Education for All Handicapped Children Act See LEGAL RIGHTS.

education of deaf children Deafness itself does not affect either a person's intellectual capacity or the ability to learn. Since most deaf children have hearing parents, it is important to begin exposing these children to communication as early as possible. But often, a child's hearing loss—or his parents' acceptance of it—might not come until the second year of the child's life. Even if the parents are willing to learn American Sign Language at that point, it takes time to learn before they become proficient. Crucial early interaction with some form of language has been lost.

Because deaf children of hearing parents are not exposed to a continuous language flow, they miss out on an enormous amount of language stimulation. Language delays can be offset by exposing deaf children to early, consistent visible communication methods (sign language, fingerspelling or cued speech) together with amplification and aural/oral training, if desired.

Only a small percentage of deaf children have deaf parents, but those who do have the great advantage of learning AMERICAN SIGN LANGUAGE (ASL) from the beginning. Studies show that these children progress in language development and acquisition at the same rate as hearing children learn English and outdistance their deaf peers who did not learn ASL from infancy.

Type of School The first problem facing parents of a school-age deaf child is where to get the best education. In the past, deaf children were educated primarily in residential schools, which provided maximum exposure to the latest technology in deaf education but limited the child's family relationship.

Today, the trend is growing in favor of MAINSTREAMING the child at least part of the day at the local public school, enabling the child to live at home and remain in touch with the neighborhood. This change reflects the popularity of the mainstreaming movement and also the Education for All Handicapped Children Act of 1975, which mandates a free public education for all ''handicapped'' children in the least restrictive environment and sets specific guidelines to protect their rights. The act also requires each child to receive nondiscriminatory testing and an individualized educational plan that is renewed each year. (See also LEGAL RIGHTS.)

As a result, parents have many more educational options today than they did prior to the 1960s. There are four major choices: residential school, special day school, special day classes, or regular classes supplemented by special services. Each of these options is described below.

Residential schools These schools board deaf students full time, although most programs allow the students to spend weekends at home with their families. These schools offer instructional, recreational and social programs designed for their deaf pupils. Students who live nearby may attend these residential schools as day pupils.

Day school programs Deaf students in these programs go to a school exclusively for deaf youngsters but return home in the afternoon like other school children.

Self-contained day classes Many neighborhood public school systems offer special classes for deaf students. Under this program, deaf students may join hearing students for physical education and art or be ''mainstreamed'' (put in classes with hearing students) with interpreters for some classes. Usually, these special programs provide a resource room to help deaf students get information for classes they attend with hearing students.

Regular classes This choice, known as mainstreaming, allows deaf students to attend regular classes with hearing students for most or all of the day. Often, the deaf child may be provided interpreters, tutors and resource room teachers.

In addition, some school districts may design their own programs for deaf students, utilizing some or all of the above methods.

In high school, deaf students can choose to enter a vocational training program or take academic courses with an aim to attending college, either at a regular university or a college for deaf students, such as GALLAUDET UNIVERSITY in Washington, D.C. or the NATIONAL TECHNICAL INSTITUTE FOR THE DEAF in Rochester, New York. In addition, there are many community colleges and technical schools in the United States with special programs for deaf adults.

Manual vs. Oral Approach In addition to the type of school, parents must make another important—and historically far more controversial—decision. There has been no issue in deaf education more bitterly disputed over the past 200 years than the question of how students and teachers should communicate in the classroom.

The problem was made more difficult by a misunderstanding of American Sign Language by linguists in the first part of the 20th century, who insisted only a spoken language was a real language. Today, linguists accept that American Sign Language is indeed a language with its own syntax and grammar and all the richness and complexity of any other language.

The manual approach was brought to this country by educator THOMAS HOPKINS GALLAUDET, who, thwarted in learning the oral English method, studied the French manual method instead. Trained at the famous Paris Institute (Institut National de Jeunes Sourds) in this method, Gallaudet introduced the manual approach to America at the first public school for deaf students in Hartford, Connecticut.

Other methods from Europe soon followed. In 1867, Bernard Engelsmann, a teacher of deaf Viennese students, introduced the German method—the oral approach—in a school for deaf children in New York City, now known as the Lexington School.

In 1878, Zenas Westervelt introduced the ROCHESTER METHOD at a school for deaf students in Rochester, New York based on a system in which deaf students are taught to speak and fingerspell English simultaneously while written English is also being emphasized.

Gradually, schools in this country began to rely on the oral approach of communication until almost all preschool and elementary classes for deaf children were oral-only and forbade the use of signs or fingerspelling. Schools emphasized oral education based on the theory that any type of manual communication would interfere with English and speech development and would keep the deaf child isolated from the larger hearing world.

But as the skills of deaf students—who have the same intelligence range as hearing children—lagged behind, educators began to question whether all-oral schools were failing large numbers of deaf people. This growing doubt was fueled by studies showing that deaf children of deaf parents outperformed deaf children of hearing parents in academic achievement, social adjustment, reading and written English skills. These studies seemed to show that not only did ASL not inhibit English fluency but apparently enhanced its acquisition. Today, few schools use an oral approach.

Manual approach supporters also argue that many children do not have the aptitude for oral instruction and that the time spent on trying to speak could better be spent developing the child's mental abilities. Further, some advocates of a manual education believe that deaf people prefer to associate with other deaf people and therefore have no need to be able to speak.

Some oral approach supporters, on the other hand, still believe that training in speech and speech reading help the child adjust to a speaking world. By learning to speak, they reason, the deaf child will not be confined to the deaf community or to those willing to

ST. THOMAS AQUINAS COLLEGE
LOUGHEED LIBRARY
SPARKILL, NEW YORK 10976

use sign or a pad and pencil. They further point out that a person who can speechread and speak may find it easier to land a job. In general, oral supporters believe that orally-trained youngsters are likely to do better as more teachers are trained in this field.

All organizations of deaf educators believe that deaf children should be given the opportunity to learn to speak, but there is often heated debate as to what constitutes "fair opportunity."

Total Communication Today, programs for deaf students are moving toward a more inclusive form of education called Total Communication, which supports a deaf child's right to be exposed to any form of communication that is effective. This includes speech, speechreading, gestures, reading, writing, FINGERSPELLING, manual codes of English, ASL and use of residual hearing.

Most programs today use a manual code of English together with spoken English.

How much the child's inability to hear will affect school performance depends on many things—the degree and type of hearing loss, the age of onset, additional handicaps, the quality of the school and support the child receives.

Typically, deaf children from ages one to three begin their education in a clinical program featuring extensive support from parents. Because 85% to 90% of deaf children are born to hearing parents, these programs often emphasize the implications of deafness and teach parents how to cope with problems. At age three, the child can attend preschool sessions with other deaf children, and by age four many deaf youngsters attend special nursery and kindergarten classes full time.

In order to learn, deaf children must devise a way to communicate. A child's hearing may be helped by hearing aids, but hearing may still be quite limited. In order to develop a consistent, two-way means of communication, many deaf children and their parents learn sign language.

EEG audiometry See ELECTROENCEPHALOGRAPHY AUDIOMETRY.

eighth cranial nerve This nerve, also called the auditory, hearing or cochlear nerve, is really two separate nerves, one responsible for transmitting sound and the other with sending balance information to the brain from the inner ear. The two parts of this nerve are intertwined as they pass through the bony canal leading from the inner ear to the brain.

This nerve is the only connection between the hair cells of the COCHLEA and the cochlear nucleus of the brainstem and is essential for good hearing. The nerve is about 25 millimeters long and contains about 32,000 nerve fibers.

electrocochleogram An electrophysical hearing test that measures impulses in the cochlear nerve by inserting a thin electrode through the EARDRUM into the promontory of the basal turn. This indicates how well the COCHLEA is functioning. (See also AUDIOMETRY.)

electrodermal response audiometry (EDR) A special hearing test procedure that measures sweat changes on the hands or feet in response to sound or speech and records these changes on a graph.

This test is one of the nonspecific electrophysiologic hearing tests used to estimate the auditory threshold in people who cannot respond voluntarily to auditory stimuli—such as newborns, infants and people with nonorganic hearing loss. (See also ELECTROPHYSIOLOGIC AUDIOMETRY.)

electroencephalogram (EEG) The measure of the brain's constant low-voltage electric signals. During the 1930s, scientists discovered that sudden loud sounds caused sudden changes in the EEGs of sleeping research subjects. These changes in the EEG were called auditory evoked potentials, since they were evoked, or caused, by a sudden sound.

When several sounds were presented at the same time, however, the evoked potentials became too small to differentiate on the EEG. It was not for another 20 years before the averaging computer was invented, allowing researchers to identify the brain's slight response to a series of sounds.

These auditory evoked potentials can provide information about how the brain responds to sound and also about how healthy the ear is. (See also AUDITORY BRAINSTEM RESPONSE TEST.)

electroencephalography audiometry A special hearing test that measures brain waves changes in response to sound or speech; it is particularly useful in testing the very young.

In this test, a brief pure tone causes a small variation in the baby's brainwave, which can be measured through the scalp by an electroencephalogram (EEG). During the test, an OTOLOGIST repeats a stimulus up to 100 times and then uses a computer to average the brain's response to these tones, eliminating the effects of background noise. This averaged response establishes the auditory threshold almost as accurately as the more standard audiometric tests in older children. (See also AUDIOMETRY.)

electromagnetic induction A process used in HEARING AIDS that replaces normal reception of sound by the microphone and picks up transmitted speech through a direct connection in telephones and many public buildings that have been equipped for that purpose. The benefit of electromagnetic induction is that it significantly reduces amplified background noise.

electronic mail An electronic mail network allows a subscriber to communicate with other members of the mail network, using a computer or ASCII-equipped TELECOMMUNICATIONS DEVICE FOR THE DEAF (TDD). The system works by transferring a message from one subscriber through a central computer to a receiver who subscribes to the same system.

The message is delivered in seconds to the recipient's ''mailbox'' (user's name or number), where it remains until that person picks it up by calling the system to retrieve messages. With electronic mail, the same message can be sent to several different mailboxes, saving time and money.

People use electronic mail because it is fast, convenient and inexpensive. Many organizations also use this service to conduct business meetings and limit travel expenses.

Many electronic mail services also offer ''bulletin boards,'' which usually focus on a specific topic of interest, such as cooking, religions, TDDS and computers, education, health and so forth. (See also DEAFTEK.USA; BAUDOT CODE.)

electronystagmography A test to determine the presence of damage to the body's balance system, which can help determine damage to the inner ear, by recording the electrical changes caused by eye movement. This technique has been used successfully for more than 50 years. (See also AUDIOMETRY.)

electrophysiologic audiometry Hearing tests that measure changes in the electric properties of the body as a response to auditory stimuli. Because the client cannot control these responses, electrophysiologic AUDIOMETRY is considered to be a completely objective test of hearing sensitivity.

There are two types of electrophysiologic audiometric tests. The first type measures specific auditory response systems, which respond only to auditory stimulation, including the COCHLEA, the AUDITORY NERVE and certain auditory pathways within the brainstem and the brain. Electrodes are placed on the promontory of the middle ear or in the external ear canal, and instruments pick up the evoked potentials of these systems, which are amplified and extracted from background brain activity.

The second type of test measures nonspecific electrophysiologic response systems, which respond to more than auditory stimulation and are only indirectly related to the auditory stimulation. The cortex, central autonomic centers or spinal autonomic mechanisms are excited by auditory stimuli, which in turn stimulate neural activity or motor reflexes that alter the electrical activity of other mechanisms, including electric recordings of heart rate, electric potential or resistance of the skin as influenced by sweat glands and ongoing electroencephalic activity.

The first electrodermal response tests were developed in the late 1940s to record changes in the electric properties of the skin as influenced by sweat glands. Sweating is an autonomic response that is set in motion when the listener is aroused in anticipation of a coming event. Using classical conditioning, a listener is conditioned to anticipate sensing a shock upon hearing a sound. Although popular up to the 1960s, it fell from favor by the 1970s. It was least effective among very young infants and retarded children.

The heart's response to auditory stimulation is usually identified by computing the difference in electric activity of the heart before and after an auditory stimulus.

By the mid-1960s, scientists began studying evoked response audiometry using a computer to extract an auditory evoked response from ongoing brain activity. Today, it is possible to get a reliable estimate of auditory sensitivity in the very young by using brainstem evoked response audiometry or electrocochleographic audiometry (which uses electric responses from the cochlea to estimate auditory thresholds and gain information about the integrity of the cochlea.) (See also AUDITORY BRAINSTEM RESPONSE TEST.)

El Mudo See NAVARRETE, JUAN FERNANDEZ DE.

employment of deaf people Deaf people work in the same jobs as hearing people, and their deafness in itself does not prevent them from doing most jobs. In fact, according to the NATIONAL INFORMATION CENTER ON DEAFNESS at GALLAUDET UNIVERSITY, more and more deaf people have been moving into professional, administrative, managerial and technical careers. Today, they are working as physicians, dentists, lawyers, physicists, engineers and computer analysts and programmers in addition to other technical and professional positions. Prior to the 1970s, however, most deaf people were employed mainly as factory workers, craftspeople and unskilled laborers.

The movement of deaf workers into all job levels can be credited to improved educational opportunities, antidiscrimination laws, a better understanding of deafness by the general public and an increased assertiveness in the deaf community.

Unfortunately, salaries have not kept pace with the upward movement of deaf employees; the average salary of deaf workers has been somewhat less than the salary of hearing workers in similar jobs, although this gap is closing due to antidiscrimination laws.

In the 1972 National Census of the Deaf Population, employed deaf workers' median incomes ranged between 72% and 76% of that of the general population. Of these workers, 71% were in crafts, operative or clerical jobs. A 1982–83 survey of managerial, professional and technical workers with hearing problems (from mild to profound) found a median salary of $21,957—about $1,700 less than the salary of workers in similar jobs.

Many experts in the field of deafness believe deaf people still tend to be underemployed, which was certainly true prior to the 1970s. Still, the picture is changing; one study found that in 1960 profoundly deaf people were working in 28 different types of professional jobs in the hearing sector. By 1982–83, this number had almost doubled to 54.

encephalitis An inflammation of the brain itself, encephalitis can cause a large variety of symptoms of brain injury, including central hearing problems. The impairments are usually neurological, not audiological, although sometimes there is a cochlear impairment.

Encephalitis is usually caused by an infective organism; viruses are the most common, although the disease can be caused by many different kinds of organisms, including bacteria, protozoa or worms, or by chemicals. There are two types of viruses that cause encephalitis: viruses (like rabies) that invade the body and do no harm until they are carried by the blood to the brain cells, and other viruses (herpes simplex and zoster, yellow fever) that first harm nonnervous tissues and then invade brain cells. The most common viral cause is herpes simplex Type I (which also causes cold sores). In the United States, mosquitos carry St. Louis encephalitis, and increasingly cases of encephalitis are caused by infection with HIV (human immunodeficiency virus), responsible for AIDS. Chemicals that can lead to encephalitis include lead, arsenic, mercury, ethyl alcohol, chlorinated hydrocarbons, morphine and barbiturates.

Children often contract the demyelinating encephalitis type, which develops as a complication of viral diseases such as measles or chickenpox, or as a result of vaccination against these diseases. In this case, damage is not done to the cell itself but to the sheath (myelin) around the nerve cell.

Meningoencephalitis is an inflammation of the brain, the meninges (outer layer of the brain) and the spinal cord; symptoms include fever, headache, vomiting and neck and back stiffness.

Common symptoms of most types of encephalitis include fever, headache, drowsiness, lethargy, tremors and coma. Convulsions may occur in patients of any age, but they appear most often in infants. Other symptoms include uncoordinated movements, weakness and unusual sensitivity of the skin to stimuli.

Encephalitis can be diagnosed from a spinal tap (insertion of a needle into the lower part of the back to extract a small sample of cerebrospinal fluid, the liquid that surrounds the entire central nervous system) and from the results of CT scans and EEG (which records electrical activity of the brain). The cause of encephalitis can be determined by a culture for the particular virus involved or by isolating the virus through a brain tissue biopsy. Sometimes, however, the cause of the disease remains unknown and makes treatment difficult. But even if the virus is discovered, there is often no treatment. There are no specific antiviral agents other than those used in the treatment of herpes simplex.

Treatment may be used to relieve some symptoms that remain after the brain inflammation subsides. Intensive medical treatment is required to monitor heart and respiratory function and to manage fluid and electrolyte balances. Survival depends on the type of virus and the age and health of the patient.

The most common problems following encephalitis include hearing loss, speech problems, paralysis and mental retardation. Any form of encephalitis in young children may damage the brain and prevent proper development.

Human infection from equine encephalitis (carried by mosquitoes) can cause irreparable brain damage in half of those who contract it. The only prevention lies in vaccinating horses and controlling mosquitoes. (See also VIRUSES AND HEARING LOSS.)

endolymph A viscous fluid contained in a small canal called the SCALA MEDIA. It is a triangular structure made up of the spiral lamina, the spiral ligament and the BASILAR MEMBRANE, located in the labyrinth of the inner ear.

endolymphatic hydrops See MÉNIÈRE'S DISEASE.

ENT physician A physician who specializes in conditions of the ear, nose and throat. An ENT physician has earned a medical degree with further study in the ear, nose and throat field combined with residency at a hospital.

These physicians are also known as head and neck surgeons or as otorhinolaryngologists ("oto"—ear, "rhino"—nose, "laryngo"—throat). They are highly trained in ear pathology and surgical procedures, but they may not necessarily be experts in aural rehabilitation (therapy that helps a person with hearing loss communicate better).

l'Epée, Abbé Charles Michel de (1712–1789) Born in 1712, de l'Epée was a French cleric who, upon meeting two deaf daughters of a Parisian family, saw the children's deafness in spiritual terms and wanted to teach the girls about the Catholic church in order to save their souls. Making up his methods as he went along, the cleric eventually taught the girls to read and write.

Following this experience, he opened a school in Paris in 1760 for deaf students; this became the first school that taught only deaf children and the first large community of deaf people anywhere in the world. Today it is known as the INSTITUT NATIONAL DES JEUNES SOURDS.

As he worked with his pupils, de l'Epée discovered that many of these children—especially those whose parents were deaf—communicated with each other by using systematic gestures. Suspecting that these gestures might be the "mother tongue" of deaf people, de l'Epée collected these signs and added his own "methodical" signs for gender, tense and number.

Although de l'Epée recognized the importance of speech and taught it to some of his pupils, he realized that in his classes (some as large as 60) signing was more practical. He believed that it was better to give many deaf children some idea of language—albeit a silent one—rather than teach only a small number to speak. His critics argued that SIGN LANGUAGE condemned deaf people to isolation, but de l'Epée believed it was important to allow deaf students to have their own identity. This tension between the value of sign versus the ability to speak is the core of a controversy over educational methods for deaf students that has lasted for more than 200 years. (See also SICARD, ABBÉ ROCH AMBROISE CUCURRON; SPEECHREADING.)

Episcopal Conference of the Deaf This group, affiliated with about 50 Episcopal congregations in the United States, promotes ministry to deaf people though the Episcopal Church.

Originally called the Conference of Church Workers Among the Deaf, the group was founded in 1881 at St. Ann's Church for the Deaf in New York City to support church members working with deaf people. The organization holds annual meetings and publishes a newsletter, *The Deaf Episcopalian.*

The Episcopal Church was the first religious group in the United States to establish a congregation specifically for deaf members—St. Ann's Church for the Deaf in New York City, founded in 1852 by Thomas Gallaudet, the eldest son of THOMAS HOPKINS GALLAUDET.

Soon, a second church for the deaf was established in 1859 in Philadelphia (All Soul's Church) with help from St. Stephen's Church, which had been holding special services for deaf members. All Soul's Church also became known for allowing the ordination of the first deaf Episcopal priest in 1876 in the United States. Contact: Episcopal Conference of the Deaf, 1616 Calle Santiago, Pleasanton, CA 94566.

epitympanum Also called the attic, a smaller but continuous extension of the middle ear cavity that contains the bulk of the incus and malleus.

eustachian tube The canal that connects the middle ear and the back of the nose. It acts as a drainage passage from the middle ear and maintains hearing by opening to regulate air pressure.

From the middle ear, the tube runs forward, downward and in toward the middle of the head, ending at the back of the nose just above the soft palate. The lower end opens during swallowing and yawning to allow air to flow up to the middle ear and equalize air pressure on both sides of the eardrum.

A person with a blocked eustachian tube who undergoes rapid change in air pressure may suffer from barotrauma (pressure damage to the eardrum or other structure). When a head cold blocks this tube, pressure cannot be equalized, causing severe pain and interference with hearing. (See also AERO-OTITIS MEDIA; EUSTACIO, BARTOLOMEO.)

Eustachio, Bartolomeo (1510?–1571) Roman anatomist and great pioneer of otology who described the air passage from the throat to the ear now known as the EUSTACHIAN TUBE.

Eustachio studied in Rome, becoming the personal physician to the duke of Urbino. When he returned to Rome as the personal physician to the pope, he soon became famous as an anatomist, physician, philosopher and linguist.

His discoveries span the entire field of anatomy, although his greatest contribution was the description of the shape and course of the structure that bears his name. Although the existence of the eustachian tube had been vaguely known, it was left to Eustachio to explore it fully.

Exact English See MANUAL ENGLISH.

expressive skill The ability to express oneself in the language of signs and FINGERSPELLING.

external auditory canal Also known as the ear canal or meatus, this inch-long curved tube extends from the floor of the external ear (auricle) inward to the EARDRUM (tympanic membrane) and can be partly straightened by pulling on the external ear itself.

The outer third of the ear canal is cartilage and lined with fairly thick skin. There are fine hairs and modified sebaceous and ceruminous glands embedded in this skin. The sebaceous glands open into the hair follicles, and the ceruminous glands are found deeper under the dermis. These glands produce earwax (cerumen), which protects the inner portions of the ear against dirt and insects. The canal cleans itself by shedding skin cells.

The inner two-thirds of the canal is bone covered by very thin skin with no hairs or glands.

external auditory meatus See EXTERNAL AUDITORY CANAL.

external ear See OUTER EAR.

external ear diseases and hearing loss In general, blocks in the external ear canal that cause hearing loss involve IMPACTED EARWAX, a foreign body lodged in the canal or a narrowing of the canal because of disease.

Impacted earwax blocking the ear canal can prevent sound from reaching the middle ear, causing a mild conductive hearing loss, especially in higher frequencies.

Foreign objects that block the ear canal (usually found in children) do not usually cause a serious hearing loss unless they totally block the ear canal or perforate the eardrum. Foreign objects that disrupt the LABYRINTH can cause a sensory hearing loss.

If the ear canal is sufficiently inflamed and swollen due to chronic bacterial, viral or fungal infection or allergic reaction, a temporary hearing loss can result if the chronic infection causes a narrowing of the ear canal.

PERICHONDRITIS (infection of the connective tissue covering the cartilage of the external ear) may destroy the cartilage and deform the ear, narrowing or closing the ear canal. Narrowing of the ear canal could also occur after surgery or a bad burn.

Cancer is also sometimes found in the external ear, and the resulting tumor can destroy the adjacent tissue and spread to nearby lymph nodes. (See CANCER OF THE OUTER EAR.)

external otitis See SWIMMER'S EAR.

eyeglass hearing aid Typically, eyeglass hearing aids enclose all the components of the hearing aid—microphone, amplifier and receiver—that inside a case fits into an eyeglass frame. They are useful for those whose hearing loss ranges from mild to severe. Bone conduction hearing aids are also available in the eyeglass model. In most states, they are fitted by a licensed specialist (either a dealer, dispenser or dispensing audiologist). (See HEARING AIDS.)

F

facioscapulohumeral muscular dystrophy (FSH MD) One of the mildest forms of muscular dystrophy, some recently reported cases of FSH MD have involved SENSORINEURAL HEARING LOSS in both ears. However, not enough cases have been documented to clearly define the incidence of hearing loss associated with this condition.

This is an autosomal dominant condition, which means it can be transmitted genetically to other offspring in 50% of all cases. (See GENETICS AND HEARING LOSS.)

Falloppio, Gabriele (1523–1562) One of the foremost Italian anatomists of his time, Falloppio of Modena was the founder of the Italian School of Anatomy and was among the first to describe the anatomy of the ear, ACOUSTIC NERVE and tympanic cavity.

fast auditory fatigue A hearing problem that occurs in patients with a tumor on the auditory nerve in which continuous loud sounds decrease in intensity.

During a continuous sound, a normal listener hears the tone loudly at first, then less loudly because of adaptation, but the tone remains audible and at a fairly steady loudness after the first 15 or 20 seconds.

However, if the auditory nerve is partially compressed—by a tumor, for example—the loudness continues to fall until the tone is inaudible. If the intensity is increased, the tone becomes audible again but then fades out again. (See ACOUSTIC NEUROMA.)

feedback, acoustic A loud squeal from the amplifier of a hearing aid caused by a loud sound escaping around an ill-fitting earpiece and then being picked up and amplified. The squeal is unpleasant and may drown out the sound the wearer wishes to hear.

A hearing aid can deliver much louder sound without squeal if the earpiece fits well, but even so, some sound inevitably escapes through the back of the receiver. A very sensitive instrument with high maximum output squeals too easily.

It is possible to lessen squeal in a number of ways: making sure the earpiece fits well in the ear, reducing the volume of the hearing aid, moving the microphone farther away from the receiver or adjusting the tone control. (See also HEARING AIDS.)

fenestra cochlea See ROUND WINDOW.

fenestra ovalis An opening in the inner wall of the middle ear into which the footplate of the STAPES is imbedded; also called OVAL WINDOW.

fenestration This name for an operation on the ear literally means "opening a window." Fenestration was once the treatment of choice for OTOSCLEROSIS, a familial form of deafness corrected only by surgery.

In 1938, American otologist Julius Lempert discovered and first performed a fenestration, which can relieve deafness by creating a new route for sound to travel from the outer ear to the cochlea. By removing most of the bone in the middle ear, Lempert extended the outer ear canal and created a new OVAL WINDOW (or fenestra) through which sound waves could be sent to the inner ear. After a fenestration, sound bypasses the entire chain of bones (OSSICLES) in the middle ear, and although the otosclerosis is still present, the new window is located in the horizontal semicircular canal of the LABYRINTH—an area rarely affected by otosclerosis.

For 20 years, fenestration was the only surgical way to treat otosclerosis, but it was never performed casually since afterwards hearing can never again be completely normal. Although patients had a good chance for some improvement of their conductive hearing at first, most patients experienced a deterioration in hearing afterwards. Since both the eardrum and ossicles (which usually help magnify sound waves) were removed, patients experienced a hearing loss of at least 25 decibels. Many experienced unpleasant side effects, including facial paralysis, VERTIGO and suppurative (draining) ear infections. The patient must be careful of his ears for the rest of his life. Even a small amount of water in the ear can cause a serious infection; baths, showers and hair-washing can be a major problem.

Because of this, fenestration has not been the treatment of choice in otosclerosis since 1951, except for a few patients. These would include someone whose disease has progressed to the point of solidifying the entire oval window, people who have already had more than one STAPEDECTOMY (an operation to free the fixed stapes) because of closure of the oval window from otosclerosis or people born without an oval window or stapes.

For everyone else—and for those for whom fenestration did not work—stapedectomy gives more satisfactory results.

fenestra vestibuli See OVAL WINDOW.

fetal alcohol syndrome This combination of birth defects is caused by excessive alcohol consumption by a pregnant mother. It has been reported that fetal alcohol syndrome causes either a sensorineural or conductive deafness in 64% of children born with the disorder.

Although even small amounts of alcohol may be harmful to a developing fetus, fetal alcohol syndrome appears only in the presence of persistent alcohol use—two mixed drinks or two to three bottles of beer or glasses of wine a day.

Symptoms of fetal alcohol syndrome include an abnormally short baby with small eyes, vertical folds of skin extending from the upper eyelid to the side of the nose and a small jaw. There may be a small brain, cleft palate, heart defects and joint deformities. About one-fifth of affected babies die during the first weeks of life. (See also PRENATAL CAUSES OF HEARING LOSS.)

fingerspelling This system of communication involves spelling out words in an alphabetical language by using the letters of the manual alphabet—with handshapes and positions corresponding to each letter of the written alphabet.

Manual alphabets are found throughout the world, although the systems in Continental Europe and the Americas are quite different from the one used in Great Britain, where manual English uses both hands.

Manual alphabets differ from sign languages in that they are not a natural language but a method invented by educators and derived from a written language.

Fingerspelling can either be used by itself or together with sign language, when it is generally employed to spell out proper names or technical words. The alphabet can be modified for use with deaf-blind people by making handshapes and movements on the palm of the receiver of the message.

Fingerspelling: The American Manual Alphabet. *Courtesy of Gallaudet University*

(Signs shown as they appear to the person reading them.)

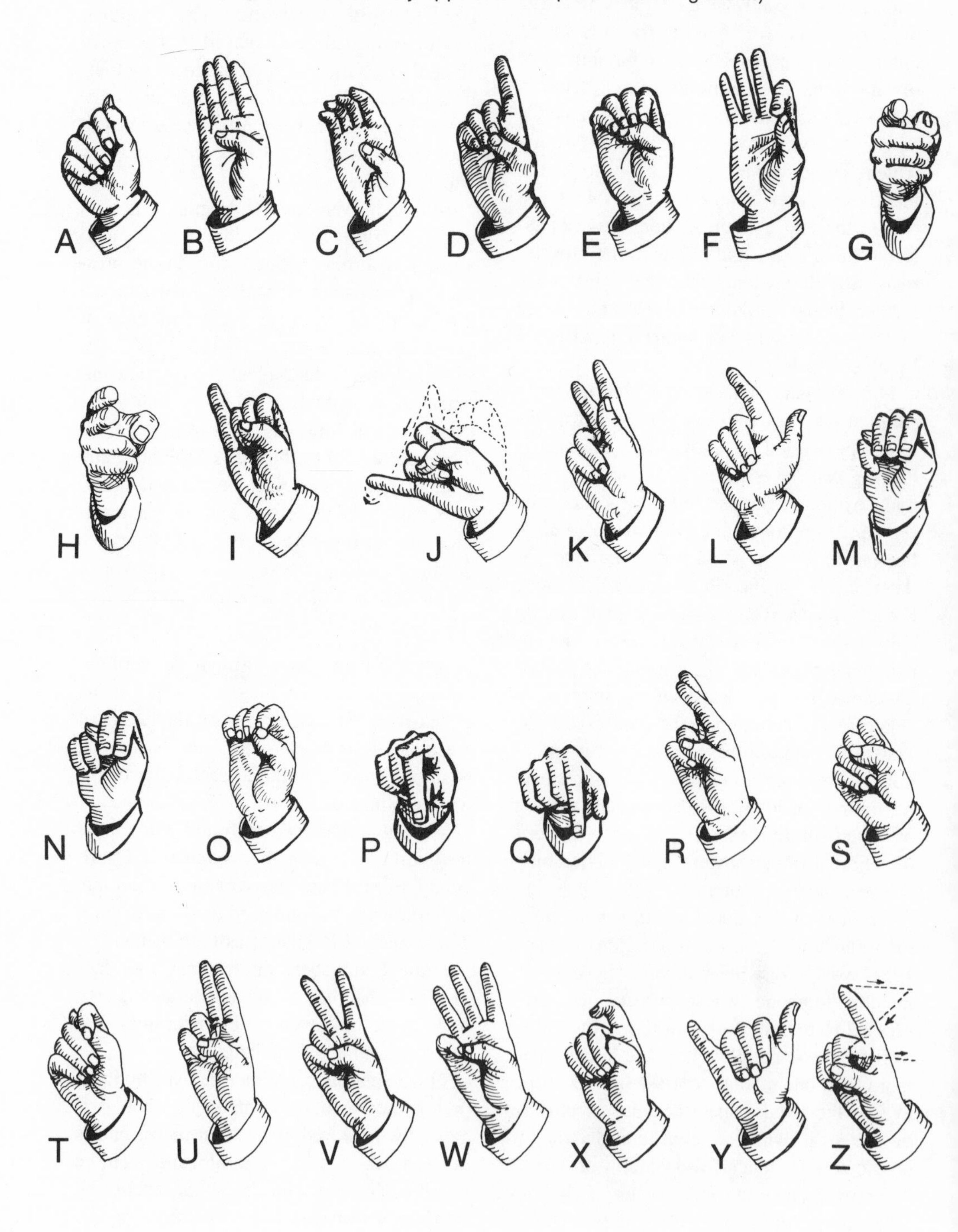

It is thought that the earliest manual alphabet was developed by PEDRO PONCE DE LEON in the 1500s and first published by JUAN PABLO BONET in 1620, and its roots can still be seen in many of the one-handed alphabets used today throughout the world. Even countries that do not use the Latin alphabet—such as Israel, which uses the Hebrew alphabet, or the Soviet Union, which uses the Cyrillic alphabet—still use a manual alphabet related to Bonet's.

Unrelated to Bonet's alphabet is the British two-handed system, which is used throughout the British commonwealth countries. A third type is the Swedish manual alphabet invented by Per Borg and exported to Portugal. It is the parent alphabet of the Swedish and Portuguese manual alphabets used today.

Still, other types of manual alphabets developed in countries without written alphabetic systems, such as Japan and China. Japan uses a fingerspelling system based on syllables instead of single sounds, and although a Chinese manual alphabet is being developed, most deaf Chinese draw the outline of the Chinese characters in the air or on palms.

In the American manual alphabet, conversations can be entirely fingerspelled, but among deaf individuals, fingerspelling is more often used in conjunction with AMERICAN SIGN LANGUAGE for proper names and terms for which there are no signs. Fingerspelling alone is used more often among people who are both deaf and blind, presented either at close distance or inside the hand.

It takes only a few hours to learn the individual hand shapes, but becoming fluent as a fingerspeller is quite difficult. The drawback to the method is its relative slowness; for people very experienced in its use, the average fingerspelling rate is about 60 words a minute, which is only about 40% as fast as the normal speaking rate.

Although very rarely used as the primary mode of communication in schools for deaf students today, fingerspelling combined with spoken English is known as the ROCHESTER METHOD.

Finnish Sign Language There are two major dialects of Finnish Sign Language (FinnSL), one used by the Finnish-speaking majority and the other by the Swedish-speaking minority. (Finland has three official languages: Finnish, Swedish and Lappish). About 5,000 of the 8,000 deaf Finns use one of the two forms of FinnSL.

By far, the majority of Finns speak the Finnish dialect; 16 of the 17 schools for the deaf are Finnish. Signing is not forbidden in any of the Finnish schools for deaf students, and teachers used Signed Finnish, a pidgin type of FinnSL using the syntax of Finnish and the vocabulary of FinnSL. As is typical in many other countries, congenitally deaf Finns can use Signed Finnish, but they ordinarily do not communicate among other deaf Finns in anything other than FinnSL.

There are 37 handshapes in FinnSL: 31 are distinctive, although six of these are rarely used. Handshapes are classified into three groups: fist, one-finger and multi-finger. Further, every multi-finger handshape must include at least one finger that appears in a one-finger handshape. There are 12 locations of signs and 24 movements. In addition, the international manual alphabet has replaced the Swedish manual alphabet for spelling out place names and proper names.

Fitzgerald Key A printed system to help deaf children learn to speak, read and write syntactically correct English sentences. The Fitzgerald Key was developed in 1929 at the Texas School for the Deaf by Edith Fitzgerald, a deaf supervising teaching.

Its set of six words and symbols help children analyze the relationships between units of connected language, enabling them to write good sentences and correct their own errors. Under the system, a child places individual words under the headings of subject, verbs and predicates, indirect and direct objects, phrases and words telling where, other word modifiers of the main verbs and "when" words and phrases.

The system is still widely used today. (See also EDUCATION OF THE DEAF.)

flat hearing loss A hearing loss that is about the same at all important frequencies.

Flourens, Marie-Jean-Pierre (1794–1867) This 19th-century French experimental neurologist was the first scientist to find evidence that the vestibular labyrinth is the organ of equilibrium. His experiments with pigeons showed, among other things, that hearing was not affected by destroying the nerves to the vestibular organs, but it was destroyed by cutting the cochlear nerve.

fluoride and hearing Fluoride is chiefly used in this country to combat tooth decay, but it is believed to strengthen the bones of the body as well.

Research suggests that the COCHLEA—the strongest bone in the body—may also benefit from fluoridation of public water systems. These studies suggest that just as tooth decay decreases in areas of fluoridated water, the incidence of OTOSCLEROSIS (softening and overgrowth of bone within the middle or inner ear) decreases in those same areas.

However, if otosclerosis is already present, fluoride does not appear to have any effect.

footplate In the ear, the base of the stirrup, or STAPES, that rests on the oval window.

Fourier analysis A mathematical principle in which any complex sound may be represented as the sum of a series of pure tones (a single frequency) whose frequencies increase in the ratio of the natural numbers 1, 2, 3 and so forth.

France This country, with its long history of education for deaf students, has about 3.5 million people with hearing problems; between 50,000 and 100,000 of these use sign language as their primary means of communication. With a deafness rate at 47 out of 100,000 France has one of the lower proportions of deafness in the world.

One of the most famous schools for the deaf is the Institut National de Jeunes Sourds founded in 1790 as a school favoring the manual education philosophy. It was to this school that THOMAS HOPKINS GALLAUDET came to learn sign language and, together with French instructor LAURENT CLERC, returned to America with the manual method.

Since the early 1960s in France, physicians emphasized the early identification of hearing problems together with immediate use of hearing aids and preschool education beginning in infancy. The four largest public national institutes for the deaf are primarily residential and were founded in the 19th century or before; most private schools for the deaf are religious institutions and today make up the Federation of Institutions of the Deaf and of the Blind of France. This private group of 40 schools, mostly residential, stresses vocational training. Finally, there is a group of private nonresidential centers that teaches students from preschool age up. These centers use more innovative techniques than the older schools and take a medical approach to deaf education.

Although the history of education for deaf students stressed vocational training, there were a few students who chose instead a more academic curriculum. Today, one private institution prepares students to take the special "baccalaureate," an exam required of 18-year-olds for many jobs and for acceptance to a university. Very few deaf students pass the exam, however, and even fewer go on to university training.

MAINSTREAMING has also been introduced in France on a very limited basis; in 1980, only 346 deaf and 1,326 hard-of-hearing students attended public schools.

The oral approach in education became accepted in France following the Congress of Milan of 1880 and endured in all schools until the late 1970s.

FRENCH SIGN LANGUAGE (FSL) began making a return to popularity in the wake of the WORLD FEDERATION OF THE DEAF Congress in Washington, D.C. in 1975, where French delegates were impressed at how AMERICAN SIGN LANGUAGE was accepted. As organizations have gathered to fight for the use of FSL, demand for classes and interpreter services has risen dramatically. The National Association of France of Interpreters for the Hearing Impaired was created in 1979. (See also SICARD, ABBÉ ROCH AMBROISE CUCURRON; L'EPÉE, ABBÉ CHARLES MICHEL.)

free field test A method of measuring auditory sensitivity by lowering sound intensity to the threshold of perception and then measuring the actual intensity of the sound after the patient has been removed from the field. (See also AUDIOMETRY.)

French Sign Language The primary method of communication among deaf French people and the first sign language to earn acceptance as a separate, complete language of its own. Called LSF (langue des signes Francaise), this language was made famous by the ABBÉ CHARLES MICHEL DE L'EPÉE, leading educator of deaf students in the 19th century.

By the 18th century, LSF was a fully integrated sign language among the deaf French populace; at the beginning of the 19th century l'Epée and the ABBÉ ROCH AMBROISE CUCURRON SICARD borrowed signs from LSF, added some of their own and created their "methodical signs." This system, which included signs representing French grammatical structure, was the first attempt at applying the structures of a spoken language to a sign language.

It was during the 19th century that the great debate between oralists and manualists took place; as the debate between the French manualists and the German oralists raged, disciples of the French method were sent all around the world. As a result, traces of LSF can be found internationally, especially in the sign languages of the United States. In fact, some say more than half the signs of ASL have been borrowed from the French.

By the 1820s, French educators were arguing that deaf students should be educated in LSF, not the artificial "methodical sign" language. For the next 50 years, LSF was used in schools as a primary communication method. With the Milan Congress of 1880 came the triumph of the oral approach over sign, however, and sign language was banned in French schools by the government. But in the late 1970s, the sign language movement gathered steam again around the world.

Today in France, LSF is taught by deaf people outside the educational system, as deaf schools have not been quick to welcome back sign language. It is estimated that up to 100,000 deaf people in France use LSF.

Research suggests that LSF is grammatically similar to ASL; handshapes are quite similar between the two. Like AMERICAN SIGN LANGUAGE, there are three categories of LSF verbs: verbs that don't use personal pronouns, verbs that change direction with the use of personal pronouns ("you give me") and classifier verbs. Many similar facial expressions are also shared between the two to indicate negative sentences, questions and conditional and relative clauses. (See also FRANCE; MANUALISM; ORAL APPROACH.)

frequency The number of sound waves that pass a fixed point in a certain period of time. It is also a measure of the number of cycles or vibrations during a period of time. Frequency is generally expressed as a HERTZ (Hz), named after the 19th-century German physicist HEINRICH HERTZ. One hertz is equal to one cycle per second; one kilohertz (kHz) is 1,000 hertz; and one megahertz (mHz) is 1,000,000 Hz.

frequency range A term used to describe the measure of power that exists in certain pitch ranges and how far the amplification ability of a hearing aid extends into the high and low pitches. For example, if a person has a high-frequency hearing loss, that person would need an aid that boosts high frequencies. (See also HEARING AIDS.)

functional hearing loss (nonorganic) Functional hearing loss exists when there is no organic reason for the patient's apparent inability to hear. It is also known as psychogenic hearing loss or hysterical hearing loss.

Instead, the person's hearing loss is primarily a result of psychological or emotional factors; the hearing mechanism itself may be completely normal. Sometimes, there is some slight damage in the ear, but the recorded hearing loss is much less than the patient reports.

Functional hearing loss is often caused by anxiety resulting from emotional conflicts and is beyond the control of the patient. In many cases, a functional hearing loss may occur at the same time as a true organic hearing problem. Called functional overlay, the problem in this case is to recognize the two different components of the hearing problem using a patient history and otologic exams.

A person with unilateral functional deafness may have a complete absence of bone conduction on the side of the bad ear and normal acuity on the side of the good ear. Such a person may even claim not to hear a shout on the bad side in spite of good hearing on the opposite side. It is these inconsistencies that help establish a functional loss.

furuncle Another name for a boil in the skin, this is a staphylococcus infection of a hair follicle that can occur in the outer ear canal. A boil in this location can be particularly painful because the skin of the ear canal is closely attached to the cartilage beneath it. There is usually swelling, redness and tenderness without fever.

Treatment includes the application of heat (hot water bottle or electric heating pad) to help the ear drain together with eardrops and a careful cleaning of the outer canal to prevent infection of other follicles.

G

Gallaudet, Edward Miner (1837–1917) This leading educator of deaf people established the first college for deaf students in the United States and fought to introduce a combined educational system integrating oral methods with the MANUAL APPROACH dominant at that time throughout the country. At a time when the rest of the world had changed to oral instruction in the wake of the Milan Congress of 1880, he clung resolutely to his belief in retaining the ''natural'' language of deaf people, although he did recognize the strong appeal ORAL APPROACH held for many people.

The son of a deaf mother and THOMAS HOPKINS GALLAUDET, cofounder of the first public school for deaf students in the United States, Edward Gallaudet felt a profound sensitivity toward deaf people. His understanding of their educational potential made him a leader in the field.

Although young Edward did not start out intending to focus on education of deaf children as a career, he changed his mind after his father died. He began teaching at the AMERICAN SCHOOL FOR THE DEAF in 1855 but, unhappy at the school, he left and was on the verge of heading to Chicago when he received a letter from philanthropist Amos Kendall of Washington, D.C.

Kendall, a multimillionaire, wanted Gallaudet to take over the Columbia Institution for the Deaf. Gallaudet saw this as his chance to establish his dream: a university for deaf students.

He began his job there in 1857 when he was only 20 years old, and in 1864 he asked Congress to allow the institution to grant degrees after a six-year course of study.

Gallaudet went to Europe in 1867 to study the ORAL APPROACH just being introduced in the United States, and upon his return, he submitted a plan to introduce oral instruction in combination with the MANUAL APPROACH then being taught at the school. He strongly believed in an equal emphasis on the manual approach and offered oral instruction as a separate course at the school. Other courses were taught manually, with additional classes in speechreading and speech.

In his career of educating deaf students, Gallaudet became an implacable opponent of oralist ALEXANDER GRAHAM BELL. Although the two initially disagreed politely, over time their enmity deepened. In 1895, Gallaudet accused Bell of fanaticism over the oral approach, calling him an outsider before a CONVENTION OF AMERICAN INSTRUCTORS OF THE DEAF. Bell and Gallaudet did not speak for the next five years.

Gallaudet lived to see the 100-year celebration of the American School of the Deaf, the institution founded by his father. He died in Hartford, Connecticut, in 1917.

Gallaudet Preschool Signed English system An invented sign system based on the spoken English language and including English spelling, pronunciation and meaning. The signs used in this system feature letter initialization and compounding. (See also MANUALLY CODED ENGLISH.)

Gallaudet Research Institute This eight-unit research group, located at GALLAUDET UNIVERSITY in Washington, D.C. is the largest institute in the world dedicated to investigating the immediate and long-range concerns of deaf people.

The institute has a multiple mission of research, teaching and service and supports broad-based research involving collaborations among scientists from many disciplines. The group brings together individuals from around the world to discuss deafness-related research and shares its information through conferences, seminars, lectures, training and consultation.

As part of its dedication to service, the institute offers a wide range of resources through its eight units, including:

- genetic counseling
- communications networks for teachers and administrators
- technological device referral
- monograph series
- demographic statistics
- projections/recommendations on needs of deaf elderly people
- ''working paper'' series in a wide variety of topics
- advice and consultation for researchers
- published proceedings of major deafness-related events
- technical assistance to businesses developing new devices for people with hearing losses

Firmly believing in the importance of outreach and service, institute staffers often give lectures and presentations to various groups, consult on deafness-related topics, serve on advisory boards, review and edit manuscripts and participate in peer review for funding agencies. A national advisory committee helps guide the institute's choice of research priorities, and the Office of the Dean of Graduate Studies and Research administers the institute.

The eight units in the institute are:

Center for Assessment and Demographic Studies This unit analyzes national databases containing information on deaf and hard-of-hearing people and advises governmental agencies on national policy. Since 1968, this unit has conducted its own annual survey of hard-of-hearing children. In addition, the unit monitors hard-of-hearing students receiving special services and studies national test standardizations for hard-of-hearing students.

Center for Studies in Education and Human Development This unit was established in 1981 to conduct research in the field of deafness. Today, ongoing research studies include how deafness affects parent-infant interaction, the earliest stages of language development and reading and writing processes. In addition, scientists are trying to develop models of the best educational environments for deaf children.

Center for Auditory and Speech Sciences Researchers in this unit investigate ways of improving the speech perception of deaf and hard-of-hearing people through auditory, visual or tactile means. Through auditory experiments, researchers try to discover the exact types of distortions hearing problems impose on the perception of specific speech sounds. Researchers are currently developing tactile devices to aid speechreading and are investigating certain types of hearing deficits common to the elderly.

Genetic Services Center This center was established by the institute in 1984 to explore the more than 200 known genetic forms of hearing problems as well as certain other kinds of deafness acquired through environmental means. The primary function of this center is to provide genetic evaluations and counseling sessions to help deaf people and their families understand the causes and effects of hearing loss. Staffers also consult with and train AUDIOLOGISTS, geneticists, parents, consumers and the medical community.

Technology Assessment Program Established in 1985, this program produces information for industrial, government and consumer groups interested in improving access to technology for people with hearing problems. The unit collaborates with several technical centers to develop devices that can, for example, alert deaf drivers to approaching emergency vehicles, convert speech to text, allow deaf people to communicate in sign language or speechread over telephone lines and provide deaf-blind people with robotic fingerspelling as an alternative to braille or personal interpreters.

Culture and Communication Studies Program This unit analyzes and compares the processes involved in acquiring language and forming cultural identities in the United States and other countries. Presently, the program's cross-cultural studies involve Spain, Italy, Mexico and some countries of Central and South America.

Mental Health Research Program The cause and effect of mental health problems among people with hearing problems is explored by this unit, which is also working to develop better ways of testing and treating these problems. Researchers are currently studying differences in cerebral organization among hearing and deaf children, personality characteristics of deaf college students and depression among deaf adults. The program also provides information on coping strategies for people who lose their hearing in adulthood and psychologists are involved in translating standard psychological tests into AMERICAN SIGN LANGUAGE.

Scientific Communications Program This program was created in 1987 to intensify the institute's efforts to communicate results of deafness-related research to others. In addition to its publication *Research at Gallaudet* and the institute's annual report, the group publishes research monographs, conference proceedings and working papers to help publicize results of selected studies. Contact: Gallaudet Research Institute, 800 Florida Ave. NE, Washington, D.C. 20002; telephone: 202-651-5400 or 800-451-8834.

Gallaudet, Thomas Hopkins (1787–1851) This Connecticut theologian was a pioneer in U.S. education for deaf people and opened the American School for the Deaf, the first permanent school for deaf students in the United States at Hartford, Connecticut.

The eldest of 12 children, Thomas Gallaudet was born in Philadelphia, the son of a merchant family of deep religious convictions. A brilliant child, Thomas entered Yale at age 14 and graduated first in his class three years later; within five years, he had apprenticed with a law firm, studied literature and earned a master's degree from Yale. He graduated with a divinity degree from Andover Theological Seminary in 1814 and intended to become an itinerant preacher until a chance meeting with a young deaf girl changed his life forever.

While visiting his parents in 1814, the 27-year-old Gallaudet met ALICE COGSWELL, nine-year-old deaf daughter of Dr. MASON FITCH COGSWELL, a prominent Hartford physician. Gallaudet began trying to teach young Alice some reading and the manual alphabet and succeeded in breaking through the communication barrier by teaching her the word "hat." With the enthusiastic backing of her father, who did not want to have to send young Alice to Europe to be educated, Gallaudet was persuaded to learn the European methods of teaching deaf students so he could return and set up a school in Connecticut.

When Gallaudet's informal census of deaf children suggested there were about 80 in Connecticut, he guessed there might be at least 400 in New England and perhaps 2,000 in the entire country.

It is probable that when Gallaudet set out, he intended to study both the British method of oral instruction and the French manual style in order to develop a combined approach to education. But when Gallaudet arrived in Great Britain, the developers of the British method—the THOMAS BRAIDWOOD family—were unwilling to share their methods. Gallaudet spent some time studying educational philosophies in Scotland and then went to Paris to interview ABBE ROCH AMBROISE CUCURRON SICARD, head of the Institut Royal des Sourds-Muets, (now called the Institut National de Jeunes Sourds) who welcomed Gallaudet. At the school Sicard allowed Gallaudet to observe methods used at each level and personally taught him the manual method used at the school. Gallaudet also studied sign language with JEAN MASSIEU and LAURENT CLERC at the school.

With Sicard's permission, Gallaudet took Clerc, one of Sicard's best pupils and a master teacher himself, back to Connecticut with him in 1816 to help organize a school for deaf students. In order to garner support for the school, Gallaudet, Clerc and Mason Cogswell toured New England, presenting demonstrations at town meetings, churches and public gatherings. Clerc's presence at Gallaudet's side was proof of the possibility of educating a deaf person and their fund-raising tours were very successful.

Within six months after returning to America, Gallaudet opened the country's first permanent school for the deaf in Hartford, Connecticut. The school featured the manual (French) method of education. Soon Gallaudet's Asylum for the Education and Instruction of the Deaf and Dumb (now the AMERICAN SCHOOL FOR THE DEAF) began enrolling students from other states.

Because the school was on its way to becoming a national institution, Gallaudet was granted financial aid from the U.S. Congress to continue his programs.

By the middle of the 19th century, there were schools for the deaf in 12 states and a national college for the deaf in Washington, D.C. run by Gallaudet's son, EDWARD MINER GALLAUDET.

Most of the schools that began during the 1800s used the French method of manual instruction, a trend established with Gallaudet's American School for the Deaf in Hartford.

Gallaudet College, renamed after Thomas (formerly the Columbia Institution for the Deaf), was officially chartered by an act of Congress in 1864 and signed into law by Abraham Lincoln. It has now operated for more than 100 years as the only liberal arts college for deaf students in the world.

Gallaudet's position as leader of the movement for deaf education was helped by his talents as preacher, orator and writer, which were useful in his push for educational reform from the pulpit and the podium.

He died on September 10, 1851, in Hartford, but his interest in education for deaf students was continued by his deaf wife Sophia Fowler, a graduate of the Hartford School, and by two of their children. Their oldest child, Thomas Gallaudet, was a minister to a deaf congregation at St. Ann's Church in New York City; EDWARD MINER GALLAUDET was the first president of Gallaudet College, now GALLAUDET UNIVERSITY, in Washington, D.C.

Gallaudet University Located in Washington, D.C., Gallaudet University is the only liberal arts university specifically for deaf students in the world.

The school was established in 1864 on land donated by Amos Kendall, a well-known journalist, politician and philanthropist, who had become interested in the welfare and education of deaf children. Called the Columbia Institution for the Deaf and Dumb and Blind when it was incorporated by Congress in 1857, it was granted a charter in 1864 to operate a collegiate division at the request of its first superintendent, EDWARD MINER GALLAUDET. Gallaudet was the son of THOMAS HOPKINS GALLAUDET, who founded the first public residential school for deaf children in the United States.

The National Deaf Mute College opened with 13 male students, one professor and one instructor; in 1887 it admitted six women as part of a two-year experiment. Although criticized for this decision, Dr. Gallaudet allowed the women to remain, letting them live in the president's house until the experiment was considered successful and a woman's dormitory could be built.

A Normal Department was begun in 1891 to train hearing teachers of deaf students, and three years later the school's name was changed to Gallaudet College to honor Edward Miner Gallaudet's father, Thomas.

Today, Gallaudet has a student body of more than 2,200, including a limited number of hearing undergraduate students. The school includes two campuses: the original 99-acre Kendall Green campus in northeast Washington and a newer nine-acre Northwest Campus seven miles from Kendall Green. Students are accepted upon recommendation from local school districts or special schools and must have graduated from high school and have passed the Gallaudet entrance exam. Of the more than 1,400 students who take the exam, usually only half qualify for admission; of these, about 70% must take up to one year of preparatory work before they can be admitted to the first-year class.

About two-thirds of the student body have a profound hearing loss and more than one-fourth have a severe loss. Almost all students lost their hearing before school age; since 1970, most students have been congenitally deaf.

In 1988 the university elected King Jordan as its first deaf president after a one-week mass protest and demonstration initiated by the deaf community, faculty and students. The successful protest is considered by deaf people to be a historic event, and profoudly important to the deaf community.

Gallaudet continues its commitment to education, research and service and houses the world's most complete collection of materials related to hearing loss, deafness and deaf people. Its library archives contain written, visual and audio materials on deafness dating back to 1546.

Gallaudet's MODEL SECONDARY SCHOOL FOR THE DEAF opened on 17 acres on the northwest part of the Kendall Green campus in 1976, and a KENDALL DEMONSTRATION ELEMENTARY SCHOOL began in 1980 on six acres in the northeast part of campus.

Gallaudet's 288 faculty members, of whom 35% are deaf and hard-of-hearing, teach in more than 40 undergraduate and graduate programs offered through the following schools: College of Arts and Sciences, School of Communication, School of Education and Human Services, School of Management and

School of Preparatory Studies. Educational programs are also offered through the College for Continuing Education.

The university grants bachelor of science or arts degrees in 26 major fields of study; its graduate school offers hearing students a two-year program leading to a master of science in audiology and both hearing and deaf students a master of arts in education, rehabilitation counseling, school counseling, educational technology and linguistics.

The Ph.D. degree in the administration of special programs is offered by the graduate school in conjunction with the Consortium of Universities in the Washington area, of which Gallaudet is a member. About one-third of these doctoral candidates have hearing problems.

Gallaudet also offers extensive noncredit courses, workshops, seminars, internships and an associate of arts degree in interpreting for hearing people who wish to become certified sign language interpreters.

The university maintains an active student government and publishes a school paper *(The Buff and Blue)*, an annual literary magazine *(Manus)* and a yearbook *(Tower Clock)*. Plays are produced twice a year and are presented in signs and voice; they are open to the public. The college has three sororities and three fraternities and a varied sports program that includes football, soccer, rugby, track, volleyball, basketball, baseball, field hockey, tennis and golf.

Gallaudet also maintains the NATIONAL CENTER FOR LAW AND THE DEAF, the International Center on Deafness, GALLAUDET RESEARCH INSTITUTE, the NATIONAL INFORMATION CENTER ON DEAFNESS and the Management Institute.

The university's Center on Deafness also features educational extension centers in cooperation with local colleges and universities. These include Ohlone College in Fremont, CA; Northern Essex Community College in Haverhill, MA; Flagler College, St. Augustine, FL; Kapiolani Community College, Honolulu, HI; Johnson County Community College, Overland Park, KS; Eastfield College, Dallas, TX; Gallaudet University Regional Center, Washington, DC; and University of Puerto Rico; San Juan, PR. (See also GALLAUDET UNIVERSITY ALUMNI ASSOCIATION.) Contact: Gallaudet University, 800 Florida Ave., NE, Washington, DC 20002.

Gallaudet University Alumni Association Representing more than 4,000 deaf people, the Gallaudet University Alumni Association members include about half of all alumni from the four-year college.

Founded in 1889 in Washington, D.C., the association meets twice a year and is open to graduates, past attendees of the college and people who have received an honorary degree from the school. It is an associate member of the WORLD FEDERATION OF THE DEAF and maintains more than 55 chapters throughout the United States and Canada. Local chapters raise money for student loans, scholarships and awards, athletic uniforms, and so forth and have provided money for memorials, endowment funds and travel for students participating in leadership conferences.

In addition, the association publishes the *Gallaudet Alumni Newsletter* twice a month, coordinates reunions and special events on campus and assists in recruiting, fundraising and public relations.

genetic mechanisms of deafness Most cases of genetic deafness are congenital and unchanging and occur in about half of all cases of deafness in children.

There are several ways in which genes can influence the ability to hear. Each child receives half his or her genetic material from each parent. All cells in the human body have 23 pairs of chromosomes (for a total of 46); because the chromosomes are paired, each segment in one chromosome has a corresponding segment in its partner. The genes—a chemical coding system of the actual units of inheritance—are also paired, one on each chromosome. Each gene provides information for the development and functioning of various organ systems.

There are many different gene locations that affect the process of hearing and many different varieties of genes. Different forms of deafness may involve different gene locations. The different types of genetic mechanisms that can result in a hearing loss are listed below:

Autosomal Recessive Inheritance This accounts for 75% to 85% of hereditary deafness. (Autosomes are the chromosomes other than the two sex chromsomes.)

"Recessive" genes are genes that must come from both parents before a trait it controls will result. In a person whose deafness is caused by an autosomal recessive gene, both parts of the gene pair must be abnormal. Both parents usually have normal hearing and are not affected, but each carries a recessive gene for deafness. Usually there is no family history of deafness.

If both parents have this recessive gene, the risk of having a child with this type of genetic deafness is one in four—25% for each pregnancy. The odds of having a child who is not a carrier are also one in four. The remainder (one in two) will carry a recessive gene, like the parents, but will not be deaf.

Autosomal Dominant Inheritance This pattern of inheritance accounts for about 20% of hereditary deafness. A gene is dominant if it is expressed when only one gene of the pair is present. Usually, in this pattern of genetic deafness, at least one parent is deaf and the deafness appears in each generation, affecting about the same number of boys and girls.

The risk of having another deaf child is 50%. None of the hearing children will be carriers because if they had the deafness gene they would be deaf themselves. The children of these hearing children would have no increased risk of having a deaf child.

In the rare case that *both* parents are deaf from the same type of autosomal dominant gene, they would have a 75% chance of having a deaf child with each pregnancy and a corresponding 25% chance of having a child without the gene.

With this type of inheritance, the deafness gene is sometimes created from a mutation in a sperm or egg cell without any prior family history. Once the gene has mutated, it will have the same effect on future generations as if it had been passed down through the family.

Often this type of inherited deafness varies so much within the family that it can be difficult to be sure of the pattern without careful study. (For example, one person in the family might be profoundly deaf while another is only mildly hard-of-hearing.)

X-Linked Inheritance This is an unusual cause of deafness in which the abnormal gene is located on the X chromosome.

Out of all the chromosome pairs in the human body, one pair determines sex: a female has two X chromosomes in this pair (an XX pattern) and a male has one X and one Y chromosome (an XY pattern). When the 46 chromosome pairs divide in making sperm, half of the resulting sperm cells will have an X, half a Y.

In X-linked genetic hearing disorders, the abnormal gene is located on the X chromosome. Females are usually protected by having another normal gene on their other X chromosome. But the male, having only one X, is not protected if he receives the abnormal gene. Thus, females are carriers and have a one in two chance of giving the abnormal gene to any one son, who will be deaf, or to a daughter, who will be a carrier. Affected males cannot pass the deafness on to their sons, because they only give them the Y chromosome, but all their daughters will be carriers because their daughters must receive the damaged X chromosome from their fathers. This results in a "skipped" generational pattern: one normal (carrier) mother may have deaf sons, but all the children of that deaf son will be apparently normal.

Chromosomal Disorders This hearing disorder results from a problem when the 46 chromosomes are being reduced to 23 in the formation of egg or sperm cells. The best-known example of a chromosomal disorder is Down's syndrome, a form of mental retardation, which is often associated with some degree of hearing loss. These genetic accidents are not usually passed on. (See GENETICS AND HEARING LOSS.)

genetics and hearing loss There are about 200 different types of genetic hearing problems ranging in degree from mild to profound. A large proportion of hearing problems that occur at birth or during the first few years of life are hereditary, as are many kinds of progressive hearing losses that occur later in life.

Although some kinds of hearing loss are associated with other physical characteristics or medical problems (changes in the eye or hair color, kidneys or heart), most types of genetic hearing loss do not involve other physical changes.

Hearing ability is only one of many different physical traits that are handed down genetically in families. Every person has 23 pairs of chromosomes, tiny rod-shaped structures made up of deoxyribonucleic acid (DNA), half inherited from the mother and half from the father. Inside each chromosome are thousands of genes, each one carrying the genetic building blocks for everything from eye color to bone structure. These genes also govern the way in which the ear structures are formed. Any change in a gene can result in a hearing problem.

Because hearing problems are so often genetic, it is common to refer a family with a deaf member to a genetic counselor or genetic team. Such a team may include a genetic associate (a person with a master's degree in genetic counseling), a genetics physician and sometimes a genetics nurse or social worker.

There is currently no blood test that can diagnose a "hearing loss gene," but a medical geneticist can often tell whether someone's hearing problem has been inherited. Genetic counseling for hearing loss always includes a detailed family history, a medical history of the deaf person and a pregnancy history of the mother of that person. The individual or family is then seen by the medical geneticist for a physical examination to uncover clues in the appearance that might suggest a basis for the hearing problem, including checking the head, eyes and ears and looking for changes in the skin, hair or kidneys.

In cases where it is possible to determine the cause of the hearing problem and how a gene has passed through the family, the team meets with the individual or the family and explains how the hearing loss was inherited and what the implications and possibilities are for future generations inheriting the gene(s).

It is possible for someone to have a genetic hearing loss and be the only person with that problem in the family, but if there is more than one person in the family with a hearing loss, then the problem is almost always genetic. Unfortunately, geneticists can not often predict which members of a family will receive the gene for a hearing problem. (See GENETIC MECHANISMS OF DEAFNESS.)

German measles See RUBELLA.

German Sign Language In the former Federal Republic of Germany (West Germany), almost all prelingually deaf Germans use Deutsche Gebardensprache (DGS), a sign language with many dialects arising from various schools for deaf students.

A traditionally oral country, there has been little research into DGS, which has not generally been used in educational settings, although it is a natural communication mode among deaf people outside the classroom. When manual approaches are mentioned in schools, the reference is to Signed German.

Although similar to AMERICAN SIGN LANGUAGE in some ways, DGS—as many other European sign languages—uses more lip movements. FINGERSPELLING, using a manual alphabet similar to the American one, is also used with DGS, although older DGS users do not know the manual alphabet. More popular is a manual system called PMS (Phonembestimmtes Manualsystem), which represents phonemes instead of letters. This system is used in schools for deaf students to teach articulation.

gestuno The first "international" SIGN LANGUAGE, developed by members of the WORLD FEDERATION OF THE DEAF in an attempt to overcome the problem of communication at international meetings.

Gestuno is a collection of about 1,500 signs chosen for ease of use to build a basic international vocabulary. The problem of syntax was simply ignored.

The problem with this international sign language is that few people are willing to learn the new signs, the communication it allows is often too limited, and there are not enough occasions to use it to make learning gestuno worthwhile for most people.

gestural language See SIGN LANGUAGE.

GLAD An acronym for Greater Los Angeles Council on Deafness; this nonprofit group, founded in 1969, is a comprehensive service center and umbrella agency for more than 45 California groups and agencies in the field of deafness, including social, recreational and service clubs for the deaf community and educational, professional, health and religious organizations. It serves more than 1,500 hearing and deaf members.

GLAD sponsors community workshops and educational lectures and links traditional social service agencies with the deaf community. It also offers employment referral services, interpreter referrals, telephone/TDD relay services, peer counseling and advocacy. Under a grant from California's rehabilitation department, GLAD also offers the first sign language interpreter pool free of charge to deaf people. With this pool, deaf people in California have access to more than 200 qualified interpreters.

The council consults with police, hospitals, school districts and the state legislature in support of deaf services. Located as it is in the heart of the entertainment business, the council also works with producers on projects that involve deaf subjects or actors to ensure that deaf characters are honestly portrayed and that deaf actors are hired as often as possible to play deaf roles.

The council produces an extensive resource book, the *Directory of Resources Available to Deaf and Hearing Impaired Persons in the Southern California Area* and the journal *GLAD News Magazine* and maintains a bookstore carrying volumes on deafness. The council is a member of the NATIONAL ASSOCIATION OF THE DEAF. Contact: GLAD, 616 South Westmoreland Ave., Second floor, Los Angeles, CA 90005; telephone: 213-383-2220 (voice/TDD).

glue ear See SEROUS OTITIS MEDIA.

grammar The structure of language. Grammar consists of a number of elements: *morphology* (how sounds go together to form words or (in a signed language) how the elements of position, shape and movement combine to form signs); *syntax* (how words or signs are organized in sentences); *semantics* (how to interpret the meaning of words, signs and sentences); *pragmatics* (how to participate in a conversation).

Greece The outlook for deaf people in Greece is not encouraging since less than half the deaf citizens in the country are given any education at all. Of those who are, only 10% get more than elementary instruction.

Although it is estimated that there are at least 1,480 deaf children in the country, only 640 receive some form of special education, and there is no state provision for their education.

The National Foundation for the Protection of the Deaf and Dumb provides six educational facilities for deaf children, serving about 400 residential and day students (most in elementary schools). There are two other schools for deaf children. The schools all favor an oral approach, with an emphasis on speechreading and auditory training and no signing in class. Despite this, Greek Sign Language, with its roots in American and French sign languages, is used by more than 30,000 adult deaf Greeks.

Since there is no provision for deaf teacher training, specialists either are educated abroad or are trained simply as regular classroom instructors. There are currently no adult or higher education programs specifically for deaf people.

Although at present deaf citizens have few choices and fewer services, there is hope for the future: In 1983 a national committee began developing a comprehensive educational program for all children with hearing problems between ages 12 and 18.

group amplification systems See ASSISTIVE LISTENING DEVICES.

H

hair cells More than 15,000 microscopic hair-like cells are located inside the inner ear in an area smaller than a fingernail. They cover the ORGAN OF CORTI—the actual part of the ear that allows a person to hear.

There are about 3,400 inner hair cells in the human cochlea that extend in a row from the base to the apex of the cochlea. In much the same way, close to the lateral surface of the organ of Corti are three or four rows of about 12,000 outer hair cells. These inner and outer hair cells incline toward each other, and cilia emerge from the upper surface of the inner and outer hair cells to penetrate the tectorial membrane, which forms a roof over the organ of Corti.

When a sound wave makes the eardrum vibrate, the vibrations are carried across the middle ear by the hammer, the anvil and the stirrup, which passes the vibrations through the oval window to the fluid in the tubes of the inner ear. This makes the hairs of the organ of Corti vibrate—and the more hairs that vibrate, the louder the sound. The shorter, thinner hair cells pick up high sounds, and the longer, thicker hairs pick up low sounds. The auditory nerve picks up the messages from these hairs and sends them to the brain, where the sound is processed.

Excessive noise can overload the tiny, irreplaceable hair cells and can seriously impede the ability to hear.

hammer See MALLEUS.

hard-of-hearing A term used to describe mild to moderate hearing loss. This term is preferred over "hearing-impaired" by the deaf community.

head injury and deafness Severe head injury can cause sensorineural and conductive deafness in one or both ears.

Sensorineural deafness resulting from severe head injury can be associated with a transverse fracture of the temporal bone, which causes a complete destruction of the hearing and balance mechanism on the affected side.

This type of deafness is usually permanent, although the dizziness that can accompany it will usually subside over a period of several weeks and the unsteadiness and swaying toward the affected side may subside after several months. Sometimes a transverse fracture of the temporal bone results in a hearing loss that is incomplete, but this is uncommon.

It is possible to have hearing damage following a head injury that doesn't fracture the temporal bone, especially from a blow to the back or side of the head—although the blow is usually severe enough to cause loss of consciousness. Deafness from this type of injury is usually similar to that which comes from excess noise. An injury of this type is often accompanied by dizziness, often made worse by a change in position of the head.

Although there may be hearing loss on the side of the injury, there may also be a mild hearing loss on the opposite side due to a concussion in the inner ear.

Conductive deafness resulting from injury is caused by blood that collects in the middle ear and external canal; occasionally there is disruption of the ossicular chain (hammer, anvil, stirrup) and a ruptured eardrum. As the blood is absorbed, however, hearing usually returns to its original level, and the eardrum heals. Occasionally, conductive deafness following head injury can be permanent, but because it is conductive, the maximum degree of hearing loss is usually about 60 dB. This means that if speech is loud enough, the person can not only hear well but can understand what is being said. Surgery can sometimes restore the hearing. (See also CONDUCTIVE HEARING LOSS; SENSORINEURAL HEARING LOSS.)

hearing The sense of hearing is a complex, coordinated process involving the transmission of sound waves through the ear mechanisms into the brain, which can then interpret the message.

First, the sound waves strike the OUTER EAR (or PINNA), the part of the ear visible on the side of the head. The outer ear is designed to help gather these sound waves and funnel them down the ear canal to the paper-thin EARDRUM (tympanic membrane), which divides the outer ear from the MIDDLE EAR.

When the sound waves strike the eardrum, it vibrates and moves a chain of three small bones on the other side, called the ossicular chain (or OSSICLES), which consists of the hammer (MALLEUS) the anvil (INCUS) and the stirrup (STAPES.) These tiny bones—the smallest ones in the body—are full size at birth and are located in the middle ear cavity. Together, the three bones transfer the energy of the sound wave from the outer ear through the middle ear and into the INNER EAR.

As the sound vibrates the eardrum, which vibrates the ossicles, it also moves the last bone in the ossicular chain, the stirrup (stapes), which is also attached to a tiny membrane called the OVAL WINDOW. The oval window is the entrance to the inner ear, which contains the organ of hearing called the COCHLEA. As the stirrup moves, it makes the oval window vibrate, disturbing the fluid-filled channel of the cochlea on the other side of the oval window.

As the cochlea moves, it stimulates the thousands of microscopic hair cells inside the organ, which send electrical impulses to the brain.

There are also other structures in the ear that may not contribute to hearing but serve very important purposes nevertheless. Located in the middle ear is the EUSTACHIAN TUBE, which helps maintain the balance of air pressure on both sides of the eardrum and connects the middle ear cavity to the back of the nose just above the soft palate. The upper end of this tube is usually surrounded by bone and is open; the lower end is usually collapsed and surrounded by soft tissue. About every third time we swallow or yawn, this tube opens, allowing air to flow up to the middle ear and equalizing the air pressure in the middle and outer ear. (The ear-popping feeling during airplane rides occurs if this equalization process is large and rapid, causing pressure to build up on one side of the eardrum, pushing it inward or outward.)

Within the inner ear, the three small loops of the SEMICIRCULAR CANALS, connected to the cochlea, help maintain balance. Problems within these tiny semicircular canals may cause DIZZINESS, VERTIGO and other balance problems.

hearing aids Devices that consist of a group of tiny components worn on one or both ears to improve hearing by making sounds louder and speech easier to understand for people with certain types of hearing loss.

The first hearing aids were simple cone-shaped devices, ranging from a rolled-up tube to an elaborate EAR TRUMPET, which provided a small boost in sound. After the invention of the vacuum tube came the first "powered" hearing aids in 1921, but they were cumbersome units with large parts and heavy batteries.

Today, a hearing aid system consists of a tiny microphone that picks up sound waves and converts them into electrical signals. These impulses are fed into an amplifier, which boosts the signal to increase the output of sound and then sends it to a receiver, which converts the amplified signals back into sound and transmits them into the ear through an EARMOLD.

If it is properly fitted, the earmold provides support for the hearing aid, directing amplified sound into the ear canal. A poorly fitting earmold can cause whistles and squeals, irritation and soreness. Ready-made earmolds are available, but many wearers prefer custom-fitted molds.

Although a hearing aid can amplify sound, it does not necessarily improve clarity and cannot make hearing completely normal. Hearing aids require practice and skill to be used effectively. They are worn by both deaf and hard-of-hearing people; even profoundly deaf people can benefit from powerful behind-the-ear aids.

People with mild hearing losses may get enough improvement simply with a tiny unit that fits directly into the ear; people with more severe problems may need a larger, more powerful system, usually worn on the body. These are sturdier, less subject to distortion and easier to regulate. Still, most profoundly deaf individuals do not wear body types.

Modern hearing aids do much more than simply amplify sound: They can filter background noise, change tonal quality and control the loudness of environmental sounds. Strides in miniaturization have resulted in a much smaller, less visible aid that is of benefit to people who don't want people to know they wear an aid. In all but four states, all hearing aids may be fitted and sold only by licensed specialists, who may be called "dealers," "specialists," "dispensers" or "dispensing audiologists."

Listed below are the hearing aids that are currently available:

In-the-ear aids are lightweight devices that fit inside the ear canal with no external wires or tubes. They include tone control but no volume control and are generally useful only for mild hearing losses.

Behind-the-ear aids include a microphone, amplifier and receiver inside a small curved case worn behind the ear and connected to the earmold by a short plastic tube. Some models have a tone control, volume control and telephone pickup device. This model is useful for people whose hearing loss ranges from mild to severe.

Eyeglass models are much the same as behind-the-ear aids, except that the case fits into an eyeglass frame instead of behind the ear. Bone conduction hearing aids are also available in the eyeglass model.

On-the-body aids feature a larger microphone, amplifier and power supply inside a case carried inside a pocket or attached to clothing. The external receiver attaches directly to the earmold and its power comes through a flexible wire from the amplifier. Although larger than other aids, on-the-body hearing aids are also more powerful and easier to adjust than smaller devices. They are not popular but are still in use.

Monaural hearing aid systems include any hearing aid that provides sound to one ear alone.

Binaural hearing aid systems include two complete hearing aids, one in each ear. Some wearers find that the binaural system increases direction sense and helps separate sounds from unwanted background noise.

CROS (contralateral routing of signal) or *crossover* systems features a microphone beside the impaired ear that feeds the amplified signal to the better ear, thereby eliminating "head shadow" (the head blocking sound from the better ear). This system may help make speech easier to understand for those with a high frequency loss in both ears.

BI-CROS systems utilize two microphones (one above each ear) sending signals to a single amplifier. Sound then travels to a single receiver, which transfers it to the better ear via a conventional earmold.

The first step in obtaining a hearing aid is to have an accurate diagnosis and hearing evaluation done by an otologist, (ear specialist) OTOLARYNGOLOGIST (a specialist in ear, nose and throat diseases) and an AUDIOLOGIST. These two specialists can determine whether a hearing aid will help and can identify the type that will do the most good. This is particularly important since aids can be expensive (ranging between $275 and $1,000) and are not generally covered by private insurance.

One of the main problems with hearing aids is that they amplify not only the desired sound but extraneous noise as well. Particularly when the source of sound is far away (as on a stage or in a large building), other environmental noises can get in the way. Hearing aids favor sounds in the frequency range of speech; therefore, sounds that lie outside this range may be altered by a hearing aid.

In cases in which the hair cells, which convert vibration to nerve impulses, do not function, a hearing aid will not help. In this case, a COCHLEAR IMPLANT may be helpful. This device converts sound to electrical impulses transmitted directly through wires to the auditory nerve. Although sounds may not be clear, the implant can enhance sound and improve speech comprehension.

hearing aid dealers Hearing aids may legally be sold and fitted by either a hearing aid dealer (or dispenser) or a "dispensing AUDIOLOGIST" (an audiologist who also sells hearing aids).

The hearing aid dealer will be responsible for making the impression for the EARMOLD and making sure the aid fits properly. The dealer will also explain the general care and use of the aid and will be able to perform both minor and major repairs. Generally, the dealer can offer suggestions about using a hearing aid or about possible changes in hearing aid models and the settings in which they can be used.

Before audiologists moved into the dealership field, hearing aids were sold by people who were not required to have additional training in the field. Most learned the trade by apprenticing to an experienced dealer; for many years, no licensure or registration was required. Some hearing aid dealers call themselves audiologists, but this title should be used only by people who have earned at least a master's degree in audiology.

Today, most states have laws that prohibit anyone from selling a hearing aid before the client has been examined by a physician who can rule out the possibility of a medical problem. (Waivers are permitted for people whose religious beliefs preclude physician visits.) In addition, a license is required for dealers in most states. In order to be licensed, a person combines study with training under a licensed person and then must pass state examination.

As audiologists move into the hearing aid dispensing field, state licensing exams are already being designed with an emphasis on audiological education.

hearing aid helpline This toll-free telephone number is operated by the NATIONAL HEARING AID SOCIETY for anyone who suspects a hearing loss and is uncertain what to do or who needs information about hearing loss and hearing aids. The helpline may be used by consumers to locate qualified, competent hearing aid specialists and answer questions about hearing instruments, dispensing and service.

Callers can also obtain a consumer information kit, which includes a regional edition of the membership directory of the Hearing Aid Society plus a 22-page booklet covering topics such as how hearing works, signs of hearing loss and types of hearing aids.

Information is available on ASSISTIVE LISTENING DEVICES, requirements for entering the hearing aid profession, statistics on hearing loss and hearing instruments, federal regulations pertaining to the hearing instrument industry and so forth. The helpline does not provide medical advice, recommend specific products or quote prices.

Although direct financial assistance is not available through the helpline, the helpline can provide a list of possible financial resources. All services and materials provided are free. Callers may use the helpline numbers (1-800-521-5247; in Michigan, 1-313-478-2610) Monday through Friday, 9:00 A.M. to 4:30 P.M. EST.

hearing ear dogs Certain dogs can be trained to respond to specific sounds (a doorbell, a crying baby, a smoke alarm, an alarm clock) by making physical contact with the owner and leading him or her to the source of the sound.

The dogs, which can be any breed or size, are usually obtained at humane shelters by a nonprofit training center. At these special centers, the dogs complete a six-month program in basic obedience, specialized skills, using both voice and hand signals, and "sound keying"—zeroing in on specific noises. Most dogs are trained to alert in different ways depending on the type of sound so that the owner can distinguish a crying baby from a ringing doorbell.

After training is completed, the dog is taken to its new home, where dog and potential owner go through an intensive one-week course together. After three months of satisfactory performance by the dog, ownership is transferred and certification is granted. The dog's blaze orange collar and leash entitle dog and master to the same legal rights accorded to blind people and their dog guides.

Hearing dog programs are completely supported by donations and community service organizations; no applicant is denied a hearing dog because of inability to pay. For more information about hearing ear dogs, contact the American Humane Association, 9725 East Hamden Ave., Denver, CO 80231. (See also AMERICAN HUMANE ASSOCIATION; CENTER FOR HEARING EAR DOGS; Appendix 12.)

hearing evaluation See AUDIOMETRY.

hearing-impaired A term for hard-of-hearing or deaf persons that many in the deaf community find objectionable due to its negative connotations. The preferred term is "hard-of-hearing."

hearing loss An estimated 21 million Americans have some form of hearing loss, which can occur at any age and range from mild to severe. Although surveys by the National Center for Health Statistics can estimate numbers of people with hearing problems, there have been no recent surveys on deafness. Estimates suggest the number of hard-of-hearing and deaf people may range from 350,000 to 2,000,000.

While total congenital deafness is rare, occurring only about once in every 1,000 live births, hearing loss in young children is much more common. As many as one-fourth of five-year-olds starting school may have

Prevalence Rates per 100,000 People with Hearing Loss by Census Region—1971

Region	Prevalence Rate
United States	6,603
Northeast	5,977
North Central	6,563
South	6,807
West	7,107

Source: Schein, J., & Delk, M. *The Deaf Population of the United States*. Silver Spring, MD: National Association of the Deaf, 1974.

Prevalence Rates per 100,000 People with Hearing Problems by Age

Age	1971	1977	1978	1979	1980	1981
All ages	7,160	7,640	7,740	7,720	7,970	8,290
Under 17	1,300	1,430	1,620	1,440	1,810	1,770
17–44	4,240	4,020	4,290	4,490	4,380	4,380
45–64	11,410	12,370	12,230	11,920	12,660	14,290
65–	29,430	29,270	28,420	28,160	28,250	28,380

Source: National Center for Health Statistics.

Causes of Hearing Problems for Hard-of-Hearing/Deaf Students (Totals add up to more than 100% because of multiple etiology)

Cause	1972–73 (%)	1982–83 (%)	1985–86 (%)
Unknown	48.6	39.5	43.0
Maternal rubella	17.6	16.3	8.0
Prematurity	5.2	4.0	4.4
Pregnancy complications	3.2	3.4	3.0
Rh incompatibility	3.1	1.4	0.9
Birth trauma	2.3	2.4	2.4
Heredity	8.5	11.6	12.4
Meningitis	5.3	7.3	8.6
High fever	2.3	3.1	3.1
Measles	2.1	0.8	0.5
Otitis media	1.6	3.0	3.5
Infection	1.5	2.7	2.8
Trauma	0.9	0.8	0.7
Mumps	0.6	0.2	0.1

Source: Hotchkiss, David. *Demographic Aspects of Hearing Impairment*. Center for Assessment and Demographic Studies, Gallaudet Research Institute, 1987, p. 5.

some type of hearing loss, usually because of earlier ear infections.

Partial deafness (from mild to severe) is usually the result of ear disease, injury or breakdown of the hearing mechanisms with age. About one-fourth of people over age 65 need a hearing aid.

It is now possible to detect the presence of hearing loss in a newborn, evaluate its severity and, depending on the type of loss, correct it. A baby who is deaf from birth cannot respond to sounds and, although its crying is normal, the baby will not babble or make other sounds.

In adults, hearing loss brings an inability to hear soft sounds and distorts high tones. Speech may begin to be difficult to understand in the presence of background noise. In addition, the person may experience ringing in the ear (TINNITUS), dizziness and loss of balance (VERTIGO) or even auditory hallucinations.

There are two main types of hearing loss: conductive and sensorineural.

Conductive Hearing Loss Conductive hearing loss refers to a problem with the transference of sound from the outer to the inner ear, usually because of damage to the eardrum or the three bones of the middle ear (the OSSICLES, also called the hammer, anvil and stirrup).

In an adult, conductive hearing loss may be caused by earwax blocking the outer ear canal or by OTOSCLEROSIS (a disease in which the stapes become fixed). In a child, it is most commonly caused by ear infection with effusion (a collection of sticky fluid in the middle ear). Sometimes conductive hearing loss may be caused by damage to the eardrum or middle ear due to sudden pressure changes (barotrauma, or AERO-TITIS MEDIA) or by a punctured eardrum.

Conductive hearing loss in children with chronic media can be treated with a MYRINGOTOMY (an operation to drain the fluid from the middle ear). Excessive earwax can be removed with a syringe and warm water, and a PERFORATED EARDRUM that does not heal on its own after a few months can be

Number of Deaf Students Served under PL 94-142 and 89-313

Diagnosis	1977–78	1979–80	1981–82	1983–84	1985–86
Deaf/Hard-of-Hearing	87,146	82,873	76,387	74,279	68,413
Deaf/blind	———*	2,576	2,642	2,512	2,132

*Figures unavailable.
Source: Hotchkiss, David. *Demographic Aspects of Hearing Impairment.* Center for Assessment and Demographic Studies, Gallaudet Research Institute, 1987, p. 6.

Estimates of the Total Population and the Hard-of-Hearing Population by Age, United States, 1985

Age Group	Hard-of-Hearing	Total
Under 18	1,203,000	62,745,000
18–44	4,955,000	99,418,000
45–64	7,077,000	44,513,000
65–	7,963,000	27,044,000
Total	21,198,000	233,720,000

Source: Hotchkiss David. *Demographic Aspects of Hearing Impairment.* Center for Assessment and Demographic Studies, Gallaudet Research Institute, 1987, p. 1.

repaired during an operation called a TYMPANOPLASTY. For otosclerosis, OTOLARYNGOLOGISTS may perform a STAPEDECTOMY (replacement of the stapes).

Sensorineural Hearing Loss Sensorineural hearing loss is a general term used to describe hearing problems from a number of conditions. It occurs when sounds that reach the inner ear do not reach the brain because of damage to the AUDITORY (hearing) NERVE or the structures of the inner ear. Its effects are permanent and irreversible in almost all cases. This type of hearing loss tends to progress slowly as a person ages and can affect one or both ears.

Sensorineural hearing loss may be mild (15–30 dB loss), causing a person to strain to hear; moderate (35–55 dB loss), requiring frequent repetition and misunderstandings; or severe (60–90 dB loss), leaving the ability to hear only very loud sounds, if anything.

People with sensorineural hearing loss usually have problems understanding speech (word discrimination) even when the speech is loud—which is one reason why hearing aids often do not help. In general, difficulty understanding speech occurs because the person has trouble hearing certain frequencies of sound (or pitch). For example, a hearing problem for high-pitched sounds would mean it would be also hard to hear some consonants (such as t, k, s) because these sounds do not carry voice. People with sensorineural hearing loss may also have a problem with RECRUITMENT (an abnormally rapid increase in sound loudness). Probably because of sensory cell damage, this means a sound that is not heard at one level be-

Number of Persons with Hearing Problems per 1,000 by Age, Sex and Race, 1985

Age	Male	Female	White	Black	Total
0–45	45.4	30.5	41.3	18.1	37.9
45–64	208.0	114.3	163.3	128.4	159.0
65–up	364.2	245.9	299.6	252.5	294.0
Total	107.4	75.1	96.9	54.3	90.7

Source: Hotchkiss, David. *Demographic Aspects of Hearing Impairments.* Center for Assessment and Demographic Studies, Gallaudet Research Institute, 1987, p. 3.

comes painfully loud after only a tiny increase in volume.

Every year, about 5,000 infants are born with sensorineural hearing loss caused by genetics, birth injury (Rh incompatability or loss of oxygen during labor) or damage to the developing fetus because of maternal infection (RUBELLA, herpes or other viral diseases).

After birth, damage to the delicate hearing mechanisms of the inner ear (including the COCHLEA and LABYRINTH) may be caused by prolonged exposure to loud noise, which damages the sensory cells and nerve fibers, particularly if the exposure lasts for a long time. Other diseases causing this type of deafness include MÉNIÈRE'S DISEASE, certain drugs or viral infections. In addition, any disease that affects the flow of blood to the inner ear can also cause hearing problems, including diabetes, emphysema, heart problems, atherosclerosis and some kidney disorders.

Sensorineural hearing loss due to problems with the auditory (hearing) nerve or the hearing centers in the brain may be caused by stroke, head injury or damage from a benign tumor on the nerve (ACOUSTIC NEUROMA).

Among the elderly, the most likely cause of sensorineural hearing loss is related to changes in the ear due to aging (PRESBYCUSIS) which even today is not well understood by scientists.

In still other cases, the cause of sensorineural deafness is simply not known.

Central Hearing Loss A third, much rarer form of hearing problem is central hearing loss caused by damage to the nerve centers in the pathways to the brain, or in the brain itself. With this type of hearing loss, sound levels are not affected, but understanding of language becomes difficult. Central hearing loss can be caused by high fever, excess exposure to loud noise, OTOTOXIC DRUGS, head injury, circulation problems or tumors.

Classification Hearing loss can be classified three ways: by type, configuration and degree. Both degree and configuration refer to the range and volume of sounds that cannot be heard; type describes the part of the auditory system that has been affected.

The degree of hearing loss is the volume needed above the normal level for sounds to be heard, and is the most common way to describe a person's hearing problem (such as "profoundly deaf").

But there is more to deafness than just the degree. The configuration of hearing loss is the range of pitch or frequency at which the loss occurs, which influences the ability to hear speech.

Normally, speech varies in loudness and pitch; vowels are strong low-frequency sounds that can penetrate background noise fairly well. On the other hand, consonants tend to be both higher and weaker in pitch, fading out at a distance and obscured by background noise.

In general, hard-of-hearing people hear some frequencies better than others, which can be a problem in understanding speech that involves a broad range of frequencies—especially the higher ones.

People with mild hearing loss may lose track of conversations or have problems hearing across a crowded room. Moderate to severe loss can make speech quite difficult to understand even in the quietest room. Percent of hearing loss is strictly a medical and legal way to handle compensation. It does not deal with problems of clarity of pitch perception, loudness growth, and so forth.

Treatment Although medical and surgical techniques to correct conductive hearing loss have improved, medical correction for sensorineural deafness is more difficult. There is no treatment for central deafness, although special auditory training may provide some help.

There are various treatments for conductive deafness, depending on the cause of the problem. Otosclerosis (fixation of the hearing bones) can be treated with surgery (stapedectomy). A hole in the eardrum or missing hearing bones can be corrected with reconstructive surgery.

Sensorineural hearing loss due to Meniere's disease or other medical problems can sometimes be improved by treating the underlying condition. While there is little help for profound sensorineural hearing loss, current research on COCHLEAR IMPLANTS that provide electrical stimulation to the inner ear may lead to important improvements in the ability to correct this problem. (See also AERO-OTITIS MEDIA; GENETICS AND HEARING LOSS; HEARING; PRENATAL CAUSES OF HEARING LOSS.)

hearing tests See AUDIOMETRY.

Heinicke, Samuel (1727–1790) This 18th-century German educator is considered to be the father of the ORAL APPROACH and founded one of the first state-supported public schools for deaf students in the world.

Although others believed that speaking was important in the education of deaf children, it was Heinicke who was convinced that speech is necessary in order to develop abstract thought. He was a contemporary of ABBÉ CHARLES MICHEL DE L'EPÉE, the founder of the MANUAL APPROACH, with whom he maintained a lifelong debate over the superiority of communication modes.

Born in Nautschutz, Germany, Heinicke joined the Saxon army after a quarrel with his father. While in the army he spent most of his time studying. Eventually, he became a tutor and in 1754 began to teach one of his pupils, a deaf boy, the manual language.

With the onslaught of the Seven Years' War in 1756, Heinicke fled the Prussian troops and eventually settled in Hamburg, where he found work as a private secretary, tutor and schoolteacher. Twenty years after teaching his first deaf student, he began to teach a second, this time abandoning the manual alphabet in favor of speech. In 1775 he published the first textbook ever written for the instruction of deaf students, and his fame as a deaf teacher grew; two years later, he was asked to establish a school for deaf students in Leipzig, Germany.

This new school, the Electoral Saxon Institute for Mutes and Other Persons Afflicted with Speech Defects, opened in 1778 as the first school for deaf students in Germany. It exists today as the Samuel Heinicke School for the Deaf.

Heinicke continued to refine his beliefs in the oral approach for deaf students during his 12 years as administrator at the school. Although he kept his methods to himself, he is known to be the world's first oralist who believed that no hearing child ever learned to speak by first learning letters. Instead, Heinicke taught deaf students the way hearing children learn to speak: first came words, which were then broken down into syllables.

Because Heinicke believed that deaf people have an inner drive to speak just the way hearing people do, he believed teaching speech was not a difficult task. Heinicke was convinced that certain tastes cause the mouth to form the correct position for certain vowels and that by substituting the sense of taste for the lost sense of hearing, Heinicke believed deaf students could be taught to articulate. In his work he used a special artificial throat and tongue designed to help students produce sounds.

Heinicke condemned the practice of operating on the tongue of a deaf child to correct speech defects since he believed that a deaf child's inability to speak was because he could not hear, not because his tongue was malformed.

Although Heinicke allowed the occasional use of signs in order to explain concepts, he required his students to speak out loud to each other in his presence.

De l'Epée and Heinicke both established schools for deaf students in their respective countries, paving the way for the idea of a free public education for deaf students and emphasizing the importance of special education for everyone who needed it. Yet although both de l'Epée and Heinicke believed in the importance of educating deaf children, they differed profoundly over how to accomplish this goal.

Heinicke maintained an ongoing debate with l'Epée over the superiority of communication methods, and was severely shaken when two universities decided that l'Epee's manual approach was superior. Heinicke was particularly distressed to learn that the University of Leipzig, with which his school was affiliated, sided with l'Epée in the controversy. Critics of his method persisted, and Heinicke continued to defend his methods. It appeared that the oral approach was waning and the manual approach was gaining momentum, but Heinicke's theories were eventually resurrected, refined and popularized many years after his unexpected death of a stroke in Leipzig, Germany on April 30, 1790.

Helen Keller National Center for Deaf-Blind Youth and Adults The only national facility providing comprehensive services for diagnostic evaluation, rehabilitation and personal adjustment training and job preparation and placement for deaf-blind people.

The center also conducts extensive field service through regional offices, affiliated programs and national training teams, offers services to elderly deaf-blind people and maintains a national register of deaf-blind people. The organization designs and improves sensory aids and publishes *The Nat-Cat News*. Contact: Helen Keller National Center for Deaf-Blind Youth and Adults, 111 Middle Neck Road, Sands Point, NY 11050; telephone (voice and TDD): 516-944-8900.

helicotrema An opening in the BASILAR MEMBRANE at the apex of the cochlear canal through which the SCALA TYMPANI communicates with the SCALA VESTIBULI. Low-frequency vibrations of the oval window create waves in the perilymph of the scala vestibuli through the helicotrema, passing on into the scala tympani.

helix The curved border of the pinna (outer ear).

Helmholtz, Hermann Ludwig Ferdinand von (1821–1894) A brilliant physiologist, anatomist, mathematician and physicist, von Helmholtz developed a resonance theory that each sound wave entering the ear induced vibrations in a basilar fiber that responded to the wave's frequency. It was these vibrations, he believed, that stimulated the ORGAN OF CORTI, which transferred the vibrations to the auditory nerve. Later scientists found, however, that while the individual fibers do not resonate, the BASILAR MEMBRANE itself can create the resonance effect.

heredity and deafness See GENETICS AND HEARING LOSS.

herpes simplex type II A sexually transmitted disease that can be passed on to the fetus if the mother becomes infected while she is pregnant. Babies born to mothers infected during pregnancy or with an active lesion during birth can contract herpes, which can cause a subsequent hearing loss.

The virus can cause death in affected infants, but modern drug treatments are saving more babies, although the survivors may have hearing loss. (See also PRENATAL CAUSES OF HEARING LOSS; VIRUSES AND HEARING LOSS.)

herpes zoster See VIRUSES AND HEARING LOSS.

hertz (Hz) A unit of vibration frequency adopted internationally to replace the term "cycles per second." The term was named after German physicist HEINRICH RUDOLF HERTZ.

Hertz, Heinrich Rudolf (1857–1894) This German physicist proved that light and heat are electromagnetic radiations, and he measured the length and velocity of electromagnetic waves in the laboratory. In honor of his achievements, the unit of vibration frequency, cycles per second, was named for him.

Hertz was also the first to broadcast and receive radio waves and proved that electromagnetic waves had the same properties of susceptibility to reflection and refraction as light and heat waves. (See also HERTZ; FREQUENCY.)

high-risk questionnaire This assessment, applied to all newborns, consists of a number of factors that identify an infant at risk of a hearing loss. Because most newborns are born with normal hearing, it would not be cost-effective to test all infants for hearing loss. In order to select which newborns will be tested, a high-risk register for the identification of hearing loss has been developed.

If the child has one or more of the listed factors, physicians will recommend an AUDITORY BRAINSTEM RESPONSE TEST. This is a hearing test that can be given to infants since it measures brain wave activity in response to sound. Still, only about half of newborns with one or more of the high-risk factors can be diagnosed with the auditory brainstem response test.

High-risk newborns fall into at least one of the following categories:

Risks Before Birth Positive family history for deafness, genetic biochemical abnormality associated with deafness, blood incompatibility between mother and child, virus infection, certain OTOTOXIC DRUGS or unusual bleeding during the first trimester.

Labor Complications Premature delivery, fetal distress, prolonged labor, difficult delivery or birth injury.

Neonatal Difficulty Apnea, jaundice, multiple anomalies (whatever the cause), drugs (especially streptomycin and kanamycin).

Infants at greatest risk for hearing loss are those with a family history of hearing loss (43%) followed by those admitted to the newborn intensive care unit (24%), infants with a low APGAR rating (a well-baby assessment that tests breathing, heartrate, color, muscle tone and motor reactions of newborns) (18%) or infants affected by maternal infection (12%). (See also POSTNATAL AND PARTURIENT CAUSES OF HEARING LOSS; PRENATAL CAUSES OF HEARING LOSS.)

home sign Sometimes called homemade SIGN LANGUAGE, this refers to the gestures developed by deaf people who are isolated from the deaf community. Home sign is often the first way a deaf child communicates with hearing family members. Home signs are not the same as artificial sign languages, which are created by educators as a representation of a spoken language. (See also AMERICAN SIGN LANGUAGE; MINIMAL LANGUAGE SKILLS.)

Holder, William A 17th-century English rector interested in teaching deaf children to speak. His book *Elements of Speech,* detailed the position of all organs related to speech during the production of PHONEMES.

Holder advocated positive reinforcement and systematic speech development in which sounds are taught first, combined into syllables and then formed into words associated with objects.

homophones Words that look alike to a person who is SPEECHREADING, causing confusion.

House Ear Institute A private, nonprofit, medical research organization specializing in research into the ear—the causes of hearing loss, diagnosis and treatment—

and training ear specialists and professionals from allied disciplines.

Founded in 1946 as the Los Angeles Foundation of Otology by patients of Howard P. House, M.D., the institute is supported entirely by private funds and was renamed in 1981 to honor House and his brother, William P. House, M.D., director of research.

Research at the institute includes studies of COCHLEAR IMPLANTS, HEARING AIDS, ear disease and tumors, diagnosis, hearing tests, TINNITUS, and prosthetic devices. In addition, the institute's researchers study normal and diseased tissues removed from patients during surgery. Its labs house the world's largest documented collection of temporal bones for microscopic study.

In 1981 the institute began a cochlear implant program for children, providing rehabilitative therapy and helping parents deal with issues facing deaf children. Parents' organizations sponsored by the institute include Bridging the Gap, Family Camp, Kid Safe and the Young Adult Work Program. Contact: House Ear Institute, 256 S. Lake, Los Angeles, CA 90057; telephone: (voice) 213-483-4431, (TDD) 213-484-2642.

Hubbard, Gardiner Greene (1822–1897) This Massachusetts lawyer was passionately interested in educating deaf people, largely because his daughter Mabel (later the wife of ALEXANDER GRAHAM BELL) lost her hearing after a bout of scarlet fever at age four.

When Hubbard was told his daughter would lose her speech and could not attend school for six more years, he realized he would need to educate his daughter himself—or find a teacher who could. Aware of the success achieved by German educators of deaf students, he decided to set up a similar school in Northampton.

Hubbard was instrumental in the establishment of the Clarke Institution for Deaf Mutes, in Northampton, Massachusetts, an oral school for deaf students now called the Clarke School.

With his son-in-law Alexander Graham Bell, Hubbard founded the American Association to Promote Teaching of Speech to the Deaf, the National Geographic Society and the publication *Science,* the official magazine of the American Association for the Advancement of Science. In addition to his many entrepreneurial ventures, such as bringing gas lights and water to Cambridge, Hubbard led the presidential commission to reorganize the U.S. Postal Service and was a trustee of the Smithsonian Institution.

hypacusis Another word for hard-of-hearing.

hyperacusis An unusually acute sense of hearing.

hypoacousia See HYPOACUSIA.

hypoacusia A synonym for hearing loss.

hysterical hearing loss See FUNCTIONAL HEARING LOSS (NONORGANIC).

Hz See HERTZ.

I

identification audiometry Screening large numbers of people to identify those with hearing problems who need to be given more specific tests on an individual basis. (See also AUDIOMETRY.)

idiopathic endolymphatic hydrops See MENIERE'S DISEASE.

immittance tests See AUDIOMETRY.

immune system and hearing loss The immune system is crucial to the defense against infection of both the middle and inner ear. There is evidence that a faulty immune system can induce hearing loss and is responsible for the progression of chronic OTITIS MEDIA and possibly other disorders for which no cause has been found, such as MENIERE'S DISEASE.

In addition, certain diseases that affect the immune system—such as AIDS—can also result in hearing loss. (See AIDS AND HEARING LOSS.)

impacted earwax A hard plug of EARWAX firmly filling the ear canal, blocking the passage of sound to the eardrum and interfering with hearing. Symptoms are worsened if water enters the ear, causing the wax to swell.

Normally, earwax (or CERUMEN) is produced by glands in the skin of the outer ear canal and carried outward to the external ear. When it is produced too quickly, it builds up and forms a hard plug.

Large plugs of earwax must be removed by a physician; smaller plugs may be removed at home. A person can remove hard wax with mineral oil drops; soft wax can be removed with hydrogen peroxide drops or a commercial softener. The drops may be applied overnight and then removed by irrigating the ear with warm water from a baby ear syringe.

COTTON SWABS should not be used because of the danger of pushing wax deeper into the ear.

impedance audiometry A test to measure hearing at the level of the COCHLEA and brainstem to determine how well the cochlea and auditory pathways of the medulla are functioning. Impedance refers to the opposition to the flow of energy.

In the test, two tubes are placed into the external ear canal, and sound is sent from a small loudspeaker through one tube. The sound reflected from the eardrum is picked up by the other tube, which leads to a microphone, amplifier and recorder. When a sudden intense sound is applied to the other ear, the stapedius muscle contracts, the impedance is increased, and the recorder indicates when more sound is picked up.

This does not, however, measure the actual acoustic impedance of the ear. This is tested by using an acoustic bridge, which allows an OTOLOGIST to listen to a sound as it is reflected from the patient's eardrum. At the same time, a similar sound of the same intensity is reflected in an artificial cavity that is adjusted to equal that of the external canal of the ear.

When the two sounds are matched by changing the acoustic impedance of the cavity, the otologist can then read the impedance of the ear from the scale of the instrument. This test can uncover conductive defects of the MIDDLE EAR (including discontinuity of the ossicular chain and immobility of the malleus or stapes). (See also AUDIOMETRY; ACOUSTIC IMMITANCE.)

implantable hearing aid Still in experimental stages, this type of hearing aid would be implanted within the ear canal in the hope of overcoming many of the drawbacks of conventional in-the-ear HEARING AIDS. These in-the-ear aids have a tendency toward acoustic feedback and cause discomfort and can also worsen ear infections.

The implantable aid would effectively remove the feedback problem by eliminating acoustic coupling and should provide greater comfort and benefit to hard-of-hearing people. It would also be more acceptable to those who need amplification but cannot (or choose not) to use currently-available hearing aids. (See also COCHLEAR IMPLANT; HEARING AIDS.)

incus The middle bone of the three OSSICLES of the middle ear, also known as the ANVIL.

India It is estimated that out of India's population of more than 700 million, 800,000 are deaf; most of these live in the rural areas. Only about 5% of India's deaf children are currently in school. At a deafness rate of 66 per 100,000, India is about midway between Peru's high rate (300) and Australia's low rate (35).

Communication for India's deaf population is complicated by the fact that the country is considered trilingual, with the three languages being Hindi, English and one of the many regional languages. The education a deaf child would receive varies depending on the area in which he or she grows up.

The government is interested in helping provide services for its deaf citizens, but most resources for this purpose are limited.

India's first school for deaf students was opened in 1885; since 1900, 200 more schools have been established—none in the rural areas. Of the 200, only 14 offer secondary school education, and only a few offer vocational training. There is no school for university education for deaf students, although there are a few deaf Indian students studying at universities in the United States.

Education in India is not required, is not free and is based on an oral approach. Although most deaf Indians communicate in sign, its use in schools has been repressed.

INDIAN SIGN LANGUAGE is a highly-structured, grammatical language, and its first dictionary was just published in 1980.

Most deaf citizens are unemployed. There is no national captioning service, TELECOMMUNICATIONS FOR THE DEAF (TDDs) are not available, and there are almost no interpreters, even in large cities.

Indian Sign Language Despite the country's official languages and more than 200 dialects, Indian Sign Language (ISL) is surprisingly universal in India; there is only one sign language, and more than one million deaf Indians communicate with it.

In general, the signs of the Indian system do not relate to any of the European sign languages, although there are a few signs similar to BRITISH SIGN LANGUAGE and its FINGERSPELLING system.

Because ISL is not used in schools, most deaf speakers use the pure, natural sign language. Initial research in ISL suggests its grammar is complex and is not similar to any of languages of India.

induction coil Another name for a loop device. (See also AUDIO LOOP; AUDIO LOOP SYSTEM; ASSISTIVE LISTENING DEVICE.)

induction loop devices See AUDIO LOOP SYSTEM.

infection, ear See OTITIS MEDIA.

Ingrassia, Giovanni (1510–1580) Born in Recalbuto, Sicily, Ingrassia was one of the most well-known Renaissance anatomists, and and a contemporary of EUSTACHIO and FALLOPPIO. A professor in Padua, Naples and Palermo, and adviser to the king, he was among the first to describe the tympanic cavity and the OSSICLES and was credited with discovering the STAPES in 1546.

inner ear An extremely intricate portion of the ear deep within the skull that contains the AUDITORY NERVE and the balance mechanism of the body in a winding maze of passages called the LABYRINTH.

The front of the inner ear, which resembles a snail shell and is concerned with hearing, is called the COCHLEA. The rear part, concerned with balance, is a series of three SEMICIRCULAR CANALS at right angles to each other and connected to a cavity called the VESTIBULE.

These canals contain hair cells continually bathed in fluid, some of which are sensitive to gravity and acceleration and others to position and movements of the head. This sensory information is registered by the cells and conveyed by nerve fibers to the brain.

inner ear diseases and hearing loss

Diseases located deep within the auditory structure are difficult to diagnose, especially since it is impossible to visually inspect the COCHLEA. Inner ear diseases involve sensorineural hearing losses that are very difficult to pinpoint since they are rarely isolated problems. In fact, the cause of many sensorineural problems, such as MENIERE'S DISEASE, are often impossible to determine.

Still, the inner ear is susceptible to many of the same problems that affect the middle ear: infection and inflammation, injury and OTOTOXIC DRUGS.

Injuries Injury to the temporal bone can affect the inner ear and is a common cause of a sensorineural hearing loss since head injuries occur in more than three-quarters of auto accidents. Hitting the front or the back of the head can result in a transverse fracture, causing SENSORINEURAL HEARING LOSS, VERTIGO or TINNITUS. Severe blows to the head can also damage the ORGAN OF CORTI.

Barotrauma (sudden pressure changes in airplanes or deepsea diving resulting in unequal pressure in the ear) can damage the cochlea, membranes of the round or oval windows or REISSNER'S MEMBRANE, all causing a sensorineural hearing loss.

Infection LABYRINTHITIS (inflammation of the inner ear), carried by bacteria or viruses from the middle ear, brain or bloodstream, can result in a sensorineural hearing loss.

Ototoxic Drugs The cochlea and VESTIBULAR SYSTEM are susceptible to the effects of a range of ototoxic drugs, especially aminoglycoside antibiotics, which cause a gradual or sudden sensorineural hearing loss. Hearing loss from ototoxic drugs cannot usually be reversed because the drugs damage hair cells, which do not regenerate, and also harm the AUDITORY NERVE.

Ménière's Disease This disease, which distends the membranous labyrinth, causes sensorineural hearing loss (usually in one ear), sudden attacks of vertigo and tinnitus. Hearing loss usually causes difficulty in hearing low-frequency sounds, progressing to difficulty with high frequency sounds as well. The cause of Meniere's disease is still not known, although a wide range of factors have been suggested.

Aging As a person ages, the hair cells in the organ of Corti begin to degenerate and the BASILAR MEMBRANE stiffens. Called PRESBYCUSIS, the sensorineural hearing loss of old age is first noticed as a loss of understanding in the higher frequencies in late middle age.

Diseases Several systemic diseases affect hearing, including certain genetic syndromes. High blood pressure and other vascular disorders can result in a sudden sensorineural loss because of clots in the internal auditory artery or a hemorrhage in the cochlea, destroying hair cells because of decreased blood flow.

Diabetes can cause a sensorineural hearing loss because of degeneration of blood vessels and nerves that supply the ear and internal auditory canal. Kidney disease often causes sensorineural hearing problems in patients who undergo hemodialysis or kidney transplants.

Genetic diseases that result in sensorineural hearing loss include PAGET'S DISEASE and ALPORT'S DISEASE. COGAN'S SYNDROME is an inflammation of the cornea accompanied by vertigo, tinnitus and severe sensorineural hearing loss with unknown cause. (See also AERO-OTITIS MEDIA; DIABETES AND HEARING LOSS; GENETICS AND HEARING LOSS.)

Institut National des Jeunes Sourds

Also called the Paris Institute, this institution was founded by ABBÉ CHARLES MICHEL DE L'EPÉE in the 1700s and is today the oldest permanent school for deaf students in the world.

Begun with a grant from King Louis XVI, the school managed to stay open during the French Revolution. L'Epée began the school by teaching two sisters in his home and by the late 1760s had six students; 10 years later there were 30 students, and at the time of l'Epée's death in 1789, there were more than 60.

After the death of l'Epee, the school was run by ABBÉ ROCH AMBROISE CUCURRON SICARD, who convinced the French National Assembly that aid for handicapped students was a natural duty. In response, the assembly nationalized the school in 1791, naming it the National Institution for the Congenitally Deaf (Instit National des Sourds-Muets de Naissance).

The years of the French Revolution were difficult, and Sicard, the school's director, was imprisoned at least twice as a suspected Royalist. He was saved at last by a petition from his deaf students. Sicard directed the spartan program for 32 years until his death in 1822 at the age of 80. At that time, the school had 150 students, all whom used SIGN LANGUAGE (Old French Sign Language).

After the Catholic church was reestablished in France following the Revolution (in 1801), the school began to emphasize religion for its deaf students. Contact: Institut National des Jeunes Sourds, 254 rue Saint Jacques, 75005, Paris, France; telephone: 33-1-435-48280

intensity The strength of a sound the brain perceives as loudness; usually measured by the amplitude of its wave. It is also measured in decibels.

internal acoustic meatus A passage in the temporal bone for the facial and auditory nerves.

International Catholic Deaf Association A group promoting ministry to Catholic deaf people and responding to spiritually-related requests worldwide.

In general, Catholics have not had separate congregations for deaf members, although they do provide worship services in which an interpreter or priest signs the spoken portion of the mass. However, there are a few deaf Catholic churches in the United States, including St. Mary Magdalene Church for the Deaf (Denver, Colorado), Mother of Perpetual Help Church for the Deaf (Omaha, Nebraska), St. Francis of Assisi Catholic Church and Center for the Deaf (Landover Hills, Maryland), St. John's Deaf Center (Warren, Michigan) and the Catholic Deaf Center (New Orleans, Louisiana). (See also NATIONAL CATHOLIC OFFICE OF THE DEAF.) Contact: International Catholic Deaf Association, 814 Thayer Ave., Silver Spring, MD 20910; telephone (TDD): 301-588-4009.

International Congress on the Education of the Deaf For the past century, international meetings have been held to discuss education for deaf students, although early meetings rarely involved deaf educators or deaf persons at all.

For the first 100 years, no group administered these international meetings; a meeting could be called simply whenever a group within a country invited representatives from other countries to meet. But in 1975 in Tokyo, an International Congress Committee made up of the chairs of the three preceding congresses was finally established.

Many different topics were discussed at these meetings, but the prime controversy for almost 100 years was the debate between the ORAL APPROACH and the MANUAL APPROACH. The oral approach was the early favorite, and the second international Congress of Milan 1880 had an enormous effect on the education of deaf students around the world when convention participants decided that speech was "incontestably superior" to sign.

Further, Milan congressional delegates decided they preferred the oral approach over the simultaneous use of signs and speech as well. Milan resolutions cited the long-term benefits of oral education and devised procedures to introduce the oral approach into the schools.

The only votes against these pro-oral approach resolutions were an English delegate and the American delegates led by EDWARD MINER GALLAUDET. The oral-manual controversy continued to rage in nearly all of the congresses up until 1980, when delegates at the Hamburg congress decided the controversy was pointless and that both the oral and manual approaches could be helpful to deaf persons.

International Games for the Deaf See WORLD GAMES FOR THE DEAF.

international hand alphabet See INTERNATIONAL MANUAL ALPHABET.

international manual alphabet A manual alphabet devised by the WORLD FEDERATION OF THE DEAF and used primarily in Scandinavian countries.

International Organization for the Education of the Hearing Impaired See ALEXANDER GRAHAM BELL ASSOCIATION FOR THE DEAF.

International Phonetic Association alphabet (IPA) The most widely used phonetic alphabet, which is used to describe the segmental sound of speech. Most of the symbols in this alphabet are variations of Roman letters and can be used to describe speech in any language or dialect.

A sentence transcribed into a phonetic alphabet would allow a person to correctly speak the transcription, even if in a language that has never been heard.

A phonetic symbol represents a letter as a type of shorthand to describe how that sound is produced. For sounds that also have small differences in how they are pronounced, the alphabet uses basic and secondary symbols called diacritics, which are placed above or below (or before or after) the primary symbols. These diacritical marks indicate differences in sound.

The phonetic symbols used in dictionaries are not generally the IPA but the dictionary's own phonetic symbols, which are defined for readers using key words.

interpreters See ORAL INTERPRETERS; SIGN LANGUAGE INTERPRETERS.

interpreters and the law Since the 1960s, federal and state governments have enacted several laws requiring that a certified interpreter be provided for hard-of-hearing people during various court proceedings.

Unfortunately, although each state has some type of law guaranteeing an interpreter for a deaf person, many of the laws are vague, simple or unclear. Some laws state that courts and judges may appoint an interpreter when "necessary," but it is unclear who pays for these services, what the qualifications of the interpreter must be or what "necessary" means. Some states have comprehensive laws stating that interpreters should be appointed at the time of arrest in all civil and criminal cases, for the preparation of depositions, during commitment hearings, before grand juries, for a state exam needed for employment with the state and in juvenile proceedings.

Under state law, it is generally up to the judge to decide the qualifications for interpreters; some states do require consultation with the local or national REGISTRY OF INTERPRETERS FOR THE DEAF.

In criminal proceedings, most states will pay for an interpreter, and some states will pay for these services during civil proceedings as well.

Hard-of-hearing and deaf persons have the right under federal and state law to use the services of interpreters upon their request. When a hard-of-hearing or deaf person states a preference for an oral interpreter, the court must do its best to find one.

The situation is a little more clear in federal courts. When the federal government brings a criminal or civil action against a deaf individual, the law requires that the court appoint a qualified interpreter; in other situations, the federal court can appoint an interpreter if it so chooses. (See also COURT INTERPRETER'S ACT.)

interpreter services See ORAL INTERPRETERS; SIGN LANGUAGE INTERPRETERS.

in-the-ear hearing aid A type of hearing aid that fits completely inside the ear. These types of HEARING AIDS are becoming more popular. They are lightweight devices in a custom EARMOLD and fit inside the ear canal with no external wires or tubes. Most of the device fits into the space in the external ear leading to the ear canal.

The microphone, volume control and battery compartment are located on the outer surface and are visible. Fitted with tone control, these models are generally useful only for mild hearing loss.

intra-aural muscles The two muscles contained in the middle ear, known separately as the TENSOR TYMPANI and the STAPEDIAL MUSCLE. Their action is reflexive and bilateral and may be initiated either by intense acoustic stimulation or by irritation of the tissues of the external or middle ears.

A number of functions for these muscles have been suggested, but only two are generally accepted: The muscles assist in maintaining the OSSICULAR CHAIN in its proper position, and they act to protect the internal ear from too much stimulation by inhibiting ossicular movement.

Some research data suggest that the intra-aural muscles under moderate levels of tension and at certain frequencies slightly enhance the transmission of sound by the middle ear.

Irish Sign Language There are three sign systems used in the Republic of Ireland—two based on manual English systems and one indigenous, informal method.

The newest system, called Irish Sign Language, is a manual code for English with one vocabulary for both men and women, unlike the older system with separate styles for men and women. It was introduced in the late 1970s by the Unified Sign Language Committee.

Most signs in the new system are based on the first letter of the word in English and are grouped so that many words of similar meaning will use the same basic sign but with different handshapes. This new sign language is used in some sign language classes taught outside traditional deaf schools and in the manual classes in the oral deaf schools. However, many people in the Irish deaf community prefer the old sign language system.

This older system is also a manual code for English and uses gender-specific vocabularies. Brought over from France in the 1800s, the French signs were modified to express English grammar and also split into ''feminine'' styles for use with the deaf girls' schools and more ''masculine'' for the deaf boys' schools. Today, the two vocabularies differ as much as 30%, although boys and girls can still understand each other.

Finally, the ''informal'' sign language, known as Deaf Sign Language, is used by deaf people in informal settings and is less accepted than the first two. It is believed this informal method is derived from the old sign language used in the Irish schools, but it does not parallel English grammar. Like all natural sign languages, however, it does appear to have its own grammatical system.

To a degree, portions of Irish sign systems have been exported to both South Africa and Australia.

Israel Although there have been no definitive studies of the deaf population in Israel, estimates suggest that the incidence of deafness in Asiatic-African Jewish children and Israel's minority (predominantly Arab) group is about double that of European-American children. This unexpected incidence of hearing problems is probably due to the incidence of intermarriage within these cultures.

By age one, most of the country's deaf children are referred to one of the nationwide nonprofit institutions designed for deaf infants. Two of these centers use Total Communication; three use the oral approach. At these centers, parents are offered a range of services, including sign language classes, special discussions groups and home training. By the age of five or six, most deaf Jewish children are mainstreamed into state-supported kindergartens; about 10% attend special kindergartens designed for deaf pupils only. Once a child reaches elementary age, there are several options: a special school for deaf children, integrated classes, mainstreaming or a special school for multidisabled children.

Until 1976, all school programs used the oral approach; today educators use a combined approach (speech and ISRAELI SIGN LANGUAGE). At high school age, a student can choose to attend a vocational high school, integrated classes or mainstreaming.

In addition, the government offers its deaf citizens job placement and training services and private tutoring for deaf children in regular classes.

Israeli Sign Language was developed in the early 1900s and was eventually unified during the late 1950s with the establishment of the Association of the Deaf. In 1977, a signed Hebrew alphabet was created.

In general, Israel's heritage and comparatively concentrated number of deaf citizens has led to a wide network of services and programs for the deaf community.

Israeli Sign Language About 5,000 deaf Israelis use Israeli Sign Language (ISL), a relatively new language continually infused with new signs from other countries as immigrants come to Israel. In addition, a FINGERSPELLING system for Hebrew was adapted from the American MANUAL ALPHABET and includes 16 handshapes for Hebrew.

Still considered a very new language, ISL appears to be very flexible regarding sign order. The modifying sign follows the sign for the thing it modifies (for example, cat fat) and quantifiers precede the sign for the thing quantified (four horses) or bracket the thing quantified (four horses four). Israeli sign language also has major structural characteristics as in other sign languages, such as the simultaneity of signs.

Although deaf schools in Israel have been completely oral since the first school was founded in 1934, teachers today use some ISL signs in their oral classes.

Italian Sign Language Still widely considered to be simple gestures in Italy, research has found the sign language of deaf Italians is indeed a complete language with a complex structure and grammar.

The structural features of LIS (Lingua Italiana dei Segni) are different from other languages, and the Italian spoken language influences LIS in the use of speechreading and articulation. FINGERSPELLING is rarely used, although there is an old and a new manual alphabet. The older method, used primarily by older deaf Italians, is a two-handed system employing hands and the face. The new version, used by younger deaf Italians, is a one-handed system using only handshapes.

There is no census information available on the number of people who use ISL, and it is not used in the all-oral school systems.

Italy The exact number of deaf citizens is not known, but a 1980 survey suggests that there may be at least 70,000 profoundly deaf people in Italy, with the rate of deafness higher in the southern regions of the country. In general, hearing loss occurs in about 8–10% of the general population.

Although there is a significant lack of good services and programs for them, deaf Italians do have a strong community among themselves, including a national organization for the deaf, and promote Italian Sign Language LIS (Lingua Italiana dei Segni).

The government provides special services only for preschool through age 14, either in special, mostly residential schools or mainstreamed with hearing children. The ORAL APPROACH is generally the preferred educational mode of communication, and sign language is generally prohibited in class, although it is tolerated elsewhere. In actuality, most deaf students and adults communicate in sign.

J

Japan About 320,000 adult Japanese have hearing problems, and the programs and services for this population have improved since World War II. The presence of deafness in Japan appears to be growing, according to demographic reports. Census data from 1947 found 118 out of 100,000 to be prelingually deaf; figures rose to 225 per 100,000 in 1970.

Education is compulsory between ages 9 and 15, and in Japan deaf and hard-of-hearing children are treated separately: Deaf children are educated in special schools, and hard-of-hearing children attend special classes or are mainstreamed. Special school populations, however, are decreasing as more and more deaf students are attending regular classes and going to a university.

Most schools in Japan use the ORAL APPROACH, although more and more schools are introducing CUED SPEECH; students use sign language among themselves. Although JAPANESE SIGN LANGUAGE is not yet considered a language, since it does not match the expressive forms of the Japanese oral language, efforts are being made to make it more systematic.

The Japanese Association of the Deaf and Dumb, with 20,000 members, serves as an advocate for improved services for deaf Japanese. The association offers an annual convention and an annual sports meeting and has local branches in many areas throughout Japan. In addition, the Japanese Society for the Study of Education for the Deaf is a national network of 5,000 teachers in deaf schools. Deaf adults can expect a lower standard of living than hearing Japanese, and less than 32% of all Japanese deaf people are employed at all. Still, the outlook has improved since new laws require public agencies and private businesses to hire a certain number of physically disabled people.

Japanese Sign Language More than 95% of the 320,000 deaf Japanese are assumed to be able to understand Japanse Sign Language (JSL), called "Shuwa" (hand talk).

Since all deaf schools are officially oral except for a few that use the simultaneous method (communication combining speech, sign and fingerspelling), JSL does not play a large part in the educational system. In the classes that use the simultaneous method, teachers use Signed Japanese or manually coded Japanese. Their sign language, called simultaneous methodic signs, uses FINGERSPELLING to represent suffixes and postpositions. In general, this language is not accepted by people in the deaf community, who use Pidgin Sign Japanese in communicating with deaf and hearing Japanese. Pidgin Sign Language is also used on TV programs, lectures and so forth.

Still in the early stages of research, JSL is not yet well understood by linguists.

Jena method Developed by Karl Brauckmann in Jena, Germany, the Jena method is a system of teaching SPEECHREADING that focuses attention on the syllable and rhythm patterns in speech.

Johnston test A group pure-tone screening test for children in kindergarten through second grade. (See also MASSACHUSETTS TEST; SWEEP-CHECK TEST.)

journals in the field of deafness A wide range of professional publications are available for people who work in the field of deafness. Full addresses of publications can be found in Appendix 8 in the back of this book.

Journal of Auditory Research This publication of the C. W. Shilling Auditory Research Center, Inc., was founded in 1961 for audiologists, auditory neurophysiologists, engineers, musicologists, otologists, psychoacousticians, sensory and comparative psychologists, speech scientists and anyone interested in the study of hearing.

It includes experimental papers on a variety of topics, and its board includes otologists, audiologists, psychologists, psychoacousticians and speech scientists. Because the subject matter of the journal is so broad, this is no board of review editors.

Journal of Communication Disorders This publication discusses a broad spectrum of topics in the field of communication disorders, including pure experimental research and clinical and theoretical issues.

Its audience includes linguists, neurologists, otolaryngologists, psychologists, psychiatrists and speech and hearing specialists. Articles primarily discuss problems related to disorders of communication, including the normal communicative processes, plus the anatomical, physiological, diagnostic, psychodynamic and psychopathological aspects of communication disorders. Most issues also contain a mix of different articles and an international review of publications dealing with communication disorders.

Journal of American Deafness and Rehabilitation This official publication of the AMERICAN DEAFNESS AND REHABILITATION ASSOCIATION, begun in 1967, is published quarterly as part of the membership benefits of the association. Articles are published on the field of deafness and are reviewed by professionals in medicine-psychiatry, psychology, vocational rehabilitation and education.

Journal of Speech and Hearing Disorders Published by the AMERICAN SPEECH-LANGUAGE-HEARING ASSOCIATION, this 54-year-old journal is one of six official periodicals of the association. Published quarterly, its circulation includes more than 50,000 practitioners in the field of speech and hearing disorders. The journal accepts articles, reports and letters focusing primarily on clinical issues, including the nature and treatment of disordered speech, hearing and language. The journal does not publish articles on theoretical or experimental research in speech, hearing or language sciences, which are published by the association's *Journal of Speech and Hearing Research.*

The *Journal of Speech and Hearing Disorders* also publishes conference proceedings in its *ASHA Reports* and information on single subjects in monographs. Information on language, speech and hearing services for children (especially in school) are not included in the journal but appear in the association's *Language, Speech and Hearing Services in Schools.*

Journal of Speech and Hearing Research This publication is one of two journals published by the American Speech-Language-Hearing Association. Designed to appeal to researchers—as opposed to the *Journal of Speech and Hearing Disorders*—the journal is aimed at clinicians in the field of speech and hearing science.

This quarterly journal focuses on studies of the processes and disorders of speech, language and hearing and has more than 50,000 readers.

Journal of the Acoustical Society of America This 60-year-old monthly publication of the Acoustical Society of America publishes articles in several branches of acoustics, including general linear, nonlinear, physiological, psychological and architectural acoustics; aeroacoustics; atmospheric and underwater sound; ultrasonics, mechanical, shock and random vibration; vibration of plates and shells; noise and its control; acoustic signal processing; speech communication; music and instruments; bioacoustics; acoustical measurements and instrumentation; and acoustical transduction. In addition to research papers in these areas, the journal includes society activities, calendars of meetings of other relevant societies, book reviews and reviews of acoustical patents.

Each year, three separate supplements are published by the society; two contain abstracts of all papers presented at the two annual conventions; the third, *References to Contemporary Papers on Acoustics,* is a bibliography of recent articles on acoustics published throughout the world.

Junior National Association of the Deaf This group, affiliated with the NATIONAL ASSOCIATION OF THE DEAF, tries to develop leadership, scholarship and service among deaf high school students. The organization carries out its mandate by creating opportunities for hands-on experience through participation in various extracurricular activities and a youth leadership camp.

The first Junior NAD national convention was held in 1968 at Gallaudet University, with 120 student delegates from 36 chapters in schools for deaf students. The association also publishes the *Junior NAD Newsletter*.

Justinian Code During the reign of Justinian I from A.D. 527–565, all of Roman law was codified, including the legal rights of deaf citizens (which were basically nonexistent).

Deaf Romans could not marry, and legal guardians were appointed to handle their affairs. The code was more lenient for the adventitious deaf person, allowing those with acquired deafness to handle their own affairs if they could write.

K

Keller, Helen Adams (1880–1968) This world-famous Alabama woman, blind and deaf from early childhood, became one of the best-known advocates of the education for blind and deaf students and was hailed for her achievements as a writer and lecturer.

She was born June 27, 1880, the daughter of a former officer in the Confederate army. A severe illness at 19 months destroyed both her sight and hearing, and she quickly deteriorated from an energetic, bright child into a spoiled, rebellious youngster who was almost impossible to handle.

Aware that the Perkins Institution of the Blind in Massachusetts had successfully educated a deaf-blind girl 50 years earlier, Helen's parents—on the advice of ALEXANDER GRAHAM BELL—sought help from the institute in educating Helen.

The institute recommended a former graduate, Anne Mansfield Sullivan, then 20 and partially blind herself. Sullivan arrived March 3, 1887, and began trying to teach young Helen names of objects by pressing the manual alphabet into her hand. Eventually, Sullivan managed to break through Helen's dark and silent world when Helen finally connected the feel of the water running over her hand to its manual sign.

A remarkably bright child, Helen's vocabulary increased rapidly, and she went on to be educated at the Horace Mann School for the Deaf in Boston and the Wright-Humason Oral School in New York City, where she learned to read and write in braille. She graduated cum laude in 1904 from Radcliffe, where Sullivan spelled lectures into her hand.

Keller—a close friend of the oralist Bell—was likewise a confirmed oralist who had learned to speak by feeling vibrations in Sullivan's larynx. Although far from perfect, her voice was understood by those who knew her well. Still, aware of the controversy between oral and manual methods of communication, she tried to find a common ground, admitting that no method was perfect and that deaf people need every advantage they can get.

Although her voice required interpretation in public, she became a noted lecturer for 12 years. Eventually, she became affiliated with the American Foundation for the Blind and spent many years traveling and speaking all over the world for this group.

In addition to lectures, Keller was a prolific writer; she wrote speeches, letters, magazine articles and books, including: *The Story of My Life* (1903), *The World I Live In* (1908), *Out of the Dark* (1913), *Midstream* (1929), *Helen Keller in Scotland* (1933), *Helen Keller's Journal* (1938) and *Teacher: Anne Sullivan Macy: A Tribute by the Foster-Child of Her Mind* (1955).

Although known all over the world, Keller lived within a small, protected circle: the ever-present, possessive teacher, (Sullivan), Sullivan's husband John Macy and, later, an assistant. In her middle years she intended to marry but decided against it in the face of her mother's reluctance to "lose" her daughter.

A relentlessly kind woman, Keller was a suffragette strongly opposed to racism and war; she joined the Socialist party and ardently supported the Bolshevik Revolution.

Of her blindness and deafness, Keller considered deafness to be the greater loss, and her efforts to help those who were both blind and deaf led to the establishment of the HELEN KELLER NATIONAL CENTER FOR DEAF-BLIND YOUTHS AND ADULTS in Sands Point, New York.

Kendall Demonstration Elementary School Originating as a school for deaf pupils in the Washington, D.C. area in 1857, the Kendall school became a national demonstration elementary school in 1970 when Congress mandated it provide not only an education to local students but also conduct research into deaf education for dissemination across the country.

Public Law 91-587 set up the school as a demonstration center and emphasized that it must stress innovative auditory and visual devices, excellent architecture and works of art. Legislation also set up a new high school in 1966 for deaf secondary students located at GALLAUDET UNIVERSITY campus.

Students at Kendall range from young infants to 15-years-olds who must live in the national capital region (the District of Columbia, northern Virginia and nearby Maryland countries) and have a hearing problem severe enough to warrant placement in a special class. Among its 200 commuter students, 90% have a severe to profound hearing loss and the other 10% have a severe to moderate loss. About 30% have a disability in addition to hearing problems. The school includes a parent-infant program and a preschool, primary, intermediate and middle school. Because it was designed as a demonstration school, Kendall often serves as a product testing ground and also supports applied and basic research. (See also MODEL SECONDARY SCHOOL FOR THE DEAF.)

kernicterus A jaundiced area of the newborn brain caused by the destruction of red blood cells. An incompatibility of Rh blood factors between infant and mother causes this destruction.

Untreated, kernicterus can cause central nerve deafness. (See also HEARING LOSS; RH FACTOR INCOMPATIBILITY AND DEAFNESS.)

kidney failure and hearing loss Kidney disease requiring renal dialysis and transplantation often causes a type of SENSORINEURAL HEARING LOSS. This loss can be caused by a number of factors, including electrolyte imbalance, inadequate dialysis or drug otoxicity (diruretics or aminoglycosides), which can affect the components of the INNER EAR fluid and alter the normal function of the COCHLEA.

L

labyrinthectomy Surgical excision of the entire inner ear. This operation has been replaced by selective VESTIBULAR NERVE

SECTION, which preserves hearing in those patients with incapacitating VERTIGO.

labyrinth, inner ear This section of the INNER EAR contains the nerve endings of the vestibular nerve (the nerve of equilibrium) and the AUDITORY NERVE (nerve of hearing).

Diseases of the labyrinth may affect both nerves or only the auditory nerve, causing hearing loss, or only the vestibular nerve, disrupting balance and causing VERTIGO. Common inner ear diseases include congenital nerve deafness (a defect of the hearing nerve in the COCHLEA), viral nerve deafness (a hearing impairment caused by a virus, such as mumps, measles or flu), deafness from OTOTOXIC DRUGS, skull fracture, NOISE exposure, LABYRINTHITIS, ACOUSTIC NEUROMA, MENIERE'S DISEASE or PRESBYCUSIS.

labyrinthitis An inflammation of the LABYRINTH (the fluid-filled maze of inner ear chambers that sense balance), labyrinthitis can cause nausea, vomiting, TINNITUS, VERTIGO and deafness. Also called otitis interna, it is almost always caused by either a bacterial or viral infection that enters the inner ear from the middle ear. The main danger is spread of the infection to the meninges (the outer covering of the brain).

Bacterial labyrinthitis can result from MASTOIDITIS or an untreated acute or chronic ear infection, particularly if a CHOLESTEATOMA (infected skin debris) has developed; the bacteria enters the inner ear through the eroded labyrinthine capsule. Infection may also reach the inner ear from a head injury or through the bloodstream from elsewhere in the body. It can also occur from contamination during a STAPES operation or a MASTOIDECTOMY.

Bacterial labyrinthitis requires immediate treatment with antibiotics to treat the infection, which otherwise could lead to meningitis or profound SENSORINEURAL HEARING LOSS, violent vertigo and total deafness.

Viral labyrinthitis is usually transmitted through the bloodstream and attacks the inner ear during illnesses such as measles, mumps, CHICKEN POX, shingles or flu. With this type of sensorineural hearing loss, onset is sudden and results in a severe or profound hearing problem. Viral labyrinthitis will eventually go away on its own, although symptoms can be relieved with antihistamines.

Meningeal labyrinthitis, more common in children, results from the transmittal of an organism to the COCHLEA by way of the internal auditory meatus or the cochlear duct.

Syphilitic labyrinthitis is usually caused by congenital syphilis and results in a sudden, flat sensorineural hearing loss with poor speech discrimination or a sudden increasing fluctuation of sensorineural hearing loss. Acquired syphilitic labyrinthitis is rare. (See also VIRUSES AND HEARING LOSS; SYPHILIS.)

language Symbols, words or signs that are composed by strict rules and arranged into sentences also governed by strict rules. All languages have symbols, and all languages have rules about how those symbols are grouped together to form sentences. In spoken languages, symbols are made up of sounds in particular ways; in sign languages, symbols are made up of body movements and positions.

The study of language, called LINGUISTICS, is still a relatively new science and is often controversial, but its basic tenets are universal. All spoken languages have rules about which sounds can be put together in certain ways to form words and sentences; similarly, natural sign languages have rules as well. But in sign language, grammatical rules govern body positions, facial expressions and movements.

Languages can differ at even the smallest levels, in the way in which sounds combine to form words and in the word order used to form sentences.

In English, word order usually follows the subject-verb-direct object format ("I love you"). In other languages, this word order is different; for example, in French, word order is subject-object-verb ("I you love"). Some languages, such as Latin, have no required word order at all but discriminate subjects from objects by word endings.

Because linguistic research into sign languages is still in its infancy, studies are only beginning to provide information on its syntactic rules. The key to understanding the grammatical structure of sign languages is to study the way signers use space.

People, places or objects not in the immediate area will be assigned a spatial location (to the left or right, for example). The signer can indicate the subject and object by moving the verb from one location to another. For example, by first assigning the right location to "Sam" and the left location to "cat," the signer moving the sign "see" from right to left means "Sam sees the cat."

Contrary to the widespread assumption that infant babbling requires normal hearing and an ability to speak aloud, recent research suggests that the brain seems to possess some type of unified capacity for learning both signed and spoken language. Psychologists at McGill University in Montreal studied five infants, two of whom were deaf and whose deaf parents' first language was sign. The three hearing babies had hearing parents who did not use sign language. When researchers videotaped babies at ages 10, 12 and 14 months alone and with their parents, they found that both deaf and hearing babies engaged in their own brand of babbling. Hearing infants initially produced strings of sounds and syllables, emitting their first words by age 1. The two deaf babies babbled with their hands, starting out with basic hand shapes for letters and numbers that they saw their parents use. Hand movements and shapes gradually grew more complex until the first linguistic signs emerged also by age 1.

language development See LANGUAGE.

late-onset deafness See ADVENTITIOUS DEAFNESS; HEARING LOSS; PRESBYCUSIS.

lateralization Sound vibrations presented to one side of the head will move through the bones of the skull toward the opposite COCHLEA. Whether the sound reaches the cochlea depends on the decibel level of the sound. All sounds will lateralize, but not all will be heard by the opposite cochlea. (See AUDIOMETRY; HEARING AIDS.)

law See COURT INTERPRETER'S ACT; LEGAL RIGHTS.

Leadership Deaf Program The Leadership Deaf Program is a unique training program for grassroots leaders and is jointly developed and sponsored by the NATIONAL ASSOCIATION OF THE DEAF and GALLAUDET UNIVERSITY.

The program provides participants with opportunities to sharpen leadership skills and learn new techniques that will help their home communities. The national program is offered biennially in odd-numbered years.

legal rights A number of laws have been enacted since the 1970s guaranteeing legal rights for deaf people. They include:

Rehabilitation Act of 1973 Called the "Bill of Rights" for disabled people, this act was designed to make sure that programs receiving federal funds can be used by all disabled people. The four major sections of the act prohibit discrimination and require accessibility in employment, education, health, welfare and social services.

Section 501: This section, which applies to federal government hiring practices, requires each executive department and agency to have an affirmative action plan for the hiring, placement and advancement of qualified handicapped people.

Section 502: This section creates the ARCHITECTURAL AND TRANSPORTATION BARRIERS COMPLIANCE BOARD, which ensures compliance with a 1968 federal law regarding architectural barriers in federally-funded buildings and public transportation systems.

Section 503: This requires affirmative action for qualified handicapped persons by people who have contracts or subcontracts with the federal government worth more than $2,500 a year or who employ more than 50 people.

Section 504: This prohibits any form of discrimination against individuals with disabilities in any federally-supported program or activity, including most public and some private schools, nursing homes, museums and airports.

Public Law 94-142 Known as the Education for All Handicapped Children Act, this federal law guarantees public education to handicapped students in the least restrictive environment. It was signed into law on November 29, 1975, by President Gerald Ford.

The law provides states with funds for special education and imposes specific requirements on how such education should be provided—emphasizing special education and related services, protecting the rights of handicapped children and their parents and providing for the assessment of the effectiveness of programs.

The definition of handicapped children includes hard-of-hearing and deaf children, with "deaf" defined as: "a hearing impairment which is so severe that the child is impaired in processing linguistic information through hearing, with or without amplification, which adversely affects education performance." The law defined "hard-of-hearing" as an impairment—either fluctuating or permanent—that affects a child's educational performance.

The act defines "deaf-blind" as a "concomitant hearing and visual impairment" that causes such severe communication and other problems that these children cannot be accommodated in special education programs designed just for deaf or for blind children alone.

The act further provides that each child must have an individualized education program (IEP), a signed, written agreement renewed yearly, that includes a statement about the child's current abilities, annual goals and short-term educational objectives, specific services and the extent of participation in regular educational programs. The IEP is prepared with input from parents, teachers and school administrators.

According to information from the Department of Education, the number of hard-of-hearing students served by this law has steadily decreased over the past 10 years, due to the aging of children deafened in the RUBELLA epidemic of 1963 to 1965. Since the implementation of public laws aimed at assisting handicapped children, the number of hard-of-hearing and deaf students below 21 years of age decreased 19% between 1977–78 and 1985–86.

Public Law 97-410 The Telecommunications for the Disabled Act of 1982 addresses the issue of compatibility between hearing aids and telephones.

The law provides that all coin-operated telephones must be hearing-aid compatible; credit card phones must also be compatible unless there is a compatible coin phone nearby. Further, emergency phones (elevator phones, police and fire call boxes) and new public phones in businesses and public buildings must be compatible and an employer must supply a compatible phone on request by a deaf employee.

Hotels and motels must also specify compatibility when installing new phones until 10% of the rooms have compatible phones. Further, new phones installed after 1985 in hospitals, convalescent homes, homes for the aged, prisons and other confined areas must be compatible.

Public Law 88-565 Also known as the Vocational Rehabilitation Act, this law provides a number of direct services for deaf people and other disabled Americans. It includes funding and services for continuing education in a university or technical school and funds research and demonstration grants influencing deaf education.

The law led the way for expanded services and organizations for deaf people, including the REGISTRY OF INTERPRETERS FOR THE DEAF, the Professional Rehabilitation Workers with the Adult Deaf (now known as ADARA, the AMERICAN DEAFNESS AND REHABILITATION ASSOCIATION) and the Council of Organizations Serving the Deaf.

Amendments enacted in 1965 (PL 89-333) extended federal support even further to include education as well as rehabilitation and provided for interpreter services in a wide variety of settings.

Public Law 85-905 This important legislation for the deaf community created the Media Services and Captioned Films Branch in the Bureau of Education for the Handicapped, granting deaf people accessibility to entertainment and educational films. Additional laws (PL 87-715 and 91-230) set up a national advisory committee on deaf education, enlarged the focus of Media Service and Captioned Films and funded a National Center on Educational Media and Materials for the Handicapped to be located at Ohio State University at Columbus.

Public Law 100-533 The National Deafness and Other Communication Disorders Act of 1988 established the NATIONAL INSTITUTE ON DEAFNESS AND OTHER COMMUNICATION DISORDERS within the National Institutes of Health. The law addresses not only hearing disorders but also balance, voice, speech, language, taste and smell.

This law requires the program include investigation into the etiology, pathology, detection, treatment and prevention of all forms of disorders of hearing and other communication processes. It also requires research into diagnostic, treatment, rehabilitation and prevention techniques; prevention and early detection of these disorders; and the environmental agents that influence hearing disorders. Finally, the law establishes a data system to collect, analyze and distribute information from patients, a national information clearinghouse and multipurpose research centers.

Public Law 87-276 In response to a shortage of teachers for deaf students, this law was signed on September 22, 1961, by President John F. Kennedy to provide stipends for undergraduate and graduate study. As a result, the number of approved university teacher training centers doubled.

Public Law 88-136 This legislation set up an advisory committee on deaf education, which began in March 1964 under the leadership of Homer Babbidge. The subsequent "Babbidge Report," which highlighted and analyzed problems in deaf education, was partly responsible for the subsequent creation of the MODEL SECONDARY SCHOOL FOR THE DEAF located on the GALLAUDET UNIVERSITY campus in Washington, D. C.

Vocational Education Act of 1963 This law allowed residential schools for deaf children to qualify for supplementary funding for their vocational departments; amendments in 1968 to this law required that at least 10% of the federal funds allocated for vocational education be set aside for handicapped students.

Public Law 89-36 This law, signed on June 8, 1965, by President Lyndon Johnson, established the NATIONAL TECHNICAL INSTITUTE FOR THE DEAF and an advisory committee to administer it. Of 28 competing colleges and universities, the Rochester Institute of Technology in New York was awarded the job.

line 21 The bottom line of a television's vertical blanking system; used in this country for closed captioning.

American television signals are made up of 525 lines, which include both the picture and a black bar, made up of 21 lines, called the vertical blanking interval (these 21 lines roll up or down on the screen when the TV is not adjusted properly).

Digital information encoded on one or more of these 21 lines within the black bar can be transmitted to TV receivers, where they can be decoded and displayed on the TV screen. The 21st line is the bottom line of the vertical blanking system and is used in this country for closed captioning.

Line 21 was first used in 1972, after the National Bureau of Standards and ABC-TV demonstrated that it was possible to place information within this "black bar"; subsequently, the Public Broadcasting System developed a method that used this 21st line in the black bar for closed captioning. (See also CAPTION CENTER; CAPTIONED FILMS FOR THE DEAF; CLOSED CAPTIONS.)

linguist A person who uses highly-specialized skills to analyze language and associated cultural patterns in research or applied LINGUISTICS. Current research in the field of deafness includes studies of the history and development of AMERICAN SIGN LANGUAGE, comparative sign languages and language development of deaf children. Applied linguistics is especially useful in schools, where a professional can analyze language patterns of individual students and help the teacher devise strategies to develop new language skills. (See also SIGN LANGUAGE.)

linguistics The study of language as a system, involving an investigation into its nature, structure, units and modification. Theoretical linguistics tries to establish a theory of the underlying structure of language, isolating the structure of language from actual language production. It does not take into account language acquisition or usage. Applied linguistics tries to use the findings and techniques of the scientific study of language for a range of practical tasks, especially to help improve the teaching of language.

Linguistics of Visual English One of the five main manually coded English systems, this one was developed by Dennis Wampler. In this system, stress was placed on signing by morpheme (a word that conveys meaning and cannot be broken down into a smaller word). This system features the use of symbols adapted from William Stokoe's symbols in the *Dictionary of American Sign Language* to show how signs were made, rather than depending on words or pictures to depict signs. This system is not widely used.

lipreading See SPEECHREADING.

Little Theatre of the Deaf Working under its parent company, the NATIONAL THEATRE OF THE DEAF, the Little Theatre has presented stories, fables and poetry to young audiences for more than 20 years.

The theater uses body movement, sign language and hearing interpreters to bring both classic literature and original works to life. Programs are presented in schools, parks, museums, theaters and libraries throughout the United States and in other places, such as India, the Far East and Scandinavia.

Now composed of two companies of five actors each, the theater offers one-hour performances that include short stories, fables and often an introduction to sign language. The actors form living sculptures during "Your Game," a program using suggestions from the audience to illustrate ensemble performances, such as a washing machine or a videocassette player in fast forward.

In 1977, the Kennedy Center in Washington, D.C. commissioned the National Theater of the Deaf to produce Sir Gawain and the Green Knight for its Children's Arts Festival. (See also PROFESSIONAL SCHOOL FOR DEAF THEATRE PERSONNEL.)

Lombard test A special test for functional hearing loss in which masking sounds are introduced into the ears while the subject talks. The test is positive if the subject raises the intensity level of his voice in order to hear himself above the masking sound and negative if his voice remains at a fixed level. (See also AUDIOMETRY; FUNCTIONAL HEARING LOSS [NONORGANIC].)

loop diuretics These powerful drugs are fast-acting chemicals that help remove excess water from the body by increasing the flow of urine; this class of diuretics is named for the part of the kidneys they affect, called Henle's loop. They are especially powerful and fast-acting when given by injection and are helpful in the emergency treatment of heart failure.

Studies suggest that loop diuretics may cause temporary or even permanent hearing loss, TINNITUS and VERTIGO, although symptoms usually disappear between 30 minutes and one day after treatment ends. Loop diuretics include azosemide, bumetadine, ethacrynic acid, furosemide, indapamide, lasix, piretamide and triflocin.

In general, physicians are advised against giving loop diuretics to premature infants or to patients taking aminoglycoside antibiotics. They are also advised against rapid intravenous use of furosemide.

Other diuretics (such as dyazide and the thiazides) have not been found to have ototoxic effects. (See also OTOTOXIC DRUGS.)

loudness The intensity factor of sound.

low birth weight and hearing loss Premature infants with a low birth weight (3.3 lbs or below) are at risk of a SENSORINEURAL HEARING LOSS ranging from mild to severe. Approximately 5% of these low-birth-weight infants will have hearing problems.

Full-term babies who have low birth weight are not at risk for hearing loss. (See also PRENATAL CAUSES OF HEARING LOSS.)

Lutheran religion and deafness The Lutheran church was the second religious group to set up a church specifically for deaf members; Our Saviour Lutheran Church for the Deaf was organized in 1896 in Chicago. It was followed by Emanuel Lutheran Church for the Deaf in Milwaukee, Wisconsin in 1898.

Soon, there were more than 14 missions to deaf people. These missions supervised programs for deaf people in the United States and provided pastors who were often assigned to more than one city. Contact: International Lutheran Deaf Association, 1333 S. Kirkwood Road, St. Louis, MO 63122; telephone: (voice) 314-965-9000, ext. 315, (TDD) 800-433-3954.

M

macula A small sensory patch inside both the SACCULE and the UTRICLE (small sacs in the vestibule). Each macula is covered with sensory hair cells and is connected to fibers from the vestibular branch of the eight cranial (auditory) nerve. These sensory patches are part of the body's delicate balance system.

mainstreaming The process in which a student with hearing problems attends some—or all—classes in a regular school for hearing students. (See also EDUCATION OF DEAF CHILDREN.)

malignant otitis externa Progressive infection that causes osteomyelitis of the temporal bone (usually caused by *P. aeruginosa*) and which sometimes involves the soft tissue of the external ear (PINNA). This condition occurs most often in people with diabetes mellitus.

Symptoms include severe refractory OTORRHEA and pain, together with swelling and tenderness in the external ear and scalp. A computerized tomography (CT) scan is often used to diagnose malignant otitis externa.

Treatment involves debridement with antibacterial ear drops and intravenous antibiotics, together with a good control of the underlying diabetic condition.

malleus One of the three OSSICLES of the middle ear, also known as the hammer.

manual alphabet See FINGERSPELLING.

manual approach Method of communication among deaf people using sign language and fingerspelling. Those who believe in the importance of manual communication consider it is a natural mode of communication for deaf people, that deaf people should be encouraged to use signs and they should be allowed to sign in school. Opponents of the manual approach generally reject sign language, at least for the purpose of education.

There are intermediate positions between the two ends of the manual-oral spectrum. Some supporters of oral communication agree with the use of FINGERSPELLING in many settings but not in schools; others approve of mouth-hand systems of communication, such as CUED SPEECH.

Many schools in the United States today have tried to reach a compromise between the manual and oral methods by combining the two approaches.

The manual approach was referred to as the "French method" during the 19th century and was the preferred educational method of ABBÉ CHARLES MICHEL DE L'EPÉE of Paris. At the same time, German deaf educator SAMUEL HEINICKE of Leipzig was promoting the oral approach.

L'Epée, as director of the French Royal Institute for the Deaf and Dumb in Paris (now the Institut National des Jeunes Sourds), promoted the use of what he called "methodical signs" for the education of deaf students, becoming the first proponent of sign language usage in schools. Because l'Epée did not believe there was any logical connection between sounds and ideas, it did not matter to him whether a person spoke or signed thoughts—each would be equally useful. All education was taught through his methodical signs, except for proper names for which he used fingerspelling. Still, l'Epée did teach speech and SPEECHREADING as well.

It was at the Paris Institute that THOMAS HOPKINS GAULLAUDET learned how to educate deaf children, and it was therefore the French manual method he took back home to the United States. From the beginning of the first permanent school for deaf students in 1817, which Gallaudet founded, until the late 1860s, all instruction in the United States (some 26 separate schools) was based on the manual method.

But in the 1840s, educators began to tour Europe and bring back reports of the oral progress in English and German schools. Eventually, when parents of some deaf children did not want their children to learn signs, they formed a school in 1867 with the assistance of John Clarke, who donated $300,000 to start the first purely oral school in America, the Clarke School of Northampton, Massachusetts.

A more recent refinement of the manual approach is called Total Communication, which implies acceptance, understanding and use of all methods of communication. Proponents of this theory believe people with hearing loss should be exposed to all methods, emphasizing whatever enables them to learn and communicate effectively. (See also SIMULTANEOUS COMMUNICATION.)

manually coded English All artificially developed codes that try to represent the English language in sign form are known as manually coded English (MCE). Typically, these systems have been developed primarily for the educational system to help build English language skills by manually incorporating many English language features.

In the past 20 years, a number of these codes have been developed, including SEEING ESSENTIAL ENGLISH (SEE 1), SIGNING EXACT ENGLISH (SEE 2) and SIGNED ENGLISH. All were designed to improve deaf students' English scores.

These codes, also known as manual English, are just that—codes, not languages—that reflect the structure and vocabulary of English. Generally, these systems use AMERICAN SIGN LANGUAGE signs in English word order, along with new signs that have been created to represent English parts of speech normally omitted from ASL. These manually coded systems therefore parallel the word and sentence structure of English.

However, manually coded English can be confusing to those used to American Sign Language. Whereas in English (and MCE) one word can have many meanings, ASL would assign a different sign to each separate meaning of the word. For example, the ASL sign for ''run'' (meaning a gait) is different from the run in a stocking or running for office.

Preliminary studies suggest these systems may improve students' grammar, but they are cumbersome to use, taking as much as twice as long to sign a word as it would to say it. Because of this, many students and teachers began to drop required signs. In response, Harry Bornstein, the author of Signed English, in 1982 came up with a pared-down version, although he continues to advocate that teachers and parents of young children slow down and sign accurately.

Use of these manual systems outside the classroom is not popular with the majority of deaf people, who view the system as an attempt to interfere with or eliminate ASL. (See also SIGN CODES.)

Martineau, Harriet (1802–1876) This strong and independent journalist was remarkable for her outspokenness during the Victorian era; she became one of the most famous writers of her time.

Born June 12, 1802, in Norwich, England to a radical Unitarian family, her severe, painful hearing problem began at the age of 12. Within six years she was severely deafened but was reluctant to use an ear trumpet.

Extremely well-educated for her time, Martineau wrote about economics, education, sociology and philosophy for the leading periodicals of her day, making enemies for her unorthodox views along the way. A believer in mesmerism (hypnotism), her subsequent views on religion (she espoused a form of atheism) brought her even more criticism.

On a visit to the United States, she was appalled at the treatment of women and Indians, and her strong antislavery views made her a controversial speaker.

Despite this, her home in the Lake District was a beacon to other well-known philosophers and writers, including William Wordsworth, Matthew Arnold, Charlotte Brontë, Ralph Waldo Emerson and Nathaniel Hawthorne.

She also wrote widely about deafness and the problems deaf people encountered, ridiculing hearing people for meddling in the affairs of the deaf community and blaming parents and teachers for inadequate education of deaf children.

maskers See TINNITUS MASKER.

masking techniques See TINNITUS MASKER.

Massachusetts test A group pure-tone hearing test that can screen 40 students at the same time by presenting pure tones of 500, 4,000, and 6,000 Hz at 20, 25 and 30 dB respectively. (See also JOHNSTON TEST; SWEEP-CHECK TEST.)

Massieu, Jean (1772-1846) This brilliant, outgoing educator, together with the ABBÉ ROCH AMBROISE CUCURRON SICARD, helped develop the manual method of education taught at the famed Paris Institute.

Born in 1772 near Cadillac, France, Massieu was one of six children, all deaf, who communicated among themselves in the family's own system of manual signs. Sent to a school for deaf children in Bordeaux, Massieu met Abbe Sicard, who taught him how to read and write. When Sicard was named head of the Paris Institute, both men moved to Paris in 1790.

As the French revolution exploded around them, Massieu and Sicard worked to establish education for deaf people. Massieu worked as instructor at the school, together with LAURENT CLERC, and helped teach THOMAS HOPKINS GALLAUDET their manual method of education. Upon Sicard's death in 1822, Massieu was fired for sexual indiscretions and moved to Aveyron, where he became headmaster of a local school for deaf students, retiring in 1839.

mastoid bone Located behind the ear, this prominent portion of the temporal bone is honeycombed with air cells that are connected to a cavity in the upper part of the bone called the mastoid antrum, which is in turn connected to the MIDDLE EAR. OTITIS MEDIA can spread through this bone to cause acute MASTOIDITIS (inflammation of the mastoid bone). (See also MASTOIDECTOMY.)

mastoidectomy A surgical procedure to remove the mastoid portion of the temporal bone, thereby removing the infected air cells within the bone caused by MASTOIDITIS, OTITIS MEDIA or CHOLESTEATOMA. It may also be used in the repair of a paralyzed facial nerve. It is performed less frequently today because of the widespread use of antibiotics in the treatment of acute OTITIS MEDIA and acute mastoiditis. Most mastoidectomies are performed behind the ear under general anesthesia.

There are several types of mastoidectomy, including antrotomy, cortical, modified radical, radical and a combined approach.

Antrotomy Now almost obsolete, this operation involves the clearing and draining of the infected bone.

Cortical Also called a simple or Swartze mastoidectomy, this procedure is used in acute and masked mastoiditis, a severely draining ear and recurrent otitis media. It involves removal of all cells of the mastoid bone.

Modified Radical This procedure is used for cholesteatoma not involving the MIDDLE EAR but confined to the attic and mastoid, in which part of the bony wall is removed. It is also called a Bondy operation.

Radical This operation for otitis media and, rarely, cholesteatoma involves removal of the tympanic membrane (EARDRUM), the OSSICLES, the posterior wall of the external canal, the diseased tissue and the mastoid. This converts the mastoid and middle ear into a single, healthy cavity. Unfortunately, a CONDUCTIVE HEARING LOSS of up to 50 dB is usually expected because the middle ear ossicles are removed, although a TYMPANOPLASTY may offset some of the loss. There may also be a partial or complete SENSORINEURAL HEARING LOSS if the footplate of the STAPES is dislodged.

Combined This treatment for cholesteatoma, also called an intact canal wall mastoidectomy, avoids leaving a mastoid cavity by clearing the mastoid cavity and the middle ear of cholesteatoma while preserving the posterior canal wall. Unfortunately, some of the disease may be overlooked and left behind, which is why some otologic surgeons perform routine follow-up surgeries in several years.

mastoiditis An inflammation of the MASTOID BONE (the bone behind the ear), caused by a spreading infection from the middle ear to the antrum (a cavity in the mastoid bone), and from there to the air cells in the bone.

Mastoiditis causes severe pain, swelling and tenderness behind and inside the ear together with fever, creamy discharge and progressive hearing loss. The real danger is that infection may spread to inside the skull, causing MENINGITIS, a brain abscess or stroke. The infection could also spread outward, damaging the facial nerve and paralyzing the facial muscles.

Mastoiditis has become uncommon since the use of antibiotic drugs for the treatment of ear infections. Antibiotic treatment will clear the infection, although a MASTOIDECTOMY (removal of the infected air cells within the mastoid bone) may be needed if it doesn't.

measles This viral illness causes a rash and fever and can cause hearing problems or deafness from complications of ear infections and encephalitis. Measles affects primarily children, but an attack can occur at any age.

Spread by airborne droplets, measles has an incubation period up to 11 days before symptoms appear, and can be transmitted during this period and up to about one week after symptoms occur. Once very common throughout the world, measles today appears much less often in developed countries because of the availability of vaccinations that protect against the disease.

Symptoms begin with a fever, cold symptoms and cough; several days later a red rash begins on the head and neck and spreads downward. Symptoms fade after about three days if no complications develop.

In addition to encephalitis and possible hearing loss, other complications include seizure and coma, sometimes followed by retardation and death. Measles during pregnancy kills the fetus in about one out of five cases.

Treatment includes plenty of fluids and acetaminophen to reduce the fever. Antibiotics will not be helpful against the measles virus, but they may be prescribed to treat a secondary infection.

In the United States, a measles vaccination (usually combined with mumps and rubella vaccinations) is given to children over age one and affords protection against the disease in most cases. In recent years, isolated epidemics have required immunizations of infants under age one living in epidemic areas.

meatus See EXTERNAL AUDITORY CANAL.

membranous labyrinth A delicate closed system of ducts and sacs filled with a watery fluid called ENDOLYMPH, the membranous labryinth is suspended in the bony labyrinth of the otic capsule and is part of the body's balance system.

Each of its SEMICIRCULAR CANALS contains a narrow membranous semicircular duct with a rounded expansion (the ampulla) at the end. These ducts open into the tubular sac of the UTRICLE, which is in turn connected to a similar sac called the SACCULE.

Ménière's disease An inner ear disorder of unknown origin that causes hearing loss, DIZZINESS OR VERTIGO and TINNITUS (noises within the head). Ménière's disease affects more than one million Americans and can be extremely incapacitating.

First described by French physician Prosper Ménière in 1861, the disease is characterized by episodes of dizziness (in which the patient will feel either he or the surroundings are spinning) accompanied by hearing loss, nausea and vomiting, tinnitus and fullness or pressure. Symptoms can last from a few minutes to eight hours and can be profoundly disturbing. The attacks of vertigo may occur irregularly, every few weeks. Ménière's disease tends to recur and subside as symptoms get progressively worse. It usually runs its course over several years, finally declining in severity until it ceases. In general, the patient by this time is severely deaf.

Normally, only one ear is affected, and the SENSORINEURAL HEARING LOSS may progressively worsen over the years, although in a few cases hearing loss in both ears has been found.

Hearing tests usually reveal loudness RECRUITMENT and poor speech discrimination. Although there is a great variability from one person to the next, hearing loss may fluctuate at first—starting with low frequencies and then involving higher frequencies—and eventually become permanent.

Most patients experience vertigo, hearing loss and tinnitus with the disease, but there are several variations: Cochlear Ménière's disease symptoms include hearing loss and tinnitus without vertigo, and vestibular Ménière's disease causes vertigo without hearing loss.

Researchers know the disease results in a swelling of the MEMBRANOUS LABYRINTH, but the cause of this swelling is not known.

The major pathological change is the accumulation of excess fluid in the inner ear that damages delicate nerve endings. One of the biggest mysteries of the disorder is its unpredictability: Remissions come and go, lasting anywhere from six months to six years.

Some researchers believe Ménière's disease may be caused by a defect in the way the body handles carbohydrates, causing the body to overcompensate by producing too much insulin.

Drugs may have some value in the prevention of attacks, but they generally are better at easing symptoms once an attack has occurred. Drugs that may help include atropine or scopolamine to lessen nausea and vomiting, antihistamines to relieve vertigo or barbiturates for general sedation.

In the early 1970s, researchers at the HOUSE EAR INSTITUTE in California, a well-known center for the treatment of hearing disorders and research, studied 120 volunteers with Ménière's and a wide range of complexities linked to the disorder. Allergies, endocrine insufficiencies, metabolic dysfunction, structural anomalies and trauma were all found in about half the cases. Although treating the separate conditions resulted in improvement in about half the cases, others with the same conditions and treatment did not respond.

More recent research by experts at the institute have found that by severely restricting diet, some patients may find their symptoms subside and hearing increases by as much as 20 dB. The severe diet restrictions include prohibitions on wheat, flour, eggs, chocolate, corn and mayonnaise. Some patients studied at the institute who have temporarily disregarded the diet restrictions notice an immediate return of symptoms.

For most Ménière's patients—those who have abnormal insulin levels and/or impaired glucose tolerance—scientists recommend six small meals of low-carbohydrate, low-cholesterol food.

There are several surgical options to control vertigo, which is often caused by excess fluid in the inner ear that puts pressure on the delicate balance system of the body centered in that area. By surgically placing a shunt to drain away excess fluid, surgeons can sometimes ease the feeling of vertigo.

Other treatment for the disease varies. Some doctors recommend lifestyle changes, including altered diet (in addition to the above restrictions, less salt and more low-fat foods), reduced psychological stress, no cigarettes or alcohol and regular exercise.

Ménière's Network, The A national network of patient support groups administered by the EAR FOUNDATION to provide people with the opportunity to share experiences and coping strategies. Contact: The Ear Foundation, 2000 Church Street, Box 111, Nashville, TN 37326; telephone (voice and TDD): 800-545-HEAR.

meningeal labyrinthitis See LABYRINTHITIS.

meningitis This disease involves an infection and inflammation of the outer coverings of the brain (meninges) and the nerves that lead to it and can cause sudden, profound and irreversible deafness in both ears. Because the deafness is incurable, physicians generally try to prevent or catch meningitis early to head off such complications.

Meningitis can be caused by almost any infectious agent, although bacteria cause the most fatal infections. Symptoms include fever, headache, vomiting, irritability, loss of appetite and a stiff neck.

Most cases of meningitis occur in children under the age of five. Recent studies suggest that about 6% of children with bacterial meningitis are left with a SENSORINEURAL HEARING LOSS, although other researchers have reported a higher rate of occurrence.

Occasionally, when deafness occurs during bacterial meningitis, a small amount of hearing remains, and a powerful hearing aid can be of some help but only to amplify sounds, not to recognize speech. TINNITUS is not often present, although there may be a brief experience of VERTIGO. Balance problems can also occur. Mental retardation occurs in about 15% of children whose deafness is associated with meningitis.

Meningitis is diagnosed by a spinal tap (insertion of a needle in the lower back to sample spinal fluid). Any bacterial, fungal or tubercular infection must be treated immediately with antibiotics.

Death from bacterial meningitis still occurs frequently, even with prompt antibiotic treatment. On the other hand, viral meningitis does not require any specific treatment, and patients usually recover within five days without lasting symptoms or risk of hearing problems. (See also POSTNATAL CAUSES OF HEARING LOSS.)

mental health services Despite advances in mental health care, finding adequate mental health services continues to be a major unmet need for the deaf and hard-of-hearing population. The shortage of inpatient and outpatient mental health programs continues to be a chronic problem for deaf people.

This paucity of special mental health services is compounded by the shortage of qualified mental health professionals to work and communicate with deaf and hard-of-hearing people in sign language, especially AMERICAN SIGN LANGUAGE. Accurate and appropriate diagnosis and treatment requires a working knowledge of the educational, psychological, social, cultural, linguistic, communication and emotional aspects of deafness—and fluency in sign language in particular.

"Because of the shortage, deaf and hard-of-hearing people do not have access to the wide diversity of mental health services, both public and private, currently available to hearing people," according to Barbara Brauer, Ph.D., psychologist and research scientist at the Mental Health Research Program at GALLAUDET UNIVERSITY.

In fact, about 85% of deaf people who need such services are not receiving them. This problem is aggravated by the fact that mental health professionals in general are not required to get special training or certification to diagnose and treat troubled deaf and hard-of-hearing people.

Significantly, it has been demonstrated in the past 10 years that deaf people do respond to and benefit from the various methods of therapy used with hearing clients, as long as treatment is carried out using the preferred communication mode and style of the deaf individual.

People who need help in treating deaf and hard-of-hearing patients may contact Barbara A. Brauer, Ph.D., Mental Health Research Program, Gallaudet Research Institute, Gallaudet University, 800 Florida Ave., NE, Washington, DC 20002; telephone: 202-651-5647.

mental illness Research has shown that the rates of psychological disorders and mental illness are about the same for both the deaf and hearing populations. However, the lack of access to quality mental health services for deaf patients often precludes preventive mental health care.

In addition, hearing mental health professionals tend to diagnose psychological disorders and mental illness in deaf patients where none exist because they are unfamiliar with the educational, psychological, social, cultural, linguistic and communication aspects of deafness and are unable to use sign language to communicate.

To the inexperienced mental health professional, deaf people may appear to be psychologically disturbed or mentally ill when in fact they are not, according to Barbara A. Brauer, Ph.D., psychologist and research scientist at the Mental Health Research Program at GALLAUDET RESEARCH INSTITUTE. Because AMERICAN SIGN LANGUAGE and English have very different structures, styles and syntax, the English comprehension and writing levels of deaf people may appear pathological when in fact they are normal. Standardized tests are also culturally biased, as the tests are given in the context of the hearing experience, which may in many respects be different from the deaf experience. Consequently, the results often yield erroneous information about psychologically healthy deaf individuals.

For this reason, a number of psychological and personality tests have been translated by Dr. Brauer into American Sign Language on videotape as part of Gallaudet University's Mental Health Research Program. According to Dr. Brauer, preliminary findings suggest normal profiles for most deaf individuals tested.

Mercer, William (1765–1839) Little is known about the early life of this deaf American painter, other than that he was born deaf in Fredericksburg, Virginia in 1765, the first of five children. At the age of 18, he was sent to be apprenticed to Charles Willson Peale, a well-known Philadelphia artist. For three years, Mercer boarded with the Peale family and studied painting under the master artist.

Mercer's artworks include *The Battle of Princeton*, and a half portrait of his grandmother, Mrs. John Gordeon (both of which are owned by the Historical Society of Pennsylvania), and an oval miniature of a Virginian official (owned by the Virginia Historical Society of Richmond).

Although Mercer returned to Fredericksburg in 1786, where he continued to work as a painter, no other pictures by him are known to have survived.

message relay service A generic term for a one-way service in which an operator relays a message from a hearing person without a TELECOMMUNICATIONS DEVICE FOR THE DEAF (TDD) to a deaf person who has a TDD, or vice-versa. This is distinguished from a RELAY SERVICE, in which both hearing and deaf parties are on the line at the same time with an operator acting as a go-between.

methods of instruction There are currently four primary methods of instruction for deaf students used in the United States—the oral, auditory, Rochester, and simultaneous methods—as well as a more recent method—total communication.

Oral Approach Also called the oral-aural method, children learning under this system are taught through SPEECHREADING (lipreading) and amplification of sound; they express themselves by speaking. Gestures and signs are prohibited.

Auditory Method This system concentrates on helping children develop listening skills by relying primarily on hearing. Early reading, writing, and speechreading (lipreading) are discouraged. This system is generally used for people with moderate hearing loss, but it is sometimes used with profoundly deaf students as well.

Rochester Method Rarely used in this country today, this system combines the oral approach with FINGERSPELLING. Children receive input through speechreading, amplification and fingerspelling, with great emphasis placed on reading and writing.

Simultaneous Method This features a combination of the oral approach plus signs and fingerspelling. Children are taught through speechreading, amplification, signs and fingerspelling.

Total Communication In addition to the above four methods, Total Communication has received widespread attention in the past several years. According to the Conference of Executives of American Schools for the Deaf, Total Communication is a philosophy incorporating aural, manual and oral modes of communication to ensure effective communication with and among deaf people.

Mexican Sign Language Known as LSM (Lenguaje de Senas Mexicanas), this sign language is used throughout Mexico by many of its more than 1.3 million deaf citizens.

As is typical for sign language, LSM does not parallel Spanish grammar. Sign meaning can be altered by varying speed, size and duration of the sign, and placement of signs depends on context. As in written Spanish, a sign for "question" appears at the beginning of the sentence.

There are no manual codes that follow Spanish language structure, such as the manual codes for English in the United States.

Education is still widely oral in Mexico, although deaf educators are working to include LSM in the schools.

Mexico With more than 1.3 million deaf and hard-of-hearing citizens there has been growth in the number of services provided for deaf people in Mexico, although there is still much more to be done in the field of education for deaf students and in the training of deaf teachers. According to a 1940 census, the prevalence rate of deafness in Mexico was 39 per 100,000; the count rose to 46 per 100,000 in the 1974 census. Still, this represents a fairly low rate compared to those of other developed nations that report data on deafness, which range from 35 per 100,000 to 300 per 100,000

Mexico does not have any national organizations or regional groups for deaf people, although there are two deaf sports associations.

Although education for deaf Mexicans began in the late 1860s, few new schools were established until the middle of the 20th century as the educational philosophy changed from the MANUAL to ORAL approach. In 1951 the first institute for deaf people in Latin America was established, called the Mexican Institute of Speech and Hearing (IMAL). The institute, primarily oral, offers courses for teachers, audiologists, speech pathologists, technicians and deaf people, conducts research and provides social services.

microphone hearing aid See HEARING AIDS.

middle ear The small cavity between the EARDRUM and the INNER EAR that houses the three bones of the middle ear (OSSICLES). The middle ear transmits the vibration of a sound from the air outside to the fluid in the inner ear by the chain of these three tiny bones, which link the eardrum to an OVAL WINDOW in the wall on the opposite side of the middle ear cavity.

The first of the three bones, called the malleus or hammer, is joined to the inside of the eardrum. The second, called the incus or anvil, is joined to the malleus and has another delicate joint to the third bone, called the stapes or stirrup. The base of the stapes fills the oval window, which leads to the inner ear.

Although the eardrum cuts off the middle ear from the outside, it is not completely airtight. A ventilation channel, called the EUSTACHIAN TUBE, runs forward and down into the back of the nose. Although the eustachian tube is normally closed, it opens during yawning and swallowing.

middle ear cavity See TYMPANUM.

middle ear diseases and hearing loss There are a number of conditions that occur in the MIDDLE EAR and result in a CONDUCTIVE HEARING LOSS. These include injuries, inflammation, tumors and diseases of the OTIC CAPSULE.

Injuries Injuries to the middle ear that produce conductive hearing loss can include an imbalance in air pressure (such as found in a descending plane), head injury and foreign objects.

A ruptured eardrum and SEROUS OTITIS MEDIA can develop in the wake of barotrauma (when the EUSTACHIAN TUBE can't equalize the pressure during an airplane landing or deepsea dive). Severe blows to the head, auto accidents or even a slap directly on the ear can fracture the temporal bone, fracturing or dislocating the OSSICLES (usually separating the incus and stapes) and causing a conductive hearing loss.

Inflammation One of the most common causes of hearing loss in children is caused by inflammation of the middle ear. In acute and chronic suppurative otitis media, ear infection caused by bacterial or viral infection of the nasopharynx, most often by streptococcus pneumonia, staphylococcus aureus and hemolytic streptococcus, can spread to the middle ear.

In acute infections, the patient has a fever and headache with possible rupture of the eardrum and draining of fluid.

Complications include MASTOIDITIS (infection of the MASTOID BONE with pus in the air cells) which requires surgery, LABYRINTHITIS, or MENINGITIS. If the acute suppurative ear infection is not properly treated, frequent repeated ear infections can result in a resistant form of mastoiditis and in a permanently ruptured eardrum, discharge and a mild to moderate conductive hearing loss.

Another type of chronic middle ear infection features a lesion made up of skin debris called a CHOLESTEATOMA and can either be congenital or acquired. The rare congenital variety of cholesteatoma can appear in any part of the temporal bone. An acquired cholesteatoma may appear as skin migrates from the external ear canal into the middle ear through a small hole in the eardrum; as the lesion grows, it damages the middle ear structure and can cause a conductive hearing loss. Serious complications can be associated with an invasive cholesteatoma, including labyrinthitis, meningitis, brain abscess or facial nerve paralysis.

Glue ear (also called nonsuppurative otitis media or serous otitis media) is the most common cause of hearing loss in children and may be a result of an ear infection treated with antibiotics but with poor drainage of ear fluids. In adults, it may be caused by a dysfunctioning eustachian tube due to barotrauma or head colds; the resulting negative air pressure in the middle ear pulls the eardrum back, forcing fluid out of the middle ear. Glue ear can lead to the formation of a cholesteatoma.

Chronic middle ear infection can also scar the eardrum and cause it to collapse (ADHESIVE OTITIS MEDIA), adhering to the ossicles and causing hearing loss. Such chronic infection can also cause new bone to form in the middle ear lining.

OTOSCLEROSIS is a disorder involving the overgrowth of bone that immobilizes the stapes (the innermost bone of the middle ear) and prevents sound vibrations from passing to the INNER EAR, resulting in conductive deafness. Generally, both ears are eventually affected. The disease begins in early adulthood, is more common among women and affects about one in every 200 people. Hearing loss progresses slowly over a period of 10 to 15 years, often accompanied by TINNITUS and sometimes by VERTIGO.

Tumors Tumors of the middle ear, although fairly rare, include squamous-cell cancer and glomus tumor. Squamous cell cancer usually appears in middle age and spreads rapidly, resulting in a conductive hearing loss until the tumor invades the labyrinth. In later stages, pain is intense and may result in blood-stained discharge.

Glomus tumor is a slow-growing mass that occurs more often in women and causes a conductive hearing loss and tinnitus, followed eventually by a SENSORINEURAL HEARING LOSS, dizziness and nerve palsy. Surgical removal is usually required. (See also AERO-OTITIS MEDIA; TUMORS OF THE MIDDLE EAR; TYMPANOSCLEROSIS.)

middle ear effusion See SEROUS OTITIS MEDIA.

mild to moderate hearing loss Generally considered to be a 30 decibel to 55 dB loss.

minimal language skills A controversial term meaning a diminished communication repertoire of some individuals with hearing loss. This term replaced the negative "low verbal" description used before the 1970s, which was incorrectly used to label people who were proficient in AMERICAN SIGN LANGUAGE but not in spoken English.

Minimal language skills does *not* mean a person has problems with spoken language (especially English), has problems speechreading or is illiterate. A person who is not competent in sign language *or* in spoken language may be said incorrectly to have minimal language skills.

Miss Deaf America During the biennial conventions of the NATIONAL ASSOCIATION OF THE DEAF, a national competition for Miss Deaf America is held among young women who have already won their state competitions. Miss Deaf America serves as a role model for young deaf people and increases deaf awareness among the general public through her appearances around the country promoting the skills and capabilities of deaf youth.

mixed hearing loss A combination of conductive and sensorineural loss that occurs in the outer or middle plus the inner ear. Conductive deafness is often treatable, depending on cause; sensorineural deafness is seldom treatable. (See also CONDUCTIVE HEARING LOSS; SENSORINEURAL HEARING LOSS.)

Model Secondary School for the Deaf (MSSD) Established by an act of Congress on October 15, 1966, the MSSD was designed to provide an outstanding example of a secondary school program for students with hearing problems and to stimulate the development of similar programs around the country.

Congress stipulated that the school should serve as a regional high school to prepare deaf students for college or a vocational career and should upgrade education for deaf students, using the newest research in testing, methodology and curriculum development.

In the beginning, admission requirements mandated that students be at least 14 years of age and have a third-grade reading level, a hearing loss of 70 decibels or more in the better ear and no other major problems. (These criteria were loosened following the passage of PL 94-142, the Education for All Handicapped Children Act.)

Students attending MSSD come primarily from Maryland, Delaware, Pennsylvania, Virginia, West Virginia and Washington, D.C., although students from other states are admitted if there is space. In that case, preference is given to students who have no access to a full-service high school.

Today, the school—located on 17 acres in the northwest corner of GALLAUDET UNIVERSITY—includes residence halls, health facilities, dining rooms, an infirmary and playing fields and serves about 400 deaf students a year. If offers students a continually-updated curriculum of more than 180 courses, including foreign language, art and theater arts. About 75% of the students live on campus; the rest commute from nearby Washington. Approximately 70% of MSSD students continue their education after graduation.

The school also offers a wide variety of interest clubs, a yearbook and service organizations, such as the Junior National Association of the Deaf.

The school provides curriculum development, workshops, seminars and internships for professionals and graduate students. School staff publish *Perspectives,* a professional journal for teachers, and *The World Around You,* a national high school student publication.

Input is received from the Parent Advisory Council and a National Advisory Council, which helps maintain goals and direction. (See also KENDALL DEMONSTRATION SCHOOL.)

modiolus The central column of the COCHLEA in which the spiral ganglion of the eighth cranial nerve is located.

monaural Pertaining to one ear.

monaural hearing aid A single-ear hearing aid available in various styles, including the body, ear level, in-the-ear or eyeglass types. (See also HEARING AIDS.)

mouth-hand systems Mouth-hand systems are not a language but an aid to the visual transmission of spoken languages using handshapes close to the mouth to differentiate PHONEMES that look the same when spoken. (Phonemes are a family of closely related speech sounds regarded as a single sound; for example, the "r" in "bring," "red" and "car.") Used as aids for speechreading and speech training, there are two major forms of mouth-hand systems: CUED SPEECH and Danish.

Cued Speech Cued Speech was developed in 1966 as a speechreading support system which (in English) uses eight hand configurations and four hand placements near the mouth to supplement visible speech. Each "cue" (hand placement or configuration) identifies a special group of two to four speech sounds. The combination of cues and mouth movements makes all the essential speech sounds appear different from each other so that the spoken message is clarified.

The hand configurations and locations are called "cues," not Cued Speech, which is the combination of the cues with speech (the cues are not readable alone).

Each hand configuration identifies a group of consonants; each hand location identifies a group of vowels. Further, Cued Speech can be used to indicate approximate voice pitch for each syllable uttered, which is important in tonal languages (such as Thai, Cantonese, Mandarin and Igbo).

For example, in Cantonese, the syllable "ma" can mean "mother," "scold," "horse," or "right?" depending on the pitch. Tone cueing is also helpful in speech therapy. In order to cue a tone, a person changes the inclination of the cueing hand to indicate changes in pitch.

Cued Speech has been adapted to many languages, and audiocassette lessons designed for self-instruction by hearing persons are available. The system is generally the same in all languages.

Proponents believe cued speech makes spoken language visually clear and solves the communication problem at home and that it helps children learn a spoken language more easily. It is also an easily-learned system, taking only about 12 to 20 hours to master.

Initial research does suggest that Cued Speech helps make the spoken language clear, but the long-term effectiveness of the language is not known. Cued Speech is not widely used by adults in the deaf community.

Danish The mouth-hand system was invented in 1900 in Denmark by Georg Forchhammer, head of a deaf oral school, who believed that visual communication was necessary. Married to a deaf woman, he realized it would be helpful to improve SPEECHREADING capability by making similar-sounding words clear.

In the Danish system, there are 14 different hand positions, each making clear a sound that is hard to speechread. Hand positions are designed to symbolize the sound, and the most-often used sounds are the easiest to make.

Easy to use, the system is the most common visual aid in Denmark by hard-of-hearing people who don't know sign language. On the other hand, this system tends to slow down communication and is tiring to read or produce over a period of time.

Among the Danish deaf population, the mouth-hand system is used as a way to improve speech training and has also become a part of SIGN LANGUAGE in much the same way that the MANUAL ALPHABET is used in conjunction with other sign languages. In Denmark, the system is used to spell out names and words with no equivalent in Danish sign language.

This system can be used with any language, with additional shapes used for sounds that are not made in Danish. These hand positions have been developed for use in English, French, German, Swedish and Norwegian. (See also Appendix 14.)

mucous otitis media A middle ear infection caused by thick fluid in the middle ear that may be the result of improper drug treatment of a draining ear infection. The fluid that collects in the middle ear causes hearing loss, which may vary between a mild high-tone loss to a considerable loss for all tones. In the presence of thick mucus, the hearing loss is most severe and may mimic the type of hearing loss seen as a result of OTOSCLEROSIS.

Hearing is restored when the thick fluid is removed by puncturing the eardrum. If the fluid is not removed, the CONDUCTIVE HEARING LOSS will persist, and the condition may lead to the formation of adhesions in the middle ear that firmly fix the ossicular chain with fibrous tissue bands. (See also OSSICLES.)

multisensory teaching approach This method, one of two philosophies used in teaching speech to deaf and hard-of-hearing children, calls for the use of all sensory channels—hearing, sight, feel—as opposed to the AUDITORY-ORAL METHOD, which teaches the child to rely solely on the auditory system, however flawed.

The proponents of the multisensory method believe that the hard-of-hearing or deaf child has an auditory system that is inadequate for the development of good speech and that this calls for the use of other senses, including sight and touch. (See also SPEECH TRAINING.)

mumps Mumps is the most common cause of severe one-sided deafness, which is usually sudden in onset and happens without ear pain or discomfort.

The deafness often goes unnoticed for many days—or years—after onset; often a patient will claim that he only recently noticed deafness in one ear. Close examination and history will reveal, however, that the deafness has been present since an attack of mumps in childhood.

Deafness due to mumps usually causes complete loss of hearing in one ear by irreparably destroying the INNER EAR without affecting the balance mechanism. If any hearing does remain in the affected ear, the deafness does not become progressive.

Mumps is an acute viral illness that usually occurs in childhood and produces swelling and inflammation of the salivary glands on one or both sides of the face. After an incubation period of two to three weeks, symptoms of pain and swelling appear. Fever, headache and difficulty swallowing may develop, but temperature and swelling soon pass.

In people past puberty, there may occasionally be swelling of the testicles in men or swelling of the breasts and ovaries in women. One attack of mumps confers lifelong immunity.

There is no specific treatment for mumps other than painkillers and plenty of fluids. In the United States, most children at age 15 months are given a combination measles, mumps and rubella vaccination to protect against these diseases. The vaccination is given earlier in areas experiencing a measles epidemic. (See also VIRUSES AND HEARING LOSS.)

mutism The inability to speak due to deafness.

myringoplasty See TYMPANOPLASTY.

myringotomy A surgical procedure used to open the eardrum to drain the middle ear cavity. It is usually performed in children to treat persistent middle ear effusion (a sticky secretion in the middle ear cavity causing hearing loss). This hearing loss may become permanent if the condition isn't treated. Before antibiotics, a myringotomy was used to treat acute OTITIS MEDIA by releasing the pus, relieving pressure on the eardrum.

While the patient is under general anesthesia, the otolaryngologist makes a small incision in the eardrum, removing most of the fluid by suction. At the same time, a small tube may be inserted in the hole to allow any remaining fluid to drain into the outer ear. The patient can leave the hospital the next day, and the tube usually falls out several months later as the hole in the eardrum closes. A second operation may be needed to insert another tube if the condition does not clear up.

Some experts advocate the use of allergic management or decongestive therapy, which eventually allows the effusion to clear. Unfortunately, the hearing loss that occurs while the effusion exists may cause developmental problems in children. Some research suggests that long-term treatment with antibiotics may help clear some cases of effusion. (See also SEROUS OTITIS MEDIA.)

N

NABTS See NORTH AMERICAN BASIC TELETEXT SPECIFICATION.

NAD Legal Defense Fund Established in 1976 to handle lawsuits aimed at protecting the rights of deaf Americans, the Legal Defense Fund is totally funded by the NATIONAL ASSOCIATION OF THE DEAF.

The fund strives to provide protection in the areas of employment, education, physical and mental health care, welfare and social services, judicial and law enforcement and insurance. (See also NATIONAL CENTER FOR LAW AND THE DEAF.) Contact: NAD Legal Defense Fund, National Center for Law and the Deaf, Gallaudet University, 800 Florida Ave. NE, Washington, DC 20002; telephone: 202-651-5373 (voice).

name sign A sign used in the deaf community that serves as the first, middle and last name of a person.

Since most deaf children do not have deaf parents, most deaf offspring of hearing parents receive a name sign from their deaf peers or teachers once they begin school. Name signs can change in different groups of people or when a person's status changes, such as after marriage.

Name signs may be descriptive, in which they describe a person's physical characteristics; research has discovered that many of these emphasize negative physical characteristics, such as being overweight or having a scar. Arbitrary name signs (usually given by deaf parents) all have alphabetically-based handshapes affiliated with the first, middle or last name.

FINGERSPELLING is also sometimes used to spell out an abbreviated form of the name.

nasopharynx examination In order to diagnose auditory disorders, it is important to examine the nasopharynx (the passage connecting the nasal cavity behind the nose to the top of the throat behind the soft palate). Part of the respiratory tract, the nasopharynx forms the upper section of the pharynx and contains the openings to the eustachian tubes.

A nasopharynx examination is important because infections can obstruct the eustachian tubes, causing abnormalities in the middle ear. Examining the nasopharynx can uncover problems such as middle ear effusion (production of sticky fluid in the middle ear), retraction of the eardrum, chronic and acute OTITIS MEDIA (ear infection), infections of the nasopharynx, sinusitis (inflammation of the membrane lining the sinuses), allergy, adenoid enlargement and adenoiditis (inflammation of the adenoids).

The nasopharynx can be examined by looking through the mouth with a mirror placed behind the free edge of the soft palate, or a right-angle telescope can be used through the mouth to look around the soft palate into the nasopharynx. Other ways to examine the nasopharynx include using a nasopharyngoscope (a thin right-angle telescope passed through the nose) or a flexible fiber-optic endoscope to look through the nose or the mouth. Feeling with the finger can also be helpful and is usually performed under general anesthesia. Imaging techniques may also be used, especially in determining the size of adenoid tissue in children.

National Association for Hearing and Speech Action This organization was founded in 1910 in New York City to advocate and provide information for deaf and hard-of-hearing people and is the consumer affiliate of the AMERICAN SPEECH-LANGUAGE-HEARING ASSOCIATION.

The group operates a toll-free speech and hearing helpline (800-638-TALK) and has produced brochures and television public service announcements promoting healthy hearing.

The association was first called the American Association for the Hard of Hearing and was designed for people interested in teaching SPEECHREADING to hard-of-hearing people. During the 1920s, the association moved to Washington, D.C. and led an aggressive campaign to prevent hearing problems and establish screening programs in schools.

In 1966 the association was renamed the National Association of Hearing and Speech Agencies and emphasized community organization and professional service, education, diagnosis and research.

Its final name change occurred in 1972. Today, its members are involved in promoting the interests of people with speech and hearing problems and emphasizing consumer advocacy, prevention and social action.

National Association of the Deaf (NAD) NAD is a consumer advocate organization concerned about and involved with everything affecting opportunities for the more than 22 million deaf and hard-of-hearing people in the United States.

With 50 affiliated state associations and more than 22,000 members, NAD changed its orientation in 1960 from a group of individuals to a federation of state associations. The first association founded by deaf people, it was founded in 1880 by a group of deaf leaders concerned that deaf people were not included in the decision-making processes affecting their own lives.

In 1964, the group abandoned its policy of allowing only deaf people to become members, but today less than 100 of its more than 22,000 members can hear. Most of these 100 are professionals who work with deaf clients.

Today, NAD serves as a clearinghouse of information on deafness and is an advocate for the employment of deaf people. The organization promotes the use of AMERICAN SIGN LANGUAGE and supports the philosophy of TOTAL COMMUNICATION—the right of all deaf people to select and use any form of communication, including SIGN LANGUAGE, gestures, writing, reading, FINGERSPELLING, SPEECHREADING and listening with amplification.

Over the years, NAD has received a number of federal grants to conduct the first national census of deaf Americans, to set up a communication skills program and to establish the REGISTRY OF INTERPRETERS FOR THE DEAF, among others.

NAD—together with its affiliate state association in Massachusetts—operates D.E.A.F., INC., a rehabilitation facility serving the deaf population in New England, and administers a survey research organization, the Deaf Community Analysts. The organization also subsidizes the NAD LEGAL DEFENSE FUND, the International Association of Parents of the Deaf and the JUNIOR NATIONAL ASSOCIATION OF THE DEAF and holds an annual leadership camp for deaf youth.

Finally, the NAD publishes a national monthly tabloid, *The Broadcaster,* featuring columns, articles, a special sports section and advertisements of special interest to the deaf community. Its quarterly magazine, *The Deaf American,* carries full-length feature articles on topics of interest to the deaf community. NAD also publishes and sells books on deafness and sells assistive devices for deaf people.

Its home office, Halex House, is located in Silver Spring, MD, where it offers for sale more than 200 books on various aspects of deafness. The NAD is a member of the WORLD FEDERATION OF THE DEAF. (See also MISS DEAF AMERICA.) Contact: National Association of the Deaf, 814 Thayer Ave., Silver Spring, MD 20910; telephone (voice and TDD): 301-587-1788.

National Black Deaf Advocates, Inc. This organization promotes leadership, deaf awareness and active participation in the political, educational, religious and economic processes that affect the lives of deaf black citizens. Contact: National Black Advocates, Inc., P.O. Box 91166, Washington, DC 20066; telephone (TDD): 301-559-5398.

National Board for Certification in Hearing Instrument Sciences Founded in 1981, the NBC-HIS is a voluntary nonprofit organization devoted to the recognition of people who are qualified to provide competent hearing instrument services to hard-of-hearing patients.

Board certification is conferred upon hearing instrument specialists who meet specified criteria and demonstrate professional competence.

National Captioning Institute (NCI) This nonprofit corporation was founded in 1979 to develop a national closed-captioned television service for the entertainment industry in order to provide deaf and hard-of-hearing people with the words accompanying current news, drama, comedy and special events.

CLOSED CAPTIONS—hidden subtitles that appear on certain programs when a signal triggers a TeleCaption decoding device—enable even profoundly deaf people to understand television programs and movies. The decoders are available nationally through major mail order catalogs and in more than 900 stores.

After the first several demonstrations of closed captioned television in the early 1970s, the then-called U.S. Office of Education (now the Department of Education) supplied seed money to develop the captioning technology. In 1976, the Federal Communications Commission reserved LINE 21 in the vertical blanking interval of the TV signal for the closed caption signal; in 1978 the television networks agreed to participate in the service, provided it was run by a non-profit group. Consequently, the next year, the Education Department awarded a $6.9 million grant to help establish NCI.

The first closed captioning programs aired on March 16, 1980—*Once Upon a Classic* and *Masterpiece Theatre* (PBS), *The Wonderful World of Disney* (NBC) and *The ABC Sunday Night Movie* (ABC). Since it first aired closed captions, the institute's output has grown from an initial 16 hours of programming a week to almost 400 hours. All programs of the three major networks on prime time are now captioned.

NCI also captions 170 hours of cable programs weekly, 85 hours of syndicated programs and more than 60 local news programs. NCI has also captioned more than 300 home video movies and captions music videos and corporate training tapes.

Private support of the service has increased since 1982, when all federal funding of the program ceased. In addition, the NCI Caption Club was formed in 1983 to accept contributions toward expanding the number of closed captioned programming.

Although originally designed for a hard-of-hearing audience, NCI has expanded its market to include people learning English as a second language and people learning to read—especially students with learning disabilities. Similarly, the Annenberg/CPB

Project and NCI joined together to produce closed captioning for eight educational telecourses in 1984 that can be taken for college credit.

NCI is the sole developer, manufacturer and distributor of the consumer device needed to view captioned television, the TELECAPTION DECODER. Beginning in 1991, NCI supplied TV manufacturers with an integrated circuit chip that provided built-in decoding capacity for televisions.

Publications of NCI include its free newsletter, *CAPTION*, and a marketing memo sent to commercial advertisers and corporations. Contact: National Captioning Institute, Inc., 5203 Leesburg Pike, Falls Church, VA 22041; telephone (voice and TDD): 703-998-2400.

National Catholic Office for the Deaf

This group organizes workshops and provides information and teaching materials for the religious education of hard-of-hearing people. It also coordinates preparation programs for pastoral workers. (See also INTERNATIONAL CATHOLIC DEAF ASSOCIATION.) Contact: National Catholic Office for the Deaf, 814 Thayer Ave., Silver Spring, MD 20910; telephone: (voice) 301-587-7992, (TDD) 301-585-5084.

National Center for Law and the Deaf

Located at GALLAUDET UNIVERSITY in Washington, D.C., this group was the first national center designed to meet the needs of the deaf population. Today it provides a variety of legal services and programs for the deaf community.

The center provides free assistance to Gallaudet University students and low-income hard-of-hearing people in the Washington, D.C. area. The clinic primarily handles common legal problems (wills, immigration, consumer issues, landlord-tenant disagreements and so forth).

During the school year, law student interns—supervised by staff attorneys—work at the center, gaining valuable experience in meeting the legal and communication needs of deaf people. The law schools at both George Washington University and Catholic University offer courses in conjunction with the law center.

Since 1975, the center's attorneys have tried to eliminate discrimination caused by the communication barriers between deaf and hearing people in education, employment, health care, legal services and governmental programs. Efforts have included technical assistance with federal and state statutes and regulations dealing with interpreter services, civil rights of deaf people and the right to good mental and physical health care. Center attorneys also provide information to a variety of groups, including other lawyers, employers, schools and the federal government, on issues that affect deaf people.

Importantly, the center concentrates on the areas of television and telephone access for deaf people and was instrumental in petitioning the FCC to require all TV stations to present emergency information in visual form; it also helped the Public Broadcasting Service reserve LINE 21 to be used for closed captioning.

Interpreters are available for interviews at the center, and all staffers have been trained in sign language. In addition, the National Association for the Deaf's Legal Defense Fund maintains an office at the law center, where it represents deaf and hard-of-hearing people with discrimination complaints. (See also CLOSED CAPTIONS; LEGAL RIGHTS; NAD LEGAL DEFENSE FUND; NATIONAL ASSOCIATION OF THE DEAF.) Contact: National Center for Law and the Deaf, Gallaudet University, 800 Florida Ave. NE, Washington, D.C. 20002; telephone: (voice and TDD) 202-651-5373.

National Congress of Jewish Deaf (NCJD) This organization has served as an advocate for religious and cultural ideals and fellowship for Jewish deaf people since it was established in 1956. It serves as a clearinghouse for information about religious, educational and cultural programs for deaf Jews and represents them in projects involving nursing homes, interpreters, legal rights, demographic studies, education, sports and so forth.

Publications include the *N.C.J.D. Quarterly,* the book *Signs in Judaism* and local affiliate newsletters.

The congress maintains a Hall of Fame honoring well-known deaf Jews and has been active in the campaign against offensive signs and terms for the words "Jews" and "Jewish." It also participated in founding the World Organization of Jewish Deaf in 1977 to serve deaf Jewish people in Israel and Europe from its headquarters in Tel Aviv. In the 1960s, the organization established an endowment fund to provide for the education of deaf rabbis. The congress holds biennial conventions in major cities. In addition to regular panel discussions and business sessions, the conventions include a Miss NCJD beauty contest, teenage programs, entertainment and a Sabbath dinner, in which a Christian minister is often invited to encourage friendship between Jews and non-Jews. Contact: National Congress of Jewish Deaf, 4960 Sabal Palm Blvd., Bldg. 7, Apt. 207, Tamarac, FL 33319.

National Cued Speech Association The membership organization which provides advocacy, information and support on the use of CUED SPEECH. Members include both families and professionals in the field of deafness. The association's board of directors are geographically diverse and each regional director provides services for people in his or her area. Publications of the association include the *Cued Speech Journal* and newsletters *On Cue* and *On Cue News Flash.* Contact: National Cued Speech Association, P.O. Box 31345, Raleigh, NC 27622; telephone (voice and TDD): 919-828-1218.

National Foundation for Children's Hearing Education and Research (CHEAR) This nonprofit organization's main objective is to further the growth of medical deafness research. Founded in 1969, CHEAR raises money for research for a cure or alleviation of nerve deafness. The group also helps parents and the public understand deafness and works to improve education and educational facilities for deaf and hard-of-hearing students. For the past 20 years, CHEAR has made medical research grants and has awarded incentive scholarship prizes to hearing-impaired students. Contact: National Foundation for Children's Hearing Education and Research, 928 McLean Ave., Yonkers, NY 10704; telephone: 914-237-2676.

National Fraternal Society of the Deaf This group was founded in 1901 by a group of young deaf adults interested in forming a fraternal society solely for deaf people and in providing low-cost insurance protection denied to deaf individuals at that time. (Insurance was denied because at the beginning of the 20th century, insurers thought that deaf people didn't live very long and were prone to accidents.)

The society was incorporated as a mutual benefit organization by the state of Illinois in 1901, and by 1984 there were 106 divisions with assets totalling $9 million. Although it began strictly as a men's fraternal organization, by 1937 it was able to form social auxiliaries; in 1951 women were granted regular insurance membership.

Today, the society provides low-cost insurance to deaf and hard-of-hearing people, granting membership with the purchase of a life insurance policy. The society also insures deaf children, hearing children and grandchildren of deaf members and hearing adults involved in the field of deafness. The society holds conventions every four years and publishes a bimonthly newsletter, *The Frat.*

In addition to providing insurance, the society each year awards more than 50 savings bonds to outstanding deaf or hard-of-hearing graduates of deaf schools and 10 university scholarships to deaf students. The NFS gives annual All-American awards to outstanding deaf football and basketball players and an annual Athlete of the Year award to a deserving deaf athlete. The society also maintains a library of books and videos on deafness. Contact: National Fraternal Society of the Deaf, 1300 W. Northwest Hwy., Mt. Prospect, IL 60056; telephone (voice and TDD): 800-876-NFSD.

National Hearing Aid Society (NHAS) A professional association that represents hearing instrument specialists who test hearing and select, fit and dispense hearing instruments. It is a leading consumer advocate and conducts programs on competency qualification, education and training and promotes specialty-level accreditation for its members.

Founded in 1951 by a group of hearing instrument specialists, the society is active in promoting the highest possible standards for its members. Its directory lists members of the hearing health profession approved by the qualifications board of the society. The group also publishes a journal, *Audecibel* and provides consumer information through a toll-free helpline. Contact: National Hearing Aid Society, 20361 Middlebelt, Livonia, MI 48152; telephone (helpline): 800-521-5247.

National Index on Deafness, Speech and Hearing See DEAFNESS SPEECH AND HEARING PUBLICATIONS, INC.

National Information Center for Children and Youth with Handicaps This group collects and shares information helpful to handicapped youths, sponsors workshops and publishes newsletters. Contact: National Information Center for Children and Youth with Handicaps, P.O. Box 1492, Washington, D.C. 20013; telephone (voice and TDD): 703-893-6061.

National Information Center on Deafness Located on the campus of GALLAUDET UNIVERSITY, this unit provides information on several aspects of deafness and on the university itself. Information on careers in the field of deafness, assistive devices, hearing loss and aging, education, resource listings, reading lists and so forth is available to the public. The center maintains contact with a multitude of resources and experts at Gallaudet and around the country and shares information through ELECTRONIC MAIL networks. Contact: National Information Center on Deafness, Gallaudet University, 800 Florida Ave. NE, Washington, DC 20002; telephone: (voice) 202-651-5051, (TDD) 202-651-5052.

National Institute on Deafness and Other Communication Disorders This institute is one of the National Institutes of Health and was established in 1988 to conduct and support research and training on disorders of hearing and other communication processes. These disorders include diseases affecting hearing, balance, voice, speech, language, taste and smell.

The institute, which was established by the National Deafness and Other Communication Disorders Act of 1988 (Public Law 100-533), requires a wide range of research and development programs, including investigations in the etiology, pathology, detection, treatment and prevention of all forms of hearing disorders and evaluations of diagnosis, treatment, rehabilitation and prevention techniques. Emphasis is also placed in early detection of disorders in infants and the elderly and on exploring environmental causes of deafness. Contact: National Institute on Deafness and Other Communication Disorders, National Institutes of Health, Bldg. 31, Room 1B-62, Bethesda, MD 20892; telephone: (voice) 301-496-7243, (TDD) 301-402-0018.

National Institute for Hearing Instruments Studies (NIHIS) The educational division of the NATIONAL HEARING AID SOCIETY, NIHIS accredits educational programs in the hearing instrument sciences as offered by approved providers or the institute.

National Rehabilitation Information Center A rehabilitation information service and research library that provides reference, research and referral services, conducts custom database searches, publishes a quarterly newsletter *NARIC Quarterly,* and disseminates rehabilitation-related information. The center offers a database called REHABDATA, a computerized listing of rehabilitation literature. Contact: National Rehabilitation Information Center, 8455 Colesville Road, Suite 935, Silver Spring, MD 20910; telephone (voice and TDD): 301-588-9284.

National Research Register for Heredity Hearing Loss A clearinghouse for people interested in research on hereditary hearing loss. The register informs participating families of new research projects applicable to them and updates all families on the progress of ongoing research through its newsletter. Contact: National Research Register for Heredity Hearing Loss, Boys Town National Research Hospital, 555 30th St., Omaha, NE 68154; telephone (voice and TDD): 402-498-6631.

National Technical Institute for the Deaf (NTID) This school is the world's largest technological college for deaf students and was established in 1965 in Rochester, New York. It is a federally-funded institution located on the campus of the Rochester Institute of Technology (RIT).

The institute's 2,100 deaf students may select from courses in 34 programs in business, computer science, engineering technology, photography and printing. The institute is one of nine colleges of RIT, sharing campus facilities, library, bookstore and athletic areas. Students may also pursue a bachelor's or master's degree in other colleges at RIT, including the Colleges of Applied Science and Technology, Business, Engineering, Fine and Applied Arts, Graphic Arts and Photography and Liberal Arts. Nearly 20% of RIT's deaf students are enrolled in another college of RIT.

Instructors at NTID use SIGN LANGUAGE, speech and FINGERSPELLING, and students may use whatever communication mode they prefer. Although instructors in other RIT courses don't use sign language, professional interpreters and trained notetakers are available. Deaf students may also obtain interpreters for student activities, counseling, theater, sports, religious services and cultural events.

The school was established with the National Technical Institute for the Deaf Act (PL 89-36), which created the school and provided that the institute must be established within a school that already existed. The law defined NTID as a postsecondary educational and residential institution with a range of basic responsibilities. The Rochester Institute of Technology was selected as the host school by a national advisory board from among 20 applicants.

Applicants to NTID must be U.S. citizens with an overall achievement level of eighth grade with good grades and have a hearing loss of 70 dB or greater without a hearing aid in the better ear.

In addition to educating deaf students, NTID cooperates with other institutions in deafness research and offers a range of programs to improve the quality of deaf education in the United States. In addition, RIT and the University of Rochester cosponsor a graduate program that qualifies secondary school educators to work with deaf people.

A placement program is offered for NTID graduates, 95% of whom find jobs upon graduation. NTID also staffs the National Center on Employment of the Deaf, which assists both employers and deaf people seeking jobs.

national temporal bone banks This program, administered by the Deafness Research Foundation, maintains four regional centers serving more than 100 hospitals in seeking the bequest of internal auditory structures from individuals with ear disorders for research and specialist training. Contact: Deafness Research Foundation, 9 E. 38th St., New York, NY 10016; telephone: 800-535-DEAF.

National Theatre of the Deaf (NTD) A professional ensemble of deaf and hearing actors, this theater company uses mime, body language and SIGN LANGUAGE augmented by reverse interpretation of the signs for hearing audiences. Founded in 1970, the company has given more than 5,000 performances of classical repertory as well as original works in 24 countries.

The company's 14 professional actors put on a new play each fall and go on tour for 27 weeks to the major theaters of the world; it is the only theatrical company to have performed in all 50 states. The NTD has appeared on many TV specials and on *Sesame Street* and received a Tony Award in 1977 for theatrical excellence. In 1984, the group represented the United States at the Los Angeles Olympics Arts Festival, and in 1986 it became the first Western theater company to tour the People's Republic of China.

Most of the actors are deaf, and the cast takes English scripts and translates them into a theatrical form of sign language, which may also include new signs created to express a dramatic point. Two hearing actors also translate orally for the primarily-hearing audiences who come to the shows.

In addition to formal performances, the company supports the LITTLE THEATRE OF THE DEAF for young audiences and presents numerous workshops and lecture-demonstrations. The company also supports a professional theater school during the summer to teach deaf individuals basic and advanced theater skills at the company's headquarters in Chester, Connecticut.

The National Theatre of the Deaf is located at the Hazel E. Stark Center, a converted mill and residence housing offices, rehearsal space, classrooms and theater shops. Funding for the theater comes from grants, gifts, performances and the Media Services and Captioned Films section of the Office of Education. (See also PROFESSIONAL SCHOOL FOR DEAF THEATRE PERSONNEL.) Contact: The National Theatre of the Deaf, P.O. Box 659, Chester, CT 06412; telephone: (voice) 203-526-4971, (TDD) 203-526-4974.

Navarrete, Juan Fernandez de (1526–1579) Also known as "El Mudo" (the mute), Juan Fernandez de Navarrete was born in Spain and became deaf at age three from unknown causes. As a child, he began to draw as a way of communicating and received his first art lessons in his hometown of Logrono. Eventually he was sent to study art in Italy upon his teacher's recommendation.

He toured the primary cities of Italy, studying art as he went, until King Phillip II of Spain summoned him to Madrid, where he became the most important of the group of Spanish and Italian painters commissioned to work in the famed monastery and royal palace of the Escorial.

A member of the Madrid school, El Mudo painted during a time of transition in the Spanish art world. He was the first to abandon the mannerist movement, which had begun in the 16th century, and was the bridge to the naturalists of the 17th century. Almost all of his paintings are religious in nature; those that remain at the cloister of the Escorial hang in the gallery of the upper cloister.

El Mudo died on March 28, 1579, in Toledo, Spain before completing his commission to paint the pictures for 30 altars in the Basilica of the Escorial.

neonatal hearing screening programs See AUDIOMETRY.

nerve deafness See SENSORINEURAL HEARING LOSS.

Netherlands About 3.4% of this population of 14.4 million is hard-of-hearing, and about 28,000 of these are deaf, representing a fairly low rate of deafness.

There are five state educational centers for deaf students, including preschool, elementary and vocational training, with varied programs offering day and residential, oral and TOTAL COMMUNICATION approaches. Few students are mainstreamed or are educated beyond high school.

The oral approach has been the basis of social interchange in the Netherlands from preschool to adult aftercare programs, but more and more experts are beginning to acknowledge the value of the manual.

Adult deaf people communicate with a blended form of Signed Dutch, DUTCH SIGN LANGUAGE and lip movements.

neural prosthesis See COCHLEAR IMPLANT.

newborn screening programs Because the prevalence of hearing problems in newborns is low (one in 1,000), seven high-risk categories have been created to identify newborns at risk for hearing problems.

These categories include neonatal asphyxia (suffocation), bacterial MENINGITIS, infection at birth (syphilis, toxoplasmosis, bacterial infection), rubella, and various herpes viruses; defects of the head or neck (such as cleft palate or malformations of the PINNA); severe jaundice (yellowing of the skin caused by excess bilirubin) requiring transfusion; family history of childhood hearing loss; and low birth weight.

Among high-risk infants, chances of having congenital hearing problems is between one out of 20 to one out of 50. Initial screening of these infants usually includes use of the AUDITORY BRAINSTEM RESPONSE TEST (ABR). (See also HIGH RISK QUESTIONNAIRE.)

New Zealand This tiny country of only three million people includes a scattered deaf population of 1,690 deaf and hard-of-hearing students in various types of classes, programs and schools.

The first state oral school for deaf students in the world was opened in 1880 by Gerrit Van Asch, whose work was praised by ALEXANDER GRAHAM BELL. Beginning in the 1940s, a host of changes were introduced: free hearing aids, formal teacher training, nursery school and guidance programs for parents and students.

Since 1960, educators for deaf students in New Zealand have tried to develop new, expanded services, serving classes for deaf children in ordinary elementary and high schools with special teachers and for students mainstreamed in regular classes. They have also developed two state residential schools. Further, the schools for deaf students are affiliated with polytechnic colleges and community colleges; they also send deaf students to regular universities.

As in many European countries, New Zealand for many years favored the oral approach; today, it has modified this approach to include TOTAL COMMUNICATION with a standardized SIGN LANGUAGE system (the Australian or Victorian) and two-handed FINGERSPELLING.

Because of the country's small size, no one school limits itself to one communication mode but consults with parents in deciding which method to use with each individual child.

Although many deaf people in New Zealand are not hired in positions that fully utilize their abilities, the increased availability of further education has raised the standard of living for deaf people.

Because the school system relied on oral instruction for many years, no formal sign language system was developed. Most deaf New Zealanders do communicate with signs they originated, but no fingerspelling is used. With the introduction of Total Communication, two-handed fingerspelling and a wide range of signs has been introduced.

nicotine and hearing loss Nicotine, a known vasoconstrictor, inhibits the flow of blood throughout the body by narrowing blood vessels, including those to the ear.

Nicotine can cause TINNITUS in addition to hearing loss. Also, research suggests that smokers have a higher failure rate following MYRINGOPLASTY (reconstruction of the eardrum), one of the least dangerous and simplest operations of the ear.

Nigeria The exact number of deaf people in Nigeria is difficult to ascertain since there has been no census of this population, but it is estimated that there are about 70,000 deaf citizens out of a population of 80 million. About 7,000 of these are believed to be between six and 18 years of age.

Too often in this country, deafness in children is unnoticed or ignored by illiterate parents; many infants are born at home, and physicians may rarely see these children. In addition, the society looks negatively at deaf children and their parents, and therefore many are hidden away. Because most cases of deafness occur after birth and during adolescence or adulthood, many deaf Nigerians can learn to speak fairly well.

Today, there are 20 schools for deaf students in addition to special classes in regular schools, and about 50 deaf Nigerian students study in the United States each year. Most schools use the American MANUAL ALPHABET and SIGN LANGUAGE.

noise One of the most prevalent—and preventable—causes of deafness in the United States, exposure to excessive noise levels accounts for 10 million of the 28 million Americans with HEARING LOSS.

Hearing occurs when sound enters the outer ear, striking the eardrum; vibrations move deep inside the inner ear where they pass over 30,000 microscopic hair-like cells, which convert vibrations into the electrical signals the brain can interprete.

Damage to hearing from excess noise occurs primarily in the COCHLEA, overloading the tiny, irreplaceable "hair cells," and possibly resulting in a sensory hearing loss. In addition, excess noise can reduce enzymes and energy sources in the cochlear fluids and change the structure of the cochlear mechanism, which provides most of the nourishment to the hair cells.

As exposure to noise continues, stress on the hair cells increases, the tiny hairs on top of the cells become fused together, the hair cells disintegrate, and finally the nerve fibers to the hair cells disappear. At this point, since hair cells do not regenerate, damage is permanent.

In the case of acoustic trauma—a sudden, sharp, very loud noise—the entire mechanical INNER EAR system vibrates so violently that its attachments are disrupted, membranes in the cochlea may rupture, and hair cells are torn from the BASILAR MEMBRANE. The rupture of the cochlea membranes results in a mixing of ear fluids that poisons any hair cells that were not destroyed in the initial blast.

Most sounds (other than acoustic trauma) that can produce lasting damage are high-intensity noises that occur over a long period of time—eight hours a day for more than ten years, for example. Such noise-induced hearing loss is quite common, for example, among rock musicians and disc jockeys.

While it's generally true that the younger a person is, the better the hearing, almost all adults in this country notice some decrease in hearing ability by age 30; by age 65 at least one out of six Americans has a severe hearing loss.

Recent research has uncovered an astonishing loss of hearing acuity among students: 4% of sixth graders, 10% of high school students and 61% of college freshmen tested all showed hearing problems. Conversely, studies have found that natives in the African jungle—exposed to no excess noise at all—show almost no decrease in hearing acuity as they age.

Studies have indicated that hearing loss in the workplace begins once noise exceeds 80 dB, although there is not a significant effect until noise reaches 90 dB. Although studies indicate that continual exposure to 90 dB noise will result in a hearing loss of about

Range of Sounds Audible to Humans

Typical Decibel	Example
0	Lowest sound audible to the human ear.
30	Quiet library, soft whisper.
40	Living room, quiet office, bedroom away from traffic.
50	Light traffic at a distance, refrigerator, gentle breeze.
60	Air conditioner at 20 feet, conversation, sewing machine.
70	Busy traffic, office tabulator, noisy restaurant. At this decibel level, noise may begin to affect hearing if exposure is constant.
	The Hazardous Zone
80	Subway, heavy city traffic, alarm clock at two feet, factory noise. These noises are dangerous if exposure to them lasts for more than eight hours.
90	Truck traffic, noisy home appliances, shop tools, lawn mower. As loudness increases, the ''safe'' time exposure decreases; damage can occur in less than eight hours.
100	Chain saw, stereo headphones, pneumatic drill. Even two hours of exposure can be dangerous at this decibel level; with each 5 dB increase the safe time is cut *in half.*
120	Rock band concert in front of speakers, sandblasting, thunderclap. The danger is immediate; exposure at 120 dB can injure ears.
140	Gunshot blast, jet plane. *Any* length of exposure time is dangerous; noise at this level may cause actual pain in the ear.
180	Rocket launching pad. Without ear protection, noise at this level causes irreversible damage; hearing loss is inevitable.

Source: American Academy of Otolaryngology; © 1983.

15 dB, it does not mean that everyone who works in this environment at 90 dB will have the same loss; some workers' ears will remain healthy while others might incur a hearing loss of over 30 dB. This is because hearing loss is also related to noise environment outside of work, which can vary a great deal.

It is also possible that noise-induced hearing loss can be made much worse by certain OTOTOXIC DRUGS that, if taken in the presence of excess noise, could harm an ear it would otherwise leave unaffected. So far, efforts to link noise damage with smoking, diet, posture and social drugs have failed.

At this time, the only way to protect the ears against damage from noise in excess of 80 dB for eight hours a day is to wear protective ear devices, such as ear plugs or earmuffs. (See also EAR PROTECTORS; OCCUPATIONAL HEARING LOSS; NOISE CONTROL LAWS.)

noise blocker Also called an automatic signal processor, these are innovative devices operating on the theory that most noise occurs at low pitch; consequently, they are designed to pick up the low pitch sounds and automatically reduce their noise level.

However, if the wearer's speech discrimination is poor, the noise blockers may not help, particularly if the noise is coming from large groups of people talking.

noise control laws Legislation aimed at controlling noise in public, first enacted in 1968 by the U.S. Congress as part of its amendment to the Federal Aviation Act. One year later, Congress included hearing-conservation rules for plants with federal contracts as part of the Walsh-Healy Act.

Unusual in its inclusion of safety provisions for private enterprise, the regulations paved the way for the Occupational Health and Safety Act of 1970 that brought together a host of safety regulations in industry. Included in the act was section 1910.95, which applied the noise regulations of the Walsh-Haley Act to all workers in all industries.

The law required industry to define areas in their plants where noise exceeded an equivalent of 90 dBA for an eight-hour workday; each time noise level increases 5 dBA, the allowable exposure time is cut in half.

If possible, noise in areas of excessive noise should be lowered; if workers' hearing can't be protected by limiting the exposure or the level of the noise, then the law requires they be protected by provision either of protective hearing devices or annual hearing tests to identify people experiencing progressive hearing loss.

The 1970 legislation was followed two years later by the Noise Control Act, which gave the Environmental Protection Agency power over federal regulatory action in noise control. However, the labor department maintained control over the Occupational Safety and Health Administration, and the Federal Aviation Agency retained authority over aircraft noise regulatory action.

noise exposure and hearing loss See NOISE.

nonhuman signing Manual communication taught to nonhumans (typically apes) in an attempt to teach these animals language.

The earliest attempts to teach apes to communicate focused on speech rather than SIGN LANGUAGE. Although years of research occasionally produced an ape that could utter one or two words, forcing the apes to produce vocal human speech was doomed from the start because of the different vocal apparatus between the species.

The first successful attempt at teaching apes communication came in 1966, when two researchers, R. Allen and B.T. Gardner, taught their 10-month old chimpanzee, Washoe, AMERICAN SIGN LANGUAGE (ASL). They began Washoe's training by raising her in the social environment of their own family, living with humans by day and in a separate house trailer at night. In addition, Washoe could play in the back yard with a sandbox, gym and a large tree.

Since chimps lack the ability to produce speech and because in the wild they use gestures to communicate, the Gardners chose to teach Washoe ASL because it was a gestural and human language.

In Washoe's first four years, she acquired more than 130 signs, using them spontaneously and in correct context. She carried on everyday conversations, initiated conversation and commented to and questioned her human companions. She could ask about friends who were not there and generalized her signs to a variety of uses. For example, she would sign "dog" not just for a real dog but for photos of dogs and sounds of barking dogs.

Further study with Washoe looked at the capacity of chimps to use cross-modal transfer between auditory words and visual signs. Researchers also compared individual differences between chimps, generic and specific use of signs, comprehension, use of prepositional phrases and the conceptual use of signs.

Still, the Gardners' research with Washoe was criticized in the late 1970s by people who argued that the conclusions of the Gardners and others were false because the evidence was ambiguous, suggesting that the Gardners wanted to believe Washoe could sign and were therefore biased, and that scientists inadvertently cued the chimp. Critics also charged that the form and structure of the ape's signs showed no resemblance to ASL.

In 1978, researchers tried to design a study to answer critics, stopping all signs around the chimp except for seven signs: who, what, want, which, where, sign and name. Researchers believed if Washoe's infants acquired sign language, it was because they had learned it from her.

After Washoe's first infant died, a 10-month-old male was given to her to adopt. Eight days later, little Loulis used his first sign: "person." At 15 months, he started using two-sign combinations, and five years later, he used 54 different signs—all learned from Washoe and signing chimp friends. Loulis was therefore the first chimp to acquire human language from another chimp.

In 1980, three new chimps were raised in their early years at the Gardners' house, intended for testing in cross-chimp communication. To control the use of human signing, the chimps were videotaped and observed on monitors from a separate room in 20-minute segments three times a day for 15 days, thereby restricting access to their human caretakers.

In the 15 hours taped, 617 chimp conversations were recorded. Together with research from another study examining many more conversations, scientists found that almost 90% of these chimp "conversations" centered around play, reassurance and social interactions. Only 5% had to do with food.

nonmanual behaviors The features of AMERICAN SIGN LANGUAGE that are not portrayed with the hands. These include facial expression, head and body movement and posture.

nonorganic hearing loss See FUNCTIONAL HEARING LOSS (NONORGANIC).

nonsuppurative otitis media See SEROUS OTITIS MEDIA.

nonverbal communication Nonverbal communication includes tone of voice and noises, shrugs, body position, facial expressions and gestures to enrich and modify speech. Hearing people generally assume this nonverbal communication is inferior to speech, because it is less variable and not a systematic form of language.

SIGN LANGUAGE, however, is *not* a form of nonverbal communication. Deaf people use nonverbal communication in much the same way hearing people do. The reason why sign languages have often been misclassified as nonverbal systems of communication is probably because their form is visual-gestural, which is also the most common form of nonverbal communication among hearing people.

North American Basic Teletext Specification Also known as NABTS, this is the teletext system that provides CLOSED CAPTIONS similar to those offered by the LINE 21 type of closed captioning.

Teletext systems use several lines of the vertical blanking interval to send closed captions to TV sets equipped with a teletext decoder (different from the TELECAPTION DECODER needed for decoding line 21 captioning).

The only television network that offers both teletext and line 21 closed captions is CBS-TV. (See also CAPTION CENTER; NATIONAL CAPTIONING INSTITUTE.)

Northhampton vowel and consonant charts A printed system to help deaf children learn to speak, read and write syntactically correct sentences.

Devised in 1884, the system uses alphabet symbols to describe English pronunciation and was first used for teaching how sounds and words were related in reading. It is now more commonly used to help develop speech.

Norwegian Sign Language There are three major sign dialects of Norwegian Sign Language (NSL), spoken by about 4,000 deaf Norwegians, which originate with the three schools for the deaf.

In these schools, teachers use a manual code for Norwegian called Signed Norwegian, together with speech in addition to signs. As is typical around the world, Norwegian students use SIGN LANGUAGE when speaking among themselves outside of school.

In addition to NSL, the INTERNATIONAL MANUAL ALPHABET developed by the WORLD CONGRESS OF THE DEAF and considered to be the best system for deaf-blind people, has been used since 1970.

Since the 1970s, there has been a growing demand for the use of NSL in education by the deaf community.

Unlike AMERICAN SIGN LANGUAGE, NSL vocabulary uses almost no fingerspelled signs. It does, however, emphasize the use of lip movements of spoken words.

O

occupational hearing loss A number of industrial environments produce enough noise to impair hearing. In part, this occurs because although noise above 90 decibels can harm hearing, a person can work in the presence of noise up to 120 dB before it begins to be painful.

At the end of a day in the presence of 90 dB noise, there might be slight ringing or muffling of noises, but after an evening or weekend away from the noise, these symptoms would be gone. A person tested after working all day in the presence of 120 dB noise might show a slight loss of hearing, but after a few days away from the job, a retest would show hearing has returned to normal. This is called a temporary THRESHOLD shift.

After several months of this type of exposure, the hearing loss becomes permanent. A worker probably would not notice work-induced hearing loss because the deficits show up first among the high frequencies, which interferes very little with the understanding of speech. Not until the loss worsens and begins to affect the middle frequencies would a hearing loss be noticed. By that time, the loss could be permanent. A person does not become "used" to working around noise; if after some months or years the noise seems less noticeable, it is only because a hearing loss has already occurred.

Jobs that put workers at risk for hearing loss include boilermaking, weaving, aircraft maintenance, blacksmithing, chipping, riveting, blasting, machine manufacturing, metalworking and loud rock music production. Also at risk are people employed in any job involving large presses, high-pressure steam, large wood saws and heavy hammering (such as iron and steel working).

People involved in work around noisy machinery should understand that if it is necessary to raise the voice to be heard by someone less than two feet away, protective devices should be worn. A person working in an environment this noisy should have a hearing test once a year and always wear EAR PROTECTORS or find other employment. (See also NOISE; OCCUPATIONAL HEALTH AND SAFETY ACT.)

Occupational Health and Safety Act An essential requirement of this act is that any industry in which employees are exposed daily to continuous noise levels greater than 90 decibels for an eight-hour working day over many years must either reduce the noise or protect the hearing of exposed workers.

The 90 dBA level specified is the level at which conservation of hearing should begin. Occupations that pose a risk to hearing include boilermaking, weaving, aircraft maintenance, blacksmithing, chipping, riveting, blasting, machine manufacturing and metal-working, as well as any job using large presses, high-pressure steam, large wood saws or heavy hammering (such as in iron and steel works). Persons involved in the production of loud rock music are also at risk of a permanent hearing loss.

on-the-body hearing aids See BODY HEARING AID.

open captions Ordinary subtitles that appear on films (such as foreign films with English subtitles) and that are available for everyone to see. These are the opposite of CLOSED CAPTIONS, which are visible only to people with special decoding devices.

oral approach A communication method that stresses the use of speech among deaf and hard-of-hearing people together with SPEECHREADING and auditory training as a way of merging with the hearing world.

The roots of the oral approach may be traced to the 1500s, when a Spanish monk named PEDRO PONCE DE LEON taught the deaf children of nobility at his monastery. Using his own methods, he taught the children to use language, speech and speech-reading. His methods were handed on to other Spanish teachers of deaf children at the end of the 16th century, including Manual Ramirez de Carrion. At about the same time, JUAN PABLO BONET published what was the first book describing oral teaching methods for deaf students.

Gradually, the oral method movement spread throughout Europe and found a special home in Germany in the 18th century, where SAMUEL HEINICKE became its leading proponent. Heinicke, a devout oral proponent, opened the first German school for deaf students in 1778. At the same time in England, the Braidwood family headed by THOMAS BRAIDWOOD was opening oralist schools for deaf children using its own secret methods of instruction.

In 1819 American educator THOMAS HOPKINS GALLAUDET came to the Braidwoods to learn the oralist tradition. When the Braidwoods refused to reveal their methods to Gallaudet, he went on to France to learn the manual method, which he subsequently brought back to the United States.

The MANUAL APPROACH was the sole method of instruction for deaf students up until the mid-1800s, when the Clarke School opened in Northampton, Massachusetts. From then on, aided by the European success of oralist education, the tide began to change in the United States, and from 1880 to 1930 oralism replaced the manual approach as the primary method of instruction. After World War I, about 75% of American deaf pupils were taught almost entirely by the oral method.

As time went on, however, schools began combining their methods; elementary students were taught orally, with signs used in some classes in high school. But studies in the 1960s and 1970s found that the educational achievement of deaf children educated orally fell short of their hearing peers and that students taught in sign from the beginning generally functioned at a higher level.

The 200-year debate over the oral and manual methods centers on the place in society in which a deaf person should fit. Those who supported the Oral Approach in this country were generally opposed to the segregation of deaf people and did not approve of special camps, churches or social organizations. Critics of the oral approach, on the other hand, believed in maintaining deaf culture and in making accommodations in communication and social organizations.

Oral supporters (whose chief champion was ALEXANDER GRAHAM BELL) promote the use of hearing aids, speechreading and speech as the right of all deaf children and do not favor the use of sign language in schools. In fact, for many years, sign language was forbidden in oral schools. This objection to sign is primarily because proponents of the oral method believe it is too difficult to learn two languages at once (speech and sign). However, not all object to sign language as a means of communication *outside* the school.

There are also differences of opinions among oral method supporters over auditory, multisensory or CUED SPEECH teaching methods. The first method uses auditory training and specialized training that does not emphasize speechreading.

The multisensory teaching method is more traditional, encouraging students to use speechreading, body language or tactile methods to communicate. Some multi-sensory programs also permit the use of FINGERSPELLING.

Cued Speech supporters believe in the Cued Speech system, which supplements what a person hears with a hearing aid, a combined form of speechreading and hand cues. (See also TOTAL COMMUNICATION; SIMULTANEOUS COMMUNICATION.)

Oral Deaf Adults Section (ODAS) A service organization, this group was formed in 1964 as part of the ALEXANDER GRAHAM BELL ASSOCIATION FOR THE DEAF. Its members choose to communicate through spoken language and SPEECHREADING and have joined together to encourage the oral-aural approach in educating deaf children. Supporters of the oral approach believe students can learn to communicate effectively using speech, speechreading and auditory training.

The section was founded by H. LATHAM BREUNIG and ROBERT H. WEITBRECHT, the developer of teletypewriters (TTYs) for deaf people. It publishes a membership directory and a newsletter for members, offers educational scholarships and plans outings for families with deaf children.

The group maintains its own member speakers' bureau in order to portray these deaf adults as role models for younger deaf people.

oral interpreters Persons skilled in the specialized interpreting ability of translating the meaning of spoken words by silently mouthing a speaker's words for a deaf person who prefers the oral approach. Oral interpreters use no sign language and are skilled in substituting words for those that are difficult to speechread. However, oral interpreters are used by only a very few deaf people.

Oral interpreters are also available to repeat to a hearing audience a spoken message from a deaf person whose speech may not be clear. They use a variety of skills and techniques to convey the message and emotions of the speaker; these are most helpful when the person with a hearing loss does not use sign language.

An oral interpreter may not be the best interpreter for a person who uses listening skills and SPEECHREADING since it is difficult to watch an oral interpreter while listening to the speaker. Because of the delay between the sound of the speaker's voice and lip movements of the oral interpreter, the oral interpreter is always several words behind the speaker.

Oral interpreters are certified by the REGISTRY OF INTERPRETERS FOR THE DEAF, the only national professional organization in the United States that certifies both oral and SIGN LANGUAGE interpreters. The registry lists interpreters in various specialties, including legal, medical and educational interpreting. In 1979, the registry established a separate certification process for oral interpreters similar to the one for sign language interpreters. Three oral interpreting certifications are awarded by the registry: Two for different levels of accuracy by hearing candidates and one for candidates with hearing problems.

Oral interpreters are listed with local and state chapters of the Registry of Interpreters for the Deaf, local speech and hearing centers, the Office of Vocational Rehabilitation, the ALEXANDER GRAHAM BELL ASSOCIATION FOR THE DEAF, a school or college with support services for hard-of-hearing students and programs and agencies serving hard-of-hearing people.

A hard-of-hearing person does not have to pay for oral interpreters under several conditions. For example, Section 504 of the Rehabilitation Act of 1973 requires that interpreting services for hard-of-hearing people must be provided free for all meetings, classes and other group activities sponsored by an agency that receives federal funds and has 15 or more employees. In an educational setting, the Education for All Handicapped Children Act of 1975 (PL 94-142) requires that the services of an interpreter must be written into a student's individual educational plan. Such an interpreter service would then be paid for by the child's school. At the same time, hard-of-hearing or deaf parents must also be given an interpreter for parent/teacher conferences and meetings. In addition, federal law requires the federal court to appoint a qualified interpreter in criminal or civil actions against a hard-of-hearing person, and the court must provide an oral interpreter if so requested. Most states also pay for an interpreter in criminal proceedings; several pay for an interpreter in civil cases as well. (See also INTERPRETERS AND THE LAW.)

organ of Corti The organ of Corti is contained in the COCHLEA and is the most important part of the hearing process.

The organ is covered with many fine hairs arranged like the strings of a harp, with the shorter, thinner hairs picking up high sounds and the longer, thicker hairs picking up low sounds. When a sound wave makes the eardrum vibrate, the vibrations are carried across the middle ear by the hammer, the anvil and the stirrup, which pass the vibrations through the oval window to the fluid in the tubes of the inner ear.

This makes the hairs of the organ of Corti vibrate; the more hairs that vibrate, the louder the sound. The AUDITORY NERVE picks up the message from these hairs and sends it to the brain, where the sound is processed.

osseous labyrinth See LABYRINTH, INNER EAR.

ossicles The three small bones of the MIDDLE EAR (the malleus or hammer, the incus or anvil and the stapes or stirrup) that help carry sound and speech from the eardrum to the inner ear. (See also OSSICULAR CHAIN.)

ossicular chain Attached to the eardrum is a chain of three small bones called the ossicular chain. Located in the pea-sized middle ear cavity, the ossicles are the smallest bones in the human body and are full size when a child is born.

The individual bones are smaller than a grain of rice: the bone attached to the eardrum is the malleus (hammer); the second bone is the incus (anvil); and the third is the stapes (stirrup). As sound waves move the eardrum, it moves the ossicles. The three bones actually serve as a type of level that transfers the energy of the sound waves from the outer ear through the MIDDLE EAR into the INNER EAR.

ossicular interruption A separation of the three tiny ossicles that carry sound vibrations from the eardrum membrane to the fluid inside the inner ear. It is caused by an infection or by a blow to the head.

The separation usually occurs at the weakest point of the OSSICULAR CHAIN, where the anvil (incus) joins the stirrup (stapes). A partial separation causes mild hearing impairment; a more complete separation results in a severe hearing loss.

Ossicular interruption can be diagnosed by hearing tests that indicate the hearing nerve in the inner ear is normal but sound is not being conducted from the eardrum to the inner ear.

Treatment of ossicular interruption is one of the most successful operations to restore hearing—performed by an otolaryngologist, it involves repositioning the ossicles so they can again conduct sound. (See also OSSICULOPLASTY.)

ossiculoplasty Surgical repair of the middle-ear OSSICLES to treat hearing loss, usually caused by chronic OTITIS MEDIA or CHOLESTEATOMA or a temporal bone fracture. Ossiculoplasty may be combined with MYRINGOPLASTY or MASTOIDECTOMY. (See also OSSICULAR INTERRUPTION; TYMPANOPLASTY.)

osteitis deformans see PAGET'S DISEASE.

osteogenesis imperfecta A bone disorder causing the entire skeleton to have brittle bones with many fractures. About half of these patients have a syndrome called van der Hoeve's syndrome, in which there is a conductive hearing loss and a blue tinge to the whites of the eyes. It is believed that this syndrome is caused by a disease similar to OTOSCLEROSIS, which causes the STAPES (stirrup) footplate to adhere to surrounding bone. The conductive hearing loss occurs because of fractures in the stapes.

osteoma An osteoma of the ear canal is a bony knob close to the eardrum, occurring particularly in people who swim frequently in cold water. Unless the growth blocks the ear canal and therefore interferes with hearing, it does not need to be removed.

otic capsule The bony case enclosing the inner ear. Part of the otic capsule forms the inner wall of the middle ear.

otitis externa See SWIMMER'S EAR.

otitis media An infection of the MIDDLE EAR (the cavity between the eardrum and the INNER EAR) that can produce pus or fluid and cause hearing loss. The inflammation can occur as the result of an infection extending up the eustachian tube, the passage that connects the back of the nose to the middle ear. This tube may become blocked by the infection or by enlarged adenoids (often associated with infections of the nose and throat). Fluid produced by the inflammation can't drain off through the tube and instead collects in the middle ear.

Acute otitis media causes sudden, severe earache, deafness, TINNITUS (ringing or buzzing in the ear), sense of fullness in the ear and fever. Occasionally, the eardrum can burst, which causes a discharge of pus and relief of pain; a physician will sometimes incise the eardrum (MYRINGOTOMY) to relieve pressure. Chronic otitis media is usually caused by repeated attacks of acute otitis media, with pus seeping from a perforation in the eardrum together with some degree of deafness. Complications include otitis externa (inflammation of the outer ear), damage to the bones in the middle ear (sometimes causing total deafness) or a CHOLESTEATOMA (a matted ball of skin debris which can erode bone and cause further damage to the ear). Rarely, infection can spread *inward* from an infected ear and cause a brain abscess.

Otitis media can be detected by examining the ear with an instrument called an OTOSCOPE. A sample of discharge may be taken to identify the organism responsible for the infection.

Acute otitis media usually clears up completely with treatment with antibiotic drugs, although there may occasionally be continual production of a sticky fluid in the middle ear known as persistent middle ear infection. Deafness can occur, but usually disappears with treatment. Otitis media is treated with antibiotics (usually penicillins) and analgesics for pain. A physician may also remove pus and skin debris and prescribe antibiotic ear drops, if necessary. Ephedrine nose drops can help establish drainage of the ear in children.

Children, probably because of the shortness of their eustachian tubes, are particularly prone to otitis media. About one in six infants under age one suffers from this problem, and some children have recurrent attacks through age 10. Chronic otitis media is much less common because most cases of acute ear infection clear up after treatment.

otolaryngologist Also called otorhinolaryngologists, or ear, nose and throat (ENT) physicians, an otolaryngologist is a medical/surgical specialist who treats ear, nose and throat problems ranging from common conditions (such as ear infections and minor hearing loss) to more complex problems like MÉNIÈRE'S DISEASE and OTOSCLEROSIS. Otolaryngologists are also sometimes referred to as head-and-neck surgeons.

In addition, otolaryngologists are expert in the diagnosis and testing of different types of hearing loss. This specialist can advise whether a hearing aid will help, and if so, what kind would be suitable.

To qualify for the American Board of Otolaryngology certification examination, a physician must complete five or more years of post-M.D. specialty training in otolaryngology.

otolaryngology A specialty medical field concerned with treatment and surgery of the ear, nose, and throat and related structures of the head and neck.

It includes cosmetic facial reconstruction, surgery of benign and malignant tumors of the head and neck, management of patients with loss of hearing and balance, endoscopic examination of air and food passages and treatment of allergic, sinus, laryngeal, thyroid and esophaegeal disorders. (See OTOLARYNGOLOGIST.)

otologist A physician specialist primarily interested in diagnosing ear diseases, specifying causes of hearing loss and treating physical defects of the auditory mechanism. Otology is one division of the ear, nose and throat field (OTOLARYNGOLOGY) of medicine. An otologist may work together with an audiologist (a specialist in hearing tests). (See OTOLARYNGOLOGIST.)

otology The branch of medicine concerned with the ear. As in many other fields of medicine, the roots of the practice of otology began well before recorded history, although actual surgery on the ear did not begin before the 18th century.

Some of the first descriptions of early otology are found in the *Ebers Papyrus,* written about 1600 B.C., in which Egyptian priests specialized in ear treatments. These treatments might include injections into the ear of olive oil, red lead, bat's wings, ant eggs or goat's urine. By the fifth century, Pythagoras was exploring the physics of sound; he constructed a musical scale by listening to different pitches that occurred when a blacksmith struck his anvil with different hammers.

It was in the 19th century that modern otology began, with the surgical advances of Sir Astley Cooper in London who cut into the eardrum to ease certain cases of deafness. Parisian surgeon Gaspard Itard explored the diseases of the ear while MARIE-JEAN-PIERRE FLOURENS discussed the action of the SEMICIRCULAR CANALS and realized that the acoustic nerve has branches for hearing and for balance. By 1860, Prosper Meniere reported the case of a girl with VERTIGO, nausea and TINNITUS during a fatal illness, and in 1851 ALFONSO CORTI, an Italian anatomist, published his studies about the organ that now bears his name.

otorhinolaryngology The full name of the surgical specialty focusing on diseases of the ear, nose and throat. (See also OTOLARYNGOLOGY.)

otorrhea The medical term for a discharge from the ear. This is usually fluid resulting from an ear infection, although it can include blood or cerebrospinal fluid following a skull fracture. A physician should evaluate any case of otorrhea.

otosclerosis Also called otospongiosis, a disorder that occurs when an overgrowth of spongy bone immobilizes the stapes (the innermost bone of the middle ear), preventing sound vibrations from passing to the inner ear and resulting in CONDUCTIVE HEARING LOSS. In most cases, both ears are usually affected. It is caused by the absorption of bone followed by the production of new, loose "spongy" bone. Eventually, this soft bone will harden and eventually become as dense as surrounding bone.

While the problem can occur anywhere on the temporal bone, it usually begins in front of the oval window, gradually spreading to the oval window and then the footplate of the stapes. Eventually, this will imbed the stapes to the surrounding tissue, restricting stapedal movement. In addition, otosclerosis can affect the cochlea, causing a sensorineural hearing loss.

The disease, which begins in early adulthood (between age 20 and 30) and is more common among women, affects about one in every 200 people and often occurs during pregnancy. People with otosclerosis tend to talk softly and hear muffled sound more clearly when there is background noise. Hearing loss progresses slowly over a period of 10 to 15 years, often accompanied by TINNITUS and sometimes by VERTIGO. Eventually, there may be some SENSORINEURAL HEARING LOSS caused by damage spreading to the inner ear, which makes high tones hard to hear.

Hearing tests can uncover otosclerosis showing a conductive hearing loss greater in lower frequencies. HEARING AIDS can greatly help, although the conductive deafness can only be cured by a STAPEDECTOMY, an operation in which the stapes (stirrup) is replaced with an artificial substitute.

otoscope An instrument used for examining the ear that includes magnifying lenses, a light and a funnel-shaped tip that is inserted into the ear canal. The instrument can be used to inspect the outer ear canal and the eardrum, and to detect certain diseases of the MIDDLE EAR. (See also OTOSCOPY.)

otoscopy Visual inspection of the ear with an OTOSCOPE to detect ear disease. Using an otoscope equipped with a bulb, magnifying lens and speculum (a device designed to open a body orifice for examination), the client's ear pinnacle is pulled slightly upward and backward and the speculum is inserted into the outer ear canal.

Pneumatic otoscopy adds a bulb syringe attachment to alternate pressure, allowing a more accurate assessment of the position and mobility of the tympanic membrane.

otospongiosis Another name for OTOSCLEROSIS.

ototoxic drugs Certain drugs and chemicals can affect hearing and balance through functional impairment of the inner ear. The actual incidence of drugs and resultant deafness has been hard to establish because of the problems and complexity in studying the ear.

The negative effects of some ototoxic drugs are increased when taken in combination with other drugs or for long periods of time. Often, TINNITUS (ringing in the ears) is the first symptom, although some damage can occur before any symptoms appear.

A number of factors place some people at higher risk when taking ototoxic drugs, including age, earlier ear infections, SENSORINEURAL HEARING LOSS, impaired kidney or liver function, extreme drug sensitivity, simultaneous use of LOOP DIURETICS or drugs that are toxic to kidneys.

Ototoxic drugs are particularly damaging to the developing fetus, especially during the sixth or seventh week of pregnancy. Chloroquinine, streptomycin, aspirin and thalidomide are most strongly associated with ototoxic effects during pregnancy.

Other drugs that have been suspected to cause ototoxicity but are as yet unproven include antipyrine, atropine, chlordiazepoxide, cisplatinum, fenoprofen, hexadimethrine bromide, ibuprofen, morphine, naproxen, nitrogen mustard, phenylbutazone and sulindac.

Substances that may temporarily reduce hearing ability or increase tinnitus include

Families of Drugs with Documented Ototoxic Effects

1. *Aminoglycoside antibiotics*

Reaction to these drugs is most severe when therapy is extended beyond 10 days. Any patient treated for longer than this period should undergo cochlear and vestibular testing before, during and after therapy. They include: kanamycin, gentamicin, tobramycin and amikacin.

streptomycin	Onset of hearing loss can occur within five days of treatment.
neomycin	Hearing loss may continue after drug is stopped and is irreversible. It is the most cochleartoxic of all drugs. Warning symptoms: tinnitus or balance impairment (not always present).

2. *Other antibiotics*

erythromycin	All known cases of toxicity with this drug have been irreversible, usually within 24 hours after treatment has been stopped. Only large doses (more than 4 grams per day are ototoxic.
viomycin	Can cause permanent hearing impairment.

3. *Loop diuretics*

Loop diuretics should be avoided in premature infants and in those receiving aminoglycoside antibiotics. Hearing loss, vertigo and tinnitus is usually reversible, with recovery between 30 minutes to 24 hours; however, permanent hearing loss is possible.

furosemide — rapid intravenous administration increases chances of ototoxicity.
ethacrynic acid
lasix
bumetadine
piretamide
azosemide
triflocin
indapamide

4. *Salicylates*

High doses of salicylates cause tinnitus and bilateral hearing loss to 40 dB. Amount of hearing loss depends on blood concentration of drug. Both tinnitus and hearing loss are reversed 24–72 hours after the drug is stopped. Aspirin is a salicylate.

5. *Quinine derivatives*

Less than 2 grams per day may cause transient tinnitus, hearing loss, vertigo, headache, nausea or vision problems. There have been cases of permanent hearing loss and tinnitus but usually only when high doses were continued after symptoms appeared.

Quinine derivatives include quinine, chloroquine, quinidine, hydroxychloroquine.

alcohol, carbon monoxide, caffeine, oral contraceptives and tobacco.

ototoxicity Having a poisonous effect on the ear and its hearing mechanisms. High doses of certain drugs can damage the COCHLEA and the SEMICIRCULAR CANALS in the inner ear. (See also OTOTOXIC DRUGS.)

outer ear The portion of the ear that contains the external ear (the pinna, or auricle). The pinna leads into the ear canal (or meatus), which is about one inch long in adults and closed at its inner end by the eardrum. The part of the ear canal nearest the outside is made of cartilage and covered with skin that produces earwax which together with hair, traps dust and small particles. (See also EXTERNAL AUDITORY CANAL.)

oval window A tiny opening in the bony wall of the COCHLEA. It is actually an entrance to the INNER EAR.

overtone Any partial tone included in a complex tone except the lowest tone.

P

Paget-Gorman sign system (PGSS) A sign language system designed by Sir Richard Paget and further developed by Lady Grace Paget and Dr. Pierre Gorman of Great Britain.

It developed in almost total isolation from the language of the deaf community; the sign vocabulary of PGSS is not related to BRITISH SIGN LANGUAGE and is not intelligible to British deaf people. Children learning PGSS have nothing linguistically in common with deaf adults.

Paget's disease Also called osteitis deformans, this common genetic disease often occurs in middle age and affects the normal process of bone formation, weakening and deforming bones of the skull, pelvis, collarbone and long bones of the leg.

Changes in the skull can cause inner ear damage, resulting in TINNITUS, VERTIGO and a SENSORINEURAL HEARING LOSS. The disorder can also distort the face, cause pain and paralysis because of pressure on the spinal cord and cause severe arthritis of the hips.

Many people do not require treatment, but others find pain relief and normal bone formation occurs with analgesic drugs or, in severe cases, calcitonin. Surgery may be required to repair deformities.

painful hearing Painful hearing is produced by moderate or loud sounds that may be a single symptom or part of a range of problems, such as those found in MÉNIÈRE'S DISEASE.

Painful hearing may occur in cases of inflammation of the eardrum, when the additional stress of loud sound can hurt. Even with a normal, healthy ear, if the sound is loud enough (generally above 140 dB) it can cause pain, although there are wide differences among individuals as to the extent of pain experienced.

A sudden loud sound, such as an explosion, is much more painful than sound at the same level reached in successive small steps.

paracusia willisiana The ability to hear speech better in a noisy environment. Named for Dr. Thomas Willis, the English physician who described it in 1672, paracusia willisiana occurs in people with all forms of CONDUCTIVE HEARING LOSS.

Normally, a person in a noisy environment will raise his voice about 40 decibels louder in order to be heard above the background sounds. The person with a conductive hearing loss at frequencies that match the background noise won't be able to hear it but will be able to hear the speaker's voice well at an intensity level 40 decibels higher. With a pure conductive disorder, the sense organ is normal, and the speech at this louder decibel level will be completely understandable. On the other hand, a person with normal hearing hears not only the speaker's louder voice, but the entire range of background noise as well. Finally, a person with sensorineural hearing loss has more trouble hearing in noise because of the masking effect.

PB words A phonetically balanced list of words for articulation hearing tests that feature speech sounds in approximately the same relative frequency of occurrence as normal speech. (See also AUDIOMETRY.)

Penred's syndrome An autosomal recessive genetic hearing problem associated with the formation of a goiter and possibly associated with an impaired thyroid gland. The exact cause of the syndrome is not known. (See also GENETICS AND HEARING LOSS; GENETIC MECHANISMS OF DEAFNESS.)

percent of hearing loss The percent of HEARING LOSS used for medical and legal purposes can be estimated by approximating the number of damaged hair cells within the COCHLEA. Because it is impossible to count the damaged cells among the 15,000 in the ear, a percent of loss is made by using the AUDIOGRAM.

The amount of hearing loss is based on threshold levels at 500, 1000 and 2000 Hz. Hearing sensitivity better than 26 dB is not considered a loss; hearing worse than 93 dB is a total loss. Therefore, the percentage (0 to 100) of hearing loss covers a range of 67 dB. Each decibel above 26 dB is rated as a 1.5% loss. To calculate percentage of hearing loss, an audiologist averages the thresholds at 500, 1000 and 2000 Hz and subtracts 26 dB from this average. The remainder is multiplied by 1.5.

Although percentage is used to describe hearing loss, it does not give a clear picture of the actual hearing deficit. For example, a 40% hearing loss does not specify whether the loss is within the high, low or middle frequencies for speech reception. But this is important to know since *where* the damage occurs in a frequency range determines the ability to hear speech.

A group of people, all with a 40% hearing loss, will not each have the same ability to understand speech—one person's loss may be in the low frequencies, one in the high, another in the middle, with uncounted degrees in between.

Pereira, Jacobo Rodriguez (1715–1780) This 18th-century Portugese teacher is known as the first teacher of deaf students in France. Born in Berlanga, Portugal, Pereira moved to Bordeaux, where he demonstrated his techniques before the Parisian Academy of Science.

Advocating a low student-teacher ratio, Pereira accepted payment for his work depending on how quickly his pupils progressed. He used a one-handed manual alphabet that represented phonic qualities, not letters—the position of the fingers indicated the position of the speech organ used in making that sound. Similar to CUED SPEECH, this alphabet was used as a pronunciation aid.

perichondritis An unusual infection of the cartilage of the outer ear, this disorder is caused by an organism and can be contracted while swimming in polluted water or by an injury.

This microorganism, *Pseudomonas aeruginosa,* creates a greenish brown musty discharge from the outer ear canal. Perichondritis can be suspected when the outer ear is tender, red and thicker than normal. Prompt treatment will prevent a permanent deformity of the outer ear.

perilymph The fluid, almost identical to spinal fluid, that is contained in the canals of the COCHLEA. (See also PERILYMPH FISTULA.)

perilymph fistula A leak of perilymph from the oval and round window areas. It may occur spontaneously or after barotrauma (damage to the eardrum after sudden pressure changes) or head injury and may cause both hearing loss and balance problems.

Perilymph fistulas are often difficult to diagnose, and even surgical exploration of the middle ear may be inconclusive.

perinatal causes of hearing loss Several conditions during and after parturition (the birth process) may result in hearing loss in infants. These include loss of oxygen, low birth weight, excess bilirubin and infection.

During Birth About 6% of newborns experience a SENSORINEURAL HEARING LOSS ranging from mild to severe if deprived of oxygen at birth. In premature infants, about 5% will experience some type of mild to severe sensorineural hearing loss.

Extremely high levels of bilirubin (bile pigment) can cause a condition called KERNICTERUS, which damages the cochlear nuclei in the brain, causing hearing loss. In addition, several kinds of bacteria and viruses in the birth canal can transmit an ear infection (acute OTITIS MEDIA) to the newborn, which can cause hearing loss. These infections are usually caused by Streptococcus pneumoniae or Hemophilus influenzae.

At least 20% of babies born with hearing problems acquired them during the birth process. Causes can include maternal high blood pressure, prematurity, lack of oxygen (ANOXIA) or jaundice. In other cases of birth-induced deafness, the cause is unknown.

After Birth One of the most common causes of acquired sensorineural deafness in a newborn after birth is bacterial MENINGITIS. Meningitis is a disease involving an infection and inflammation of the coverings of the brain and the nerves that lead to it.

Bacterial meningitis in infants is usually caused by *Escherichia coli* (*E. coli*) bacteria, and can result in a hearing loss ranging from mild to profound. About half the infants who contract this disease will have a profound hearing loss which is usually permanent.

Often, the COCHLEA is damaged when bacteria from the covering of the brain enter the cochlea from the cochlear nerve. Prognosis for children who contract bacterial meningitis is poor; about half of those who live will have severe problems, including hearing loss, retardation and seizures.

Sometimes, children with meningitis get an ear infection with a conductive deafness; this can be cured with antibiotics.

peripheral auditory system All of the anatomic structures from the pinna or auricle (actual ear visible on the outside of the head) to the end of the auditory nerve in the brain. Generally, the system is divided into three parts: the outer, middle and inner ear structures.

Any problem with the conduction of sound in the OUTER EAR (such as excess wax) or the MIDDLE EAR (such as fluid) that blocks the transmission of sound to the INNER EAR can result in a conductive hearing loss.

If there is a problem with the sensory cells in the COCHLEA located in the inner ear, however, both the ability to hear and understand the sound will be affected; this is called a sensory hearing loss.

If a hearing problem is caused by a condition affecting the hearing nerve to the brain (also called the auditory nerve), the resulting hearing problems is called a neural loss. Since it is common for both a sensory and a neural loss to occur at the same time—or it may be impossible to tell the difference between them—such a loss is often called a sensorineural loss. A mixed hearing loss results from conditions affecting both the conductive and sensorineural structures.

pharyngotympanic tube See EUSTACHIAN TUBE.

Philippines About 300,000 people of this republic have hearing problems.

For many years, there was only one school for deaf students—the Philippine School for the Deaf, but by 1982 there were more than 2,000 deaf students enrolled in state-run educational programs. In addition, there are a number of private schools for deaf students throughout the country, serving a total of less than 400 pupils.

Communication modes vary from school to school and often change as administrators come and go. Deaf students may continue their education past high school, either with short-term vocational courses or college.

The schools may vary in their communication styles, but many graduates of deaf schools communicate as adults in sign language; those who have not gone to school use natural signs.

phonemes The essential and smallest elements of a finite number of speech sounds. They are the code signals that give meaning to speech. Phonemes are really abstractions, a bit like an averaging of the types of sounds that actually occur in speech.

For example, the phoneme "t" in the words "cat" and "tea" sounds very much the same yet is produced very differently. In "cat," the "t" sound is really just a stop made with only a very slight explosion of breath. The same "t" sound in the word "tea" is exploded with an audible breath. There are many different variations of pronouncing the phoneme "t," which are called its ALLOPHONES.

phonetics The study of the smallest units of language. (See also LINGUISTICS.)

phonology The study of how the smallest units of language (PHONEMES) can be combined to form words or signs. (See also LINGUISTICS.)

phonophobia An extreme sense of discomfort caused by sounds above the threshold of hearing.

Pidgin Sign English (PSE) A sign language system most often used by hearing people learning to communicate with deaf people. It combines the English word order and simplified grammatical structure with the vocabulary and nonmanual features of AMERICAN SIGN LANGUAGE. Signs for definite and indefinite articles are omitted, and only one sign is used for the verb "to be," unlike the MANUALLY CODED ENGLISH systems.

Another name for PSE is "Siglish." (See also SIGN LANGUAGE; SIGN LANGUAGE CONTINUUM; SIMULTANEOUS COMMUNICATION.)

pinna The part of the outer ear that we can see; also called auricle. The pinna is built to help gather sound waves and funnel them into the ear canal to the eardrum. In man, the pinna has no useful muscle and so remains relatively immobile.

pitch The perception of sound frequency, measured in terms of the number of cycles per second at which a sound wave vibrates. Pitch can vary with the intensity, duration or complexity of the sound vibration.

In music, "perfect" pitch (also called absolute pitch) is the very rare ability to identify the position of a tone within an octave (in other words, the ability to identify a note, A through G, without using a reference pitch). Perfect relative pitch is the ability to identify a note with the aid of a reference pitch. Perfect relative pitch is more common and is a skill that can be learned.

Plater, Felix (1536–1614) A 17th-century Swiss physician who published a detailed study of the bones of the ear, including the way in which sound is transmitted through the bones of the head.

In his book, Plater described both sensorineural and conductive deafness. He understood that the root of deafness was found sometimes in the brain and sometimes in the cavity of the ears. He found that if the cause of deafness is found in the brain, there is no cure. Plater is also known for his descriptions of the presence of TINNITUS in many of his deaf patients.

polyomography The process of taking x-rays of the inner ear.

Ponce de Leon, Pedro (?–1584) This 16th-century Benedictine monk is considered to be the father of education for deaf people and is thought to have been the first person to invent a method to teach deaf students.

Ponce de Leon was born in the province of Leon in northern Spain and entered a local monastery in 1526. Taking as his first pupil a man who had been denied admittance to the Benedictine order because he could neither hear nor speak, Ponce de Leon taught him to speak so he could make his confession. This student, Gaspard Burgos, went on to write several books of his own.

When transferred to a monastery in the mountains of north-central Spain, he met the two deaf sons of the wealthy Marquis of Berlanga, Juan Fernandez de Velasco. The Marquis' family was known for hereditary deafness, probably caused by intermarriage. Becoming close to Francisco and Pedro Velasco, aged 9 and 12 respectively, Ponce de Leon taught them both to speak. Pedro also learned how to write, speak and read books in Latin, Italian and Spanish before his death at age 30. Ponce de Leon also taught about 12 other deaf people to speak, including the Marquis' deaf daughters Bernardina and Catalina.

He next established a school at the Ona monastery for teaching wealthy deaf students to talk, beginning his teaching with writing and progressing to speech. Historians believe he taught speech to his students by tracing letters and indicating pronunciation with his lips. Historians also suspect that the manual alphabet he used was probably the same one published by the Franciscan monk Melchor Yebra in 1593. This alphabet is almost identical to the one used by 16th century deaf teachers JUAN PABLO BONET and Manuel Ramirez de Carrion, who also taught deaf members of the Velasco family.

Ponce de Leon is also assumed to have used signs in the education of his deaf pupils, since the Benedictines took strict vows of silence and had developed their own signs as a result.

In addition, he is said to have written a book, *Instruction for the Mute Deaf,* which was probably lost during the social upheavals common in Spanish monasteries at that time. Although books and documents from the monastery of Ona were sent to the National Archives in Spain, Ponce de Leon's book has never been found.

postlingual deafness Deafness occurring after language has been acquired. (See also ADVENTITIOUS DEAFNESS.)

prelingual deafness Deafness occurring before language skills have been acquired.

premature birth and hearing loss See POSTNATAL AND PERINATAL CAUSES OF HEARING LOSS.

prenatal causes of hearing loss Loss of hearing from prenatal causes occurs in between 7% and 20% of deaf and hard-of-hearing people. All of these prenatal causes are preventable.

There are three major threats to the hearing mechanism of a woman's unborn baby: viral diseases, ototoxic drugs and the condition of the woman's uterus during pregnancy.

The largest number of cases of prenatal deafness are a result of viral diseases contracted by the mother, including toxoplasmosis, RUBELLA, CYTOMEGALOVIRUS (CMV) and HERPES SIMPLEX.

A mother who contracts rubella during the first three months of her pregnancy may have a child who is born with some degree of hearing loss. This risk is less likely today because a vaccination is available for those women who have never had rubella but who would like to become pregnant. In fact, following the rubella epidemic of the 1960s, many states require rubella testing for women when applying for a marriage license.

Other viral diseases contracted by the mother may also cause a hearing loss in the fetus, including mumps and influenza (particularly during the first three months). An active herpes simplex Type II lesion in the genital area during a vaginal delivery can also infect the infant, causing hearing loss.

OTOTOXIC DRUGS taken by the mother during pregnancy are known to cause hearing problems in the sensorineural structures of the developing fetus, especially the developing cochlea. These drugs include the aminoglycosides, thalidomide and alcohol.

- *aminoglycosides* The incidence of prenatal deafness due to the aminoglycosides (kanamycin, neomycin, gentamicin, tobramycin and amikacin) is extremely low. These drugs have been reported to cause hearing loss in infants only when mothers who took them had kidney problems and received diuretics (ethacrynic acid and furosimide) in addition to an aminoglycoside. It has been suggested that there may be a genetic susceptibility to hearing problems associated with aminoglycosides.
- *streptomycin* When the antibiotic streptomycin is given to a pregnant mother at any time, it can cause a sensorineural hearing loss ranging from mild high-frequency to severe bilateral.
- *thalidomide* Although the drug thalidomide taken during the first trimester of pregnancy caused a large number of malformations of the ear in Europe during the 1960s, the drug was never released in the United States.
- *alcohol* It has also been reported that fetal alcohol syndrome may cause hearing loss in up to 64% of infants born to alcoholic mothers.

Infections in the mother transmitted to the infant in the blood before birth can cause pneumonia or MENINGITIS; other infections in the amniotic fluid can be swallowed by the fetus and then pumped up the eustachian tube into the middle ear, where they can create an ear infection. SYPHILIS transmitted from mother to child during pregnancy may also result in a hearing loss in the child, either during the first two years of life or at puberty.

Incompatible Rh blood factors also pose a threat to the hearing mechanism of the unborn child. When a mother with Rh negative blood has a child with Rh-positive blood, cells from the baby sensitize her and she will develop antibodies to Rh-positive blood. While this will not harm the first baby, subsequent pregnancies risk damaging the baby when the mother's antibodies attack the red blood cells of the Rh-positive fetus.

However, problems for the newborn due to Rh sensitization are becoming rare since the development of Rh (D) immune globulin (anti-D serum). When injected into the mother 72 hours before delivery, it prevents 99% of the incidences of sensitization.

A range of other conditions in the mother during pregnancy may be connected with prenatal hearing loss. These include maternal diabetes, hypothyroidism, toxemia and malnutrition. (See also NEWBORN SCREENING PROGRAMS; PERINATAL CAUSES OF HEARING LOSS; RH-FACTOR INCOMPATABILITY AND DEAFNESS.)

presbycusis More than 10 million Americans suffer from presbycusis, a type of SENSORINEURAL HEARING LOSS that comes with age. It is one of the most common chronic problems among older people.

After about age 50, most people slowly begin to lose some ability to hear. A person with presbycusis hears sounds less clearly and tones (especially higher ones) less audibly. People with presbycusis often have trouble understanding speech, particularly in the presence of background noise.

But presbycusis is not just caused by physiological aging; it may simply be a result of wax build-up in the ear or of damage to the inner ear from infection, disease, injury or a loud noise. In fact, some experts believe excessive noise accounts for more hearing loss than all other factors combined.

Medications—most commonly aspirin, antibiotics and hypertension drugs—can also cause hearing problems in the elderly.

Studies at the HOUSE EAR INSTITUTE and elsewhere have shown that as a person ages, there is a loss of nerve cells in the base of the COCHLEA where high-frequency sounds are perceived. But researchers don't know whether the degeneration of cells in the cochlear nucleus is primarily due to aging or whether it is due to a decrease in the specific frequencies supplying those cells from the cochlea.

Each person experiences the development of presbycusis differently. Generally, it involves a slow decline in hearing ability. First a person loses the ability to hear high-pitched sounds, followed by a loss of hearing in the middle frequencies and finally the lowest. Because normal speech covers all these frequencies, the ability to understand conversation may vary according to the extent of presbycusis.

A person who notices hearing loss should immediately see either an OTOLOGIST (specialist in diseases of the ear), an OTOLARYNGOLOGIST (specialist in diseases of the ear, nose and throat) or an AUDIOLOGIST (professional who often works with a physician to assess hearing loss and provide auditory training). Unfortunately, most people with presbycusis wait an average of five years before doing anything about it.

Although HEARING AIDS can help most people, not everyone will benefit from them (people who can't discriminate different speech sounds, for example). For those who can, an aid should not be prescribed or fitted before an examination and hearing test are given. (See also AGING AND HEARING LOSS.)

Professional Rehabilitation Workers with the Adult Deaf Known today as the AMERICAN DEAFNESS AND REHABILITATION ASSOCIATION, ADARA was formed in 1964 under the above name as a way to separate people who worked with deaf people from the organization for rehabilitators who worked with all disabilities.

Professional School for Deaf Theatre Personnel America's only professional theater school for deaf students has offered deaf actors a concentrated four-week session in basic and advanced theater since 1967.

The faculty includes professional stage actors, academic instructors and company members of the NATIONAL THEATRE OF THE DEAF. Courses include acting, directing, playwriting, dance, costume design, fencing, storytelling, set design and Japanese dance and theater. Deaf and hearing teachers instruct both deaf students and hearing students involved in deaf culture who are proficient in sign.

The program is accredited by Connecticut College and is supported by the U.S. Department of Education's special education program. Full scholarships for 20 deaf Americans are granted each year. The application process each year ends April 15 for the session beginning in June. Contact: National Theatre of the Deaf, Hazel E. Stark Center, Chester, CT 06412; telephone: 203-526-4971 (voice), 203-526-4974 (TDD)

profound hearing loss Generally considered to be a loss greater than 90 decibels.

Project ALAS A nonprofit service organization affiliated with D.E.A.F., INC. Project ALAS (Spanish for "wings") offers services for deaf Latinos and their families in the New England area. Contact: Project ALAS, c/o D.E.A.F., Inc., 215 Brighton Ave., Allston, MA 02134; telephone (voice and TDD): 617-254-4041.

PSYCH.NET A computer-accessed bulletin board on an ELECTRONIC MAIL system that allows professionals in the fields of mental health and deafness to communicate. This type of electronic mail service provides cheap and instantaneous access to other subscribers.

PSYCH.NET is a limited access bulletin board, part of a larger system called DEAFTEK.USA. People wishing to become a user must first join DEAFTEK, which requires an annual fee and monthly charges depending on usage. There is no charge to join

PSYCH.NET, although an application is required. (See also ASCII; BAUDOT CODE.)

psychogenic hearing loss See FUNCTIONAL LOSS (NONORGANIC).

Public Law 94–142 See LEGAL RIGHTS.

Public Law 97-410 See LEGAL RIGHTS.

Public Law 100-533 See LEGAL RIGHTS.

Puerto Rican Sign Language There are at least four varieties of Puerto Rican Sign Language (PRSL) used today on the small Caribbean commonwealth island. It is similar to AMERICAN SIGN LANGUAGE and is believed to have developed from the introduction of ASL in the early 1900s. American Sign Language was brought to Puerto Rico in 1907 by nuns who founded a deaf school; in the 1950s a Spanish teaching order of nuns introduced the oral approach and forbade SIGN LANGUAGE.

Puerto Rican Sign Language is different from ASL in that it does not use FINGERSPELLING and has many signs that are different or do not appear in ASL. Its structural characteristics, as in other sign languages, include the use of space to show relationship between objects or ideas, classifiers and size- and shape-specifiers and the use of compound signs to describe new ideas.

In addition, Signed Spanish, which uses signs in Spanish word order, is used by deaf persons in communicating with Spanish-speaking hearing people. Signed English is used by deaf Puerto Ricans who were educated in mainland United States. Of the two, Signed Spanish is more commonly used in Puerto Rico to communicate with hearing people, especially for interpreting and watching television.

pure tone average (PTA) The average level of THRESHOLDS elicited for each ear for frequencies believed by some to be essential to understanding speech—500, 1000 and 2000 hertz. The PTA is used to determine the level at which to start presenting words to find a person's speech reception threshold. (See also AUDIOMETRY.)

pure tone audiogram The graph of a person's ability to hear pure tones. (See also AUDIOGRAM, AUDIOMETRY.)

pure tone sweep-check test The most reliable method of screening large numbers for hearing loss by testing for auditory response to different frequencies presented at a constant level. It is generally possible to screen one person every two or three minutes. (See also JOHNSTON TEST, MASSACHUSETTS TEST, AUDIOMETRY.)

pure tone test A hearing test presenting pure tone sounds through a speaker or earphones. (See also AUDIOMETRY.)

Q

quinine derivatives and hearing loss Drugs derived from quinine in doses of about two grams per day may cause a combination of TINNITUS, decreased hearing, VERTIGO, headache, nausea or blurred vision. Symptoms can quickly disappear when the drugs are discontinued, although permanent hearing loss and tinnitus have been reported after high doses were continued after symptoms began.

Quinine derivatives include quinine, chloroquine, quinidine and hydroxychloroquine. (See also OTOTOXIC DRUGS.)

Quota International, Inc. A service group whose major project, Shatter Silence, helps individuals with hearing and speech handicaps. The group publishes *The Quotarian,* offers fellowships and conducts an annual Outstanding Deaf Woman of the Year program. Contact: Quota International, Inc.,

1420 21st St. NW, Washington, DC 20044; telephone (voice and TDD): 202-331-9694.

R

radio for the deaf The Pennsylvania School for the Deaf in Philadelphia established the first and largest radio network for deaf people who have specially tuned home radio receivers connected to a telecommunication device for the deaf for printout.

At the station, words are coded on a teleprinter, punched on paper tape and then converted into audible tones sent via telephone to Temple University's FM station. There, the tones are broadcast within a 30- to 50-mile radius as a type of "captioned radio."

Rainbow Alliance of the Deaf A national organization serving the deaf gay and lesbian community, this group has 17 chapters throughout the United States and two in Canada. Contact: Rainbow Alliance of the Deaf, P.O. Box 14182, Washington, DC 20044; telephone (TDD): 301-779-6459.

receiver The part of a hearing aid that carries amplified sound and speech to the earmold. (See also HEARING AIDS.)

receptive aphasia See AUDITORY AGNOSIA.

receptive skill The ability to understand what is being communicated in both FINGERSPELLING and SIGN LANGUAGE.

recruitment An abnormal, rapid increase in loudness as the strength of the acoustic signal is increased. A person with normal hearing would notice a gradual increase in loudness as the level of sound is increased; someone with a cochlear impairment would find that loudness increases more rapidly as the signal becomes more intense. Conversely, a person with a dysfunctional AUDITORY NERVE would notice loudness decruitment—as the signal level intensifies, loudness growth decreases or even declines.

Audiologists therefore find recruitment tests very useful in deciding whether a hearing problem originates in the COCHLEA or the auditory nerve.

In order to test for recruitment, audiologists use a loudness balance test—either the alternate binaural loudness balance test (ABLB) or the monaural bi-frequency loudness balance test (MLB). The ABLB is used to compare loudness growth in both ears for patients with hearing loss on one side. In the test, the client must judge the loudness of a tone at a specific frequency in both the good and poor ear.

If a patient has lost hearing in both ears, the MLB can determine recruitment, especially in high-frequency hearing loss, by presenting two different frequency tones in one ear. The reference tone is set for a frequency the person can hear normally; the variable tone is set at a frequency the person cannot hear, and the examiner notes at what frequency the variable tone is judged to be equal in loudness to the reference tone.

In an excessive case of recruitment, the range of useful hearing between the THRESHOLD and the level at which loudness becomes uncomfortable may be very narrow. Hearing aids would therefore be of limited value for such a problem.

Refsum's syndrome A rare, genetic, neurological disease associated with hearing loss.

Registry of Interpreters for the Deaf (RID) The largest national organization of interpreters in the United States. The registry maintains a national list of people skilled in the use of AMERICAN SIGN LANGUAGE and other sign systems.

The RID provides information on interpreting and evaluation and certification of interpreters for deaf people. When it was first established in Muncie, Indiana in 1964, the organization was designed simply as a way to register certified interpreters. But in the early 1970s, the registry began to expand its interests: It set up both the first national certification system and the first performance evaluation for interpreters in the world. At the same time, interpreter associations were founded at the local and state level to advocate legislative reform in the area of interpreter laws.

Today, RID consists of more than 3,000 members—most certified interpreters—who work to further the profession of interpretation of American Sign Language and English. Its national office produces the bimonthly newsletter *Views* and serves as a clearinghouse of information about interpretation. (See also COURT INTERPRETERS ACT; INTERPRETERS AND THE LAW; ORAL INTERPRETERS; SIGN LANGUAGE INTERPRETERS.) Contact: Registry of Interpreters for the Deaf, Inc., 511 Monroe St., Suite 1107, Rockville, MD 20850; telephone (voice and TDD): 301-779-0555.

Rehabilitation Act of 1973 See LEGAL RIGHTS.

Reissner's membrane The thinnest membrane in the COCHLEA with the thickness of just two cells, this separates the perilymph and endolymph fluids.

relay service A generic term for a service in which an operator relays a conversation between a hearing person without a TDD and a hard-of-hearing or speech-impaired person who has a TDD. It is also called a "dual party relay service."

The operator serves as a bridge between the two callers and uses two phones, one connected to a TDD. The caller phones the relay service; while the caller waits, a relay service operator places a call to the other party. When both parties are on the line at the same time, the operator speaks the deaf person's typed message and types the hearing person's spoken message. This term distinguishes relayed calls from a message relay service, in which a message is relayed in one direction only and not while both parties are on the line.

Most of the early relay services were staffed completely by volunteers, but as the number of TDD users rose, so did the demand for statewide relay services. Some states have already established statewide dual party message relay services, which are funded by tax revenue or a surcharge on telephone lines. In other states, the relay service is considered part of the telephone companies normal operating expenses.

The NATIONAL CENTER FOR LAW AND THE DEAF at Gallaudet University in Washington, D.C. provides information on the funding and administration of mandated state and federal dual party message relay systems. The TELE-CONSUMER HOTLINE in Washington, D.C. provides a "TDD Relay Center Comparison Chart" offering comparative information about areas served, membership requirements, fees and service limitations. (See also MESSAGE RELAY SERVICE; TELECOMMUNICATIONS DEVICE FOR THE DEAF.)

residential schools See EDUCATION OF DEAF CHILDREN.

residual hearing measurement See AUDIOMETRY.

retracted eardrum When the pressure inside the middle ear is lower than the pressure on the outside in the external canal, the eardrum is gradually pushed inward by the extra pressure from the outside. Sometimes the eardrum can be pressed so far into the middle ear that it touches the cochlea itself, almost completely obliterating the middle ear.

This retraction occurs during a head cold, an allergy attack or an infection in the back of the nose and throat, any of which force the eustachian tube closed so that no air can get into the middle ear. In such a situation, the air normally present in the middle ear becomes locked in, and some of it is absorbed by the lining of the middle ear, reducing the pressure in the middle ear.

This can reduce the efficiency of both the eardrum and the OSSICULAR CHAIN in transmitting sound to the inner ear, although the amount of retraction is no indication of the amount of hearing loss. The amount of hearing loss is determined instead by the site and type of damage in the ossicular chain, and this cannot be determined by appearance alone.

retrocochlear lesion A type of lesion located on the AUDITORY NERVE (not the cochlea) that causes SENSORINEURAL HEARING LOSS.

reverse interpreting See SIGN-TO-VOICE INTERPRETING.

Rh factor incompatibility and deafness Red blood cells carry the Rh (Rhesus) factor, an antigen present in about 85% of the population (Rh-positive) and absent in about 15% (Rh-negative). Having Rh-negative blood causes no harm unless Rh-positive blood enters the bloodstream of an Rh-negative person.

When an Rh-negative mother has an Rh-positive child, the mixture of these blood factors can cause the mother to develop antibodies against the Rh-positive blood of the child. Because it takes some time for these antibodies to develop, the first child is rarely affected by them. However, in a second pregnancy, the antibodies in the mother's blood will pass through the placenta, damaging the child's blood cells. This destruction of blood cells can cause many problems, including erythroblastosis (a disorder causing severe jaundice) and athetoid cerebral palsy; a fair number of these children also have congenital hearing loss.

Children who become deaf through Rh incompatibility have a series of similar characteristics: a nonprogressive hearing loss, the same in both ears and usually worse in the high frequencies; reduced bone conduction; hearing loss present at birth; and a frequent speech difficulty, particularly in pronouncing the letter *s*.

Rh-negative mothers are now easily identified in this country, and treatment is available to prevent or modify the damage. As a result, few children born in developed countries have this form of deafness.

Rinne test This common test compares a patient's ability to hear a tuning fork by air and bone conduction. The vibrating fork is first placed about an inch from the ear (air conduction), and the patient is asked how loud it is. Then the base of the fork is quickly pressed against the mastoid bone (bone conduction). The patient is then asked in which position the fork sounds louder. (See also AUDIOMETRY.)

People with normal hearing can hear the sound better and longer through air conduction—almost twice as long as sound through bone. This test result is called a "positive Rinne."

Although people with a sensorineural hearing loss can also hear better with air conduction, they can't hear the sound as loud or as long as people with normal hearing.

Patients with a conductive hearing loss will show a "negative Rinne"—hearing better by bone conduction, since the bone-conducted sound bypasses the conductive block and is then accurately perceived by the healthy cochlea.

Rochester Method See FINGERSPELLING.

Ronsard, Pierre de (1524–1585) This "Prince of Poets" was one of the outstanding writers during the French Renaissance and was responsible for a renewed interest in poetry. He was deafened at age 15, a loss that diverted his interests from a diplomatic career toward literary pursuits. Today he is considered to be one of the leading poets in the history of French literature.

He was born on September 11, 1524, in Possoniere castle, the son of a noble family, and embarked at a young age on a career as a diplomat in the royal household. Unfortunately, in 1540 an ear infection and high fever resulted in a severe hearing loss that eliminated further advancement as a diplomat.

Much to his father's displeasure, Ronsard turned to a career in literature. Although he took preliminary steps toward the priesthood, his heart was never in it. After the death of his father, life as a literary figure became easier, and he began to study poetry and literature more seriously.

In 1547, Ronsard joined with Joachim du Bellay, who was also deaf, in forming a group of aspiring poets. He was also frequently at the royal court, eventually earning a job administering kneeling cushions and holy water for the king.

Ronsard published his first collection of poems in 1560 and was at this time an important spokesman at court and defender of the Catholic faith. Still, he was best known for his love poetry, although it is not known to what extent he pursued these relationships in actuality.

round window An elastic membrane opening between the MIDDLE EAR and INNER EAR. Within the internal ear, the VESTIBULE and COCHLEA are filled with virtually incompressible fluid. The STAPES (stirrup) can move toward the vestibule because of the pressure relief points provided by the round window and the oval window.

rubella This viral illness (also known as German measles) causes hearing problems in about half of all infants born to mothers who contract the disease while they are pregnant. When infection occurs during the first trimester, 68% of babies will be born deaf; when infection occurred during the second trimester, 40% of babies will be deaf. There is significantly less risk to babies whose mothers contract rubella during the third trimester, although deafness is still a possibility.

Even if the mother is exposed to the disease at any time during her pregnancy but does not develop symptoms, her baby can still become deaf. For this reason, any female of childbearing age who is unsure whether she has been immunized should have her immune status checked. Vaccination is performed only if there is no chance that a woman is pregnant since there is a risk that the vaccine itself can cause rubella in the fetus.

Typically, hearing loss as a result of prenatal rubella produces a SENSORINEURAL HEARING LOSS and can be progressive during the childhood years. Less commonly, prenatal rubella infection can result in a conductive hearing disorder.

During the rubella epidemic of 1963–1965, the rubella epidemic caused 8,000 cases of prenatal deafness in the United States and was responsible for 20% of all cases of deafness during that time.

The introduction of a successful rubella vaccine has slashed the number of prenatal cases of deafness due to rubella to only 5%. (See also PRENATAL CAUSES OF HEARING LOSS.)

S

saccule One of the structures of the INNER EAR, this is a small sac located in the VESTIBULE, which encapsulates a single sensory patch called a MACULA. The macula, which resembles the letter *j*, lies against the inner wall of the vestibule directly over the bone.

The UTRICLE and the saccule together with their maculae are also called otolith organs and gravity receptors (since they respond to gravitational forces). These receptors—particularly the utricle—are important in the righting reflexes and in maintaining the contractions of the muscles that keep the body standing upright.

The role the saccule plays is less well understood, although it is believed it may respond to vibration and backwards-forwards positions of the head.

Of the two, the utricle seems to be the dominant receptor.

SAI See SOCIAL ADEQUACY INDEX.

SAL See SENSORINEURAL ACUITY LEVEL.

scala media This tube-like structure lies upon the BASILAR MEMBRANE and follows the turns of the COCHLEA. Inside the entire length of the scala media is the extremely sensitive mechanism of hearing called the ORGAN OF CORTI, which contains about 15,000 minute hair cells responsible for sending impulses on to the brain.

scala tympani A spiral fluid channel containing PERILYMPH; located in the cochlea below the basilar membrane.

scala vestibuli A spiral fluid channel containing PERILYMPH; located in the cochlea above the basilar membrane.

scarlet fever Also known as scarletina, this is an acute infectious disease caused by the streptococcus bacterium. It can lead to complications such as sinus infections, followed by abcesses of the ear and MASTOIDITIS.

Symptoms of the disease begin from two to seven days after exposure, starting with fever, sore throat, headache and (in children) vomiting. A rash appears about two or three days later on the neck, armpits, groin and chest. The throat is red with red spots on the palate and the tongue is coated and inflamed. The rash and fever can last for more than a week, sometimes followed by skin peeling.

Scarlet fever, which today is fairly uncommon in the United States, is treated with penicillin, bed rest and plenty of fluids. It is believed that the reduced threat of the disease is due to a change in the virulence of the bacteria and has nothing to do with the development of drugs to treat the condition.

Schenck, Johannes A 16th-century physician who explored the etiology of deafness.

Schenck was able to describe the idea of hereditary deafness by exploring the case of a family with several children with congenital deafness. He also discussed how a person might lose the ability to hear following an injury.

Schwabach test This test compares the patient's ability to hear a tuning fork by bone conduction through the mastoid bones with a normal hearing person's ability to hear the fork in the same position. (Generally, the listener with normal hearing is the OTOLOGIST.)

In this test, the examiner holds the vibrating tuning fork on the patient's mastoid bone, who then tells the examiner when the fork's tone ceases. The examiner then places the fork on his own bone and notes the time elapsed until the vibration is no longer heard.

If the patient hears the tone longer than the examiner (Schwabach-shortened), the hearing loss is probably conductive. If the patient hears the tone for a shorter time than the examiner (Schwabach-prolonged), than a sensorineural loss is indicated. (See also AUDIOMETRY.)

Scotland There are an estimated 4,000 deaf adults in Scotland, with another 2,000 students receiving help for some form of hearing loss.

The history of deaf education in Scotland is long, beginning in 1769 with the establishment of a school operated by THOMAS BRAIDWOOD in Edinburgh. As in the United States, deaf education in Scotland has gone through constant evolution, beginning with an emphasis on residential schools and now centering on MAINSTREAMING. Similarly, philosophies of communication have included the ORAL and MANUAL approaches and TOTAL COMMUNICATION.

Today, most deaf children attend regular schools, and about 25% go to special units or schools. The scattered deaf population in the country, together with its isolated location, has made services sometimes difficult to provide for this population.

Since the 1970s, pressure has grown to provide more schools closer to home, with a resulting growth in local clinics and programs for deaf people. But the quality and type of programs still varies considerably from town to town.

secondary tympanic membrane A membranous flap at the base of the COCHLEA that closes the SCALA TYMPANI at the ROUND WINDOW.

secretory otitis media See SEROUS OTITIS MEDIA.

SEE 1 See SEEING ESSENTIAL ENGLISH.

SEE 2 See SIGNING EXACT ENGLISH.

S.E.E. Center for the Advancement of Deaf Children The S.E.E. (SIGNING EXACT ENGLISH) Center is a nonprofit organization dedicated to improving the communication and English literacy skills of hard-of-hearing children and hearing language-delayed students.

Signing Exact English (SEE 2) is a manual communication system first published in 1972; the center was established in 1984 in response to requests for workshops, materials and information for implementing S.E.E. 2 in homes and schools across the country.

The center provides information, materials and referral services for new parents emphasizing the importance of early communication stimulation for preschool children utilizing the S.E.E. 2 approach. It also provides information for training and evaluating sign language instructors and educational interpreters in the use of S.E.E. 2.

Further, the group offers videotapes and helps educators, audiologists, psychologists and speech therapists implementing S.E.E. 2 as part of a total communication program and provides support for research assessing the impact of S.E.E. 2. Contact: The S.E.E. Center for the Advancement of Deaf Children, P.O. Box 1181, Los Alamitos, CA 90720; telephone: 213-430-1467.

Seeing Essential English (SEE 1) One of at least five separate codes for English, SEE 1 takes much of its sign vocabulary from AMERICAN SIGN LANGUAGE.

SEE 1, published in 1971, was the first MANUAL CODE FOR ENGLISH system. David Anthony, the congenitally deaf son of deaf parents born in England, originally began SEE 1 as a graduate degree project in 1962 at GALLAUDET UNIVERSITY.

The system features the sound-spelling-meaning principle: That is, each criterion is used to determine a sign for a particular word. A single sign is used when two of these three are the same. Therefore, "I have a right to vote," "It's on the right" and "you're right" would be signed the same ("right" in this case sounds and is written the same way but has different meanings), but the word "write" would use a different sign since it sounds the same but has a different spelling and meaning.

Seeing Essential English has specific signs for morphemes, suffixes and prefixes.

Self Help for Hard of Hearing People, Inc. (SHHH) A volunteer educational organization devoted to the interests of people who cannot hear. The group's activities include social activities, education, advocacy and consumer activism.

The group publishes *Shhh,* the only bimonthly journal in the United States written specifically for hard-of-hearing people and offering information on hearing loss, assistive technology, coping techniques and personal experiences for more than 200,000 readers.

The organization also offers referral and advisory services and operates an information and resource center. Contact: Self Help for Hard of Hearing People, Inc., 7800 Wisconsin Ave., Bethesda, MD 20814; telephone: (voice) 301-657-2248, (TDD) 301-657-2249.

semantics The interpretation of the meaning of words, signs and sentences. (See also LANGUAGE.)

semicircular canals Also called the LABYRINTH, this very important organ inside the inner ear is connected to the cochlea but does not contribute to the sense of hearing.

The semicircular canals are three small fluid-filled loops that help maintain balance by sending information about the position of the head through the vestibular branch of the AUDITORY NERVE to the brain. Infections or other problems in the middle or inner ear may directly or indirectly affect these canals, causing DIZZINESS or VERTIGO. Thus, some deaf children have difficulty with balance and may learn to walk later than a hearing child.

sensorineural acuity level A way of testing bone conduction hearing by using a bone-conduction vibrator to issue a masking noise at the midline of the skull and noting THRESHOLD shifts caused by the noise in pure-tone air conduction hearing. (See also AUDIOMETRY.)

sensorineural hearing loss This form of hearing loss—commonly called nerve deafness—is a general term to describe conditions of the inner ear that lead to some measure of deafness, either by injury or malfunction of the inner ear. Sensorineural hearing loss (which results from damage to the hair cells of the inner ear or the nerves that supply it) differs from CONDUCTIVE HEARING LOSS, which is caused by diseases or obstructions in the outer or middle ear. The causes are varied, but many can be treated and others improved with properly adjusted HEARING AIDS.

Every year, about 4,000 U.S. infants are born with nerve deafness from many different causes, including heredity, maternal viral infection during pregnancy and problems during the birth process. Among the elderly, nerve deafness is most often caused by changes in the ear associated with the aging process (also called PRESBYCUSIS).

Still other types of nerve deafness can be caused by injury from stroke or injury to the head that causes irreversible damage to the AUDITORY NERVE and brain. Any tumor that grows close to the auditory nerve or auditory centers in the brain can also cause nerve deafness. Even a loud noise can damage sensory cells and nerve fibers, particularly if the noise occurs over a period of time, such as in constantly listening to loud music or working in a factory or airport. Further, drugs such as aspirin, some antibiotics and diuretics can affect the structure of the inner ear. Diseases that affect the flow of blood to the inner ear can also cause nerve deafness: These include diabetes, emphysema, heart disease, hardening of the arteries and some kidney disorders. Sometimes nerve deafness occurs in the absence of any identifiable condition or injury. Almost always, it is permanent and irreversible (except in the cases of some drug effects) and tends to progressively worsen. In some people, one ear can be affected in a very different way from the other.

The degree of nerve deafness may vary. A mild loss (15–30 db) will cause a patient to strain to hear; moderate loss (35–55 dB) causes frequent repetition of conversation, much louder TV volume and misunderstood words in conversation. A severe loss (60–90 dB) usually requires a hearing aid, and a person with a profound hearing loss (90 dB or more) hears only very loud sounds, if anything at all.

In general, people with nerve hearing loss have problems understanding speech (also called word discrimination) even when the speech is loud enough to be heard comfortably. Problems in understanding speech usually depend on the frequency (or pitch) at which the hearing loss occurs. For example, if a person can't hear high pitches, he will have problems hearing consonant sounds that do not carry voice (t, p, k, s and so forth) Words such as tea, pea and key will sound alike since, without the consonant, the person hears only the vowel.

Hearing aids that are capable of amplifying some sounds more than others, especially high pitched sounds, can help resolve this problem. SPEECHREADING (lipreading) combined with this type of hearing aid can also be of assistance.

Another problem associated with nerve deafness is RECRUITMENT, that is, an abnormally rapid increase in the perception of sound loudness. Someone with this problem who can hear nothing at one level finds that the slightest increase in loudness causes a painfully loud sound.

Nerve deafness can be diagnosed with a pure tone audiogram to identify the degree to which damage has occurred, although the audiogram will not explain what caused the damage in the first place. A full audiological evaluation and IMPEDANCE measurements by an AUDIOLOGIST will determine the presence of a hearing loss, its type and its degree. This information, with a complete otological exam by an OTOLOGIST, will allow a physician to determine the need for further testing. These other tests could include blood tests, ELECTRONYSTAGMOGRAPHY (a test to determine the presence of damage to the balance system), POLYOMOGRAPHY (X-rays of the inner ear) and brain scans. (See also AUDIOMETRY; HEARING LOSS.)

sensory aid A device that provides sound information to a person with hearing problems through sight or touch. This is distinctive from devices that provide autitory sensation (such as a COCHLEAR IMPLANT).

Bell Laboratories devised the first sensory aid in the 1920s, a vibrating sound analyzer for deaf people, and during World War II, Bell's labs created a visual display of sound called a spectrograph to help unscramble coded voice messages. After the war, the first instant-display spectrograph, the "visible speech translator," was developed for use with deaf people.

Upton Eyeglass Speechreader The first visual aid that could be worn was the Upton Eyeglass Speechreader, developed by deaf engineer Hubert Upton to improve comprehension beyond speechreading alone. Upton's speechreader features a microphone and analyzer that control separate bars of red light from light-emitting diodes (LED). The LED is mounted in a small projector fitted into the corner of the eyeglass frame, aimed at a reflecting area in the rear surface of the eyeglass lens.

The images of the bar lights appear in the space between the wearer and the speaker. When lighted, each bar indicates a type of sound pattern. Six different bars are assigned by the analyzer to six different types of speech sound patterns as they are picked up by the microphone.

Autocuer This device also uses a projection display together with a computer that detects vowels and consonants and pairs a consonant with the following vowel to establish a syllable. It then flashes a symbol indicating the category on the eyeglasses of the deaf speechreader, who can decide from the lip and facial movements of the speaker which syllable was spoken.

Computer Speech Someday, scientists hope they will be able to develop a computer that can recognize spoken sentences and print them on a video screen and translate sentences typed on a keyboard into synthesized speech. While talking computers are now commonplace (for example, the mechanical voice inside your car which reminds you to buckle up)—a device which can *recognize* speech instead of generate it is much more difficult to design.

Theoretically, at least, researchers know how it should work: The interactive speaking computer of the future would convert the sound of a spoken word into a digital code and then search its vocabulary for a word with the same code. When found, the computer would print out the word on paper or on a screen. Most systems today can do this only when the speaker pronounces every word with great clarity and pauses after each one.

The problem is that natural, rapid speech is much more difficult for a computer to recognize. In order for the computer to distinguish between "I scream" and "ice cream," for example, it must be able to discern what the speaker means from the context of the message.

Because of problems like this, scientists predict it will be many years before computers are able to recognize natural speech with any degree of accuracy.

Tactile Speech Aids Since some people find visual displays distracting, researchers have developed a system that can present sound patterns through vibrations on the skin.

The Boothroyd Portapitch Aid, for example, is worn on the wrist or arm and contains eight vibrators energized by different levels of pitch of the voice received. Other tactile aids have many more stimulators that can respond to various combinations of vowels and consonants.

sensory aphasia See AUDITORY AGNOSIA.

sensory cells Located on the surface of the basilar membrane are sensory cells, which together with supporting cells form the ORGAN OF CORTI. Decades ago, it was shown that the production of sensory cells in the ears of mammals stops before birth and that these cells are produced only during embryonic development. This meant that damage to sensory cells later in life was irreparable; it became the basis for considering nerve deafness a permanent condition.

However, recent basic research with animals has shown that under certain conditions sensory cell production can be reactivated in mature damaged ears and that these regenerated cells contribute to recovery of hearing.

Scientists at the NATIONAL INSTITUTE OF HEARING AND OTHER COMMUNICATION DISORDERS believe it is reasonable to expect that within 10 to 20 years progenitors of regenerated sensory cells will be cloned from animals and will aid in the development of ways to recover hearing in humans.

serous otitis media Also called glue ear, this results in thin and watery fluid in the middle ear that reduces hearing acuity by interfering with the movement of the OSSICULAR CHAIN. It has become more common since the use of antibiotics in the treatment of ear infections.

Serous otitis media is the most common cause of hearing problems in children because of the prevalence of ear infections in childhood. Its origin is unclear, although it is believed to be caused by treatment of suppurative otitis media with antibiotics or other drugs without adequate drainage.

After diagnosis of suppurative otitis media, antibiotics are prescribed and the infection clears. But the fluid, no longer infectious, remains in the middle ear cavity, making the ear more susceptible to further ear infections and reducing hearing acuity. Usually, the person is unaware of the hearing loss until both ears are affected; by this time, the fluid has thickened and become glue-like and can cause a permanent deterioration of the bones of the middle ear.

Other causes of serous otitis media include allergy and viral infection of the middle ear. It can also occur in adults when the EUSTACHIAN TUBE does not function due to a cold or barotrauma (damage to the ear caused by unequal air pressure between the outer and middle ear, as can occur during rapid descent in an airplane).

Physicians recommend that a person recovering from an ear infection have a hearing test each time to make sure healing is complete. Otherwise, if fluid remains in the middle ear, the patient may not know it. Some OTOLOGISTS recommend surgically removing the fluid in the inner ear to prevent permanent damage.

Because some otologists deny there is any inflammation involved, they object to the suffix "itis" and prefer the term "otic transudates." Serous otitis media or glue ear is also called nonsuppurative otitis media, secretory otitis media, middle ear effusion or catarrhal otitis media. (See also AERO-OTITIS MEDIA; OTITIS MEDIA.)

severe-profound hearing loss Generally considered to be a 70 decibel to 90 dB loss.

shingles Also called herpes zoster, this is a viral infection of the nerves that supply certain areas of the skin. It is caused by the varicella-zoster virus, which also causes chickenpox. Some of the viral organisms lie dormant in certain sensory nerves many years after a chickenpox infection; in some people with damaged immune systems, it can re-emerge and cause shingles many years later.

Symptoms begin with skin sensitivity followed by pain, which can be severe. After about five days, a rash appears, which can last for two weeks. Although the blisters disappear, severe pain lasting for years follows in about one-third of patients.

Once the rash appears, little can be done to treat the disease other than giving painkillers. It is possible to reduce the severity of the active stage with antiviral drugs.

No treatment has been proven effective to eliminate the pain following a shingles outbreak. (See also VIRUSES AND HEARING LOSS.)

short increment sensitivity test See SISI.

Sicard, Abbé Roch Ambroise Cucurron (1742–1822) This pioneer of education for deaf students led the Institut National des Jeunes Sourds established by ABBÉ CHARLES MICHEL DE L'EPÉE in 1760.

Born near Toulose on September 28, 1742, little is known of his early life; he was sent to Paris to be trained by l'Epée because of his educational gifts. After l'Epée's death, Sicard succeeded him and ran the school with an iron hand for 32 years.

Sicard's early success in educating his prize pupil JEAN MASSIEU assured him fame and the position of headmaster at the Paris institute.

Sicard's educational method was based on a combination of writing and a system of "methodical signs" developed by l'Epée. This system borrowed some signs from French sign language and invented some others to represent the grammatical structure of French, which represented the first effort at linking a sign and spoken language. Sicard also emphasized extensive grammar drills for his students. In fact, Sicard was widely recognized in France for his excellence as a grammarian, winning him faculty appointments, book contracts and a role as leader of a committee to revise the *Dictionary of the French Language*.

Often dictatorial and unyielding, Sicard's strength and popularity helped him lead his institution through the stormy years of the French Revolution, a time when many clerics were imprisoned as potentially monarchistic.

side-tone Auditory signal that gives a speaker information about his own speech.

Siglish Another name for PIDGIN SIGN ENGLISH, Siglish is a form of signing using the vocabulary of AMERICAN SIGN LANGUAGE in English word order along with some FINGERSPELLING and the use of ASL features such as directionality.

signaling devices These devices add a flashing or vibrating signal to an existing auditory signal and are used for door bells, telephone ring signallers, baby-cry signals, alarm clocks and smoke alarm systems. (See Appendix 3 for information on companies that manufacture and/or distribute these devices.)

sign codes At least four codes for English have been invented, although they all adapt much of their sign vocabulary from AMERICAN SIGN LANGUAGE. Each of these codes tries to duplicate the structure of English in different ways.

Unlike PIDGIN SIGN ENGLISH, these coded English systems use invented signs that correspond directly to English grammar and vocabulary. By matching a sign to a part of English, these systems become codes for English instead of a separate language.

These sign codes were developed in the United States as a way of providing a visual representation of English to improve school performance. Codes include SEEING ESSENTIAL ENGLISH (SEE 1), SIGNING EXACT ENGLISH (SEE 2), and SIGNED ENGLISH.

Developed in the early 1970s, some of these code systems are still used in schools today, although they remain controversial among some deaf people. The invented codes have aroused hostility in the deaf population who believe their native sign languages have not been given dignity and who feel these sign codes create linguistic distortions.

The sign codes now in use are a result of the increasing acceptance of nonoral communication and the wish to teach deaf children the majority oral language by manual means. These codes have been developed as a system, very different from the native and pidgin sign languages that evolved naturally.

Sign codes were developed because it was assumed that oral language can be learned more easily this way rather than by using a native or pidgin sign language. They seem to be easier for parents to learn, since they involve only switching a mode of communication, not learning an entire new language. (See also MANUALLY CODED ENGLISH.)

Signed English This is a manually coded English system used to represent spoken English. Developed in 1973 by Gallaudet University educators Harry Bornstein, Karen Saulnier, Lillian Hamilton and Ralph R. Miller Sr., it is considered to be the least complicated of the manual systems. Signed English includes manual gestures signed in the same word order as English, used with speech, to provide a clear language environment for a hard-of-hearing child.

Signed English features two kinds of gestures: sign markers and sign words. A person using Signed English can match each spoken English word with a sign word or with a sign word and a sign marker. Each of the 3,500 sign words matches the meaning of a separate word in English, with all its various meanings. Sign words do not represent any sounds or spelling. The 14 sign markers represent the most frequent grammatical changes (such as singular, plural, possessive). With a vocabulary limited to 3,500 sign words and 14 affixes, it is not possible to represent the whole English language. But by choosing the most-commonly used English words to transcribe into sign words and affixes, the system is complete enough for most general needs. The manual alphabet can be used to supplement vocabulary.

Learning Signed English is facilitated by an extensive series of texts and posters, which include its main reference text, *The Comprehensive Signed English Dictionary,* three other texts, 50 children's books and three posters. (See also MANUALLY CODED ENGLISH.)

Sign English Another name for PIDGIN SIGN ENGLISH, which is a form of signing using the vocabulary of AMERICAN SIGN LANGUAGE (ASL) in English word order along with some FINGERSPELLING and the use of ASL features such as directionality.

Signing Exact English (SEE 2) This manual communication system is one of the most commonly used manually coded English systems in schools. It was developed in 1972 by Gerilee Gustason, a deaf teacher who lost her hearing at age five; Donna Pfetzing, mother of a deaf child; and Esther Zawolkow, daughter of deaf parents.

SEE 2 uses only one sign to represent an English word that may be expressed by several signs in AMERICAN SIGN LANGUAGE, depending on the meaning of the word in context. Hand signs for words, prefixes and endings are used to give a clear manual representation of English.

In much the same way as Seeing Essential English (SEE 1), Signing Exact English utilizes the sound-spelling-meaning principle. Although both systems define words either as basic, compound or complex, their definitions of these categories are very different. In Signing Exact English, basic words are words that can have no more taken away and still form a complete word, such as "run" or "trot." Compound words are two or more basic words put together, if the meaning of the words separately is consistent with the meaning of the words together.

Complex words are basic words with an added ending, such as dog*s* and run*ning*. Signing Exact English has signs for about 70 different endings.

According to a 1978–79 survey, the SEE 2 system is the most widely used sign method used in schools and classes for hard-of hearing students in the United States. Programs have used this system to support spoken English emphasized in a TOTAL COMMUNICATION approach.

Sign Instructors Guidance Network (SIGN) A listing of sign instructors as part of the communicative skills program of the NATIONAL ASSOCIATION FOR THE DEAF. It offers an evaluation/certification program for sign language instructors. Contact: Sign Instructors Guidance Network, 814 Thayer Ave., Silver Spring, MD 20910; telephone: 301-587-1788.

sign language Sign languages are widely used by deaf people all over the world. Although each country has its own national sign language with its own visual-gestural signs, the sign language does not conform to the grammatical rules and structure of the native language. Within each country there are also different sign language dialects that reflect racial, ethnic or geographical differences. These dialects differ mostly in idiomatic expressions rather than grammar or syntax.

sign language continuum The range in manual communication, from the completely English representation used in schools to the non-English pattern with its own grammar and syntax used by the deaf community.

sign language interpreter A person skilled in the ability to translate the meaning of spoken words into sign language as the words are spoken and to translate sign language into English as signs are formed.

Technically, sign language interpretation is only used when describing the communication process between a hearing person and a person using a true sign language, such as AMERICAN SIGN LANGUAGE. A person interpreting to or from a manually coded form of a spoken language (such as SIGNED ENGLISH) is actually "transliterating," not "interpreting."

Sign language interpreters today are trained to practice their skill in a variety of settings: the legal, educational, medical, diplomatic and business areas. They are also trained to translate from either signed to spoken language or from spoken language to sign (also called sign-to-voice or voice-to-sign). Most importantly, they try to accomplish their communication task without becoming personally involved in the activity and without adding or subtracting any information in either direction.

In addition to standard sign language interpreters, specialized interpreters may at times be necessary. A person who is deaf and blind, for example, may need a specially-trained deaf-blind interpreter. This person can spell words in the deaf person's hand rather than perform traditional sign language. Oral interpreters silently mouth the speaker's words for the deaf person without signing and are skilled in substituting words for words that are difficult to speechread.

In addition, special settings may require special knowledge or responsibilities on the part of the sign language interpreter. One of the most common places to find an interpreter is in school—from elementary to university. An interpreter is most often needed when the deaf student is mainstreamed and must communicate with many hearing students and teachers.

Interpreters in a medical setting will encounter technical terms and may find medical personnel unfamiliar with the role of an interpreter. Mental health interpreting requires sensitivity in other ways since the importance of accurately communicating in both directions can be of critical importance to treatment success. Legal interpreting also involves extensive technical language in very formal settings.

Due to a range of new legislation and educational opportunities affecting deaf people in the mid-1960s, the demand for qualified sign language interpreters suddenly exceeded the limited supply. At about this time, California State University/Northridge, the NATIONAL TECHNICAL INSTITUTE FOR THE DEAF and three regional technical vocational programs opened their doors to deaf students. In response to a much greater need, these schools also set up programs to train interpreters. At the same time, the NATIONAL REGISTRY OF INTERPRETERS FOR THE DEAF was established.

Up to that time, it was assumed that if a person could sign, he could interpret; no research had been done into exactly how interpreting was done or the best way to train an interpreter. Because of this, the first interpreter classes focused simply on teaching American Sign Language, which ended up producing a people who could converse primarily in PIDGIN SIGN ENGLISH. But in 1973, a federal grant established the Interpreter Training Consortium composed of six colleges charged with developing a curriculum for sign language interpreters.

Eventually, experts realized sign language interpreters must be both bilingual and bicultural; therefore, interpreting training courses must include comparative English/ASL linguistic and cultural analyses; text analysis; consecutive and simultaneous interpreting skills; and an overview of the profession (ethics and business practices). From a six-week course, the education of an interpreter has gradually developed into a formal four-year bachelor degree program of study, which may well progress to a graduate-level program.

All types of interpreters are listed with local and state chapters of the Registry of Interpreters for the Deaf, the only national organization that certifies both oral and sign language interpreters. (See also COURT INTERPRETER'S ACT; ORAL INTERPRETERS.)

sign-to-voice interpreting Previously called reverse interpreting, sign-to-voice interpretation is now the preferred term for translating from a signed language to speech. Reverse interpreting is no longer used because it is now recognized that one direction of interpretation is not more important than another. (See also COURT INTERPRETER'S ACT; ORAL INTERPRETERS; REGISTRY OF INTERPRETERS FOR THE DEAF; SIGN LANGUAGE INTERPRETERS.)

sign writing A method of writing down the symbols used in SIGN LANGUAGE. Many ways of sign language writing have been invented by many different researchers for many different reasons.

One of the main problems with sign writing is that the words do not convey the whole message of the sign language sentence. As a way to improve this problem, sign writers write various marks above and below the written word to stand for facial action or body position. But the fact that there is no standard system for these additional descriptors makes sign writing sometimes difficult for everyone to understand.

sim-com See SIMULTANEOUS COMMUNICATION.

simultaneous communication This communication mode combines the use of speech, signs and FINGERSPELLING and is said to offer the benefit of seeing two forms of a message at the same time. The deaf person speechreads what is being spoken and simultaneously reads the signs and fingerspelling of the speaker. In this country, users of simultaneous communication (or sim-com) at times put AMERICAN SIGN LANGUAGE signs in English word order while speaking.

Simultaneous communication is often confused with TOTAL COMMUNICATION since many people use the latter term when they mean speaking and signing at the same time. In the strictest sense, total communication actually refers to a philosophical attitude toward education using all forms of communication; simultaneous communication is one of those forms.

The communication method appeared in early 20th-century America following the oral approach as encouraged by ALEXANDER GRAHAM BELL. As educators began to argue over the importance of oral education, more and more classrooms switched from all-manual communication to a combined method using speech, signs and fingerspelling. The combined method meant that part of a student's day might be taught in sign and part in speech and SPEECHREADING. Students might also be divided according to percent of hearing loss; some might be taught orally, others manually.

Eventually, the conviction of the importance of speaking and speechreading grew to the point where most teachers decided they should speak all the time, and by 1950 most elementary school programs were completely oral. Some teachers still believed in the importance of sign, however, and therefore these instructors paired speech with signing.

But by the late 1960s, educators were disappointed with the poor results of oral-only programs and encouraged by the superior performance of offspring of deaf parents who used sign language from birth. Thus the use of simultaneous communication began an upsurge. By the late 1970s, hundreds of programs for deaf students had abandoned the oral-only approach and started to use sim-com, calling it total communication.

Today, sim-com is the most frequently-used method of communication in deaf schools across the country. It is also the standard method of communication at Gallaudet University.

Sim-com is also frequently used by a deaf and a hearing person in communication, particularly if the hearing person is not fluent in sign, or in a group of people that includes a person who cannot sign. Deaf people, however, almost never use sim-com among themselves; for many, speech had been forced on them for many years and represents a denial of their own language and culture.

Generally, it is not possible to speak English and sign in American Sign Language, since the word order and structure of ASL is fundamentally different from English. Instead, educators and proponents of sim-com have adapted ASL in order to speak English and sign at the same time. The adaptations include using a form of signing called PIDGIN SIGN ENGLISH, a manual code for English, or an older form of signing modeled after English.

Pidgin Sign English uses signs while relying on English to provide a simplified grammatical structure. The manual codes for English include a range of systems developed in the early 1970s that also use signs and English grammatical structure, together with new signs created to represent English articles, pronouns, and affixes (such as -ing, -ed, -s).

These codes include SIGNED ENGLISH, SEEING ESSENTIAL ENGLISH (SEE 1), SIGNING EXACT ENGLISH (SEE 2). Finally, older signers sometimes use modeling English in which the meaning of ASL signs are not changed and English articles or affixes are simply dropped. However, these adaptations are not strictly separated and are often used in combination, because the differences are not well understood by people not fluent in sign.

Simultaneous communication has been controversial because it satisfies neither the proponents of the oral or manual approach. Oralists, who would like to eliminate all signs, believe sim-com doesn't teach good speech skills; those who favor the manual approach counter that the English-linked manual codes usually used in sim-com are pidgin languages.

There are problems with sim-com as well. It is very difficult to speak and sign at the same time and requires such a great deal of concentration that it can inhibit communication. Further, hearing people often do not sign everything they say, which makes it hard for deaf people to follow what they are trying to communicate.

Studies of simultaneous communication have revealed that a person's oral English often deteriorates when speaking and signing; at the same time, the meaning of signs often does not match the meaning of the English words. Further, when speaking and signing together, communication tends to bog down and go much slower than when signing or speaking alone.

Studies of whether simultaneous communication actually helps deaf students learn English have reached conflicting conclusions; it is apparent that these students improve in using a manual code for English but not necessarily in English skills. Studies also do not agree on whether or not deaf students understand and learn better from teachers who use simultaneous communication.

simultaneous interpreting This form of communicating requires the interpreter to mouth and sign everything that the speaker is saying, as opposed to manual interpreting, in which not everything is mouthed. (See also SIGN LANGUAGE INTERPRETERS.)

sinus problems and hearing loss Sinusitis is an inflammation of the linings of the air spaces in the bones of the face around the nose; irritation at the back of the nose may cause swelling around the EUSTACHIAN TUBE, which can interfere with the normal function of the middle ear, resulting in a temporary hearing loss.

Nasal sprays used to treat sinusitis can aggravate a hearing problem since these sprays can actually increase swelling and irritation around the eustachian tube.

SISI A type of hearing test (an abbreviation for Short Increment Sensitivity) used by an AUDIOLOGIST to uncover certain types of nerve loss. Because individuals with cochlear lesions often are oversensitive to sound (called RECRUITMENT), a person with recruitment can also detect smaller changes in sound intensity than a person with normal hearing could.

In the test, a steady tone 20 DECIBELS (dB) above the patient's threshold is presented every two minutes. Every five seconds, the intensity is increased one dB, and the patient pushes a button each time a change is heard. A detection percentage is determined by multiplying five times the number of increments out of a maximum of 20 that are perceived. Scores over 60% suggest a cochlear disorder. (See also AUDIOMETRY.)

Smetana, Bedřich (1824–1884) The creator of the Czech national opera and composer of "My Fatherland," this Czechoslovakian musician first had hearing problems at the age of 36 and became completely deaf 14 years later as a result of the disintegration of the nervous system caused by SYPHILIS.

Still, he continued to play and compose and completed the last four of his six symphonic poems without being able to hear any of them.

Smith, Erastus (1787–1837) This Texas folk hero was the chief scout and spy for General Sam Houston, commander-in-chief of the Texas army.

Erastus "Deaf" Smith was born to a large family near Poughkeepsie, New York. A sickly, solitary child, Smith lost his hearing during early infancy and received little education thereafter.

Nineteen years later he visited what is now Texas, moving there permanently in 1821, where he was known as "el Sordo" (the Deaf One). After marrying a Spanish woman, he was granted Mexican citizenship and became fluent in Spanish despite his severe hearing problem. The two lived in San Antonio, which at the time was part of Mexico.

A loyal Mexican citizen, he never suspected Texas would one day petition to join the United States. But with the beginning of the Texas Revolution in 1835, Smith's neutrality was soon over; upon returning to his home in San Antonio one day, he found the town occupied by Mexicans and under siege by Texans. When the Mexicans fired on him and refused to let him return to his home, Smith joined General Stephen F. Austin and the Texas forces.

Because he was so familiar with the area, Smith was invaluable to the Texan army, becoming scout to Sam Houston en route to the Alamo. It was Smith who brought back the only two survivors of the massacre there, Mrs. Almeron Dickerson and her baby daughter. It was also Smith's advice to Houston that assured the Texan's victory at San Jacinto, where Santa Anna was captured and Texas gained its independence from Mexico.

Smith died from a lung problem in Richmond on November 30, 1837. Deaf Smith County in Texas is named in his honor.

smoking and deafness See NICOTINE AND HEARING LOSS.

social adequacy index (SAI) A measure of the degree to which a patient has problems in hearing and understanding speech. The SAI is computed from the results of speech reception thresholds and speech discrimination tests.

Social Security and hearing loss The Social Security Administration has two benefit programs for people with a hearing loss who meet their state's requirements for "disability": Supplemental Security Income (SSI) and Social Security Disability Insurance (SSDI). Both benefits are awarded to children or adults who meet the criteria for being disabled and—in the case of SSI—for financial need. To be eligible for SSDI, a working adult must have paid Social Security at least five of the last 10 years.

sociocusis A hearing loss caused by environmental noise.

sound conduction Sound waves move outward in all directions by back and forth movements of molecules through solids, liquids or gases.

Each complete back-and-forth movement (oscillation) is called a cycle, and the number of cycles generated by a sound source every second is known as the frequency. The term "hertz" (abbreviated Hz) represents cycles per second and is named after HEINRICH HERTZ, a famous scientist who studied sound.

Human ears can detect sounds within a frequency range of 20 Hz to 20,000 Hz; the range of speech lies mostly between 100 and 8,000 Hz. The higher the frequency, the higher the pitch or tone; almost all of the sounds we hear are combinations of many frequencies. Sounds used in hearing tests that are only one frequency are called pure tones.

A sound wave's pressure on the surface it contacts is a measure of the sound's intensity, or power. The greater the intensity of the sound waves on a person's eardrum, the louder the sound that is heard. A sound that is just barely able to be heard is the threshold intensity.

In order to test hearing, it is important to be able to measure the intensity of sounds heard; therefore, an internationally-accepted sound pressure level has been set to correspond approximately to that of a threshold intensity for a sound with a frequency of 1,000 Hz. Other sound pressures are compared to this reference pressure on a scale measured in decibels (dB), a name taken from the inventor of the telephone, ALEXANDER GRAHAM BELL. Sound intensities on this scale increase tenfold for every 20-dB difference in sound pressure.

There are two ways for sound to be conducted through our ears—air and bone conduction. Air conduction occurs when sound moves from the external ear (pinna) to the middle and inner ears. Bone conduction occurs when sound vibrations are transmitted through the skull bones directly to the cochlea.

A blockage in the external or middle ears means an overall reduction in all sound intensities but not a total hearing loss, since sound is also routed through bone. (See also AUDIOMETRY.)

soundfield testing A hearing test used with young children in which sounds are presented to both ears at once without the use of earphones. (See also AUDIOMETRY.)

sound spectrograph A device that records the continually changing intensity levels of frequency components in a complex sound wave via a filter analyzer.

sound wave A pressure area produced by vibration moving through air or water, causing reactions in the ear that the brain interprets as sound. (See also SOUND CONDUCTION.)

Spain This country, which has a deaf population of 20,000, has a deeply-rooted tradition of educating deaf students.

More than 400 years ago, a Spanish monk named PEDRO PONCE DE LEON first taught deaf people to speak. Today there is a range of special elementary and secondary schools specializing in deaf education that use a wide variety of approaches. Although some schools favor MAINSTREAMING, this method is opposed by schools who favor the oral approach.

Most deaf children begin school at age four and continue to 18; there are vocational courses open to them but no special university for deaf students. If a deaf student wishes to earn a degree at a regular university, he or she must do so without the use of an interpreter. For this reason, there are not many deaf graduates of Spanish universities.

Deaf Spaniards have a strong community, and communicate in SPANISH SIGN LANGUAGE, although dialects vary from province to province. There are special telephone devices available, but few deaf Spaniards have them in their homes. Television captioning has not yet become available.

Spanish Sign Language The origins of Spanish Sign Language are unknown, but today sign language is used by virtually all Spaniards. It has few dialects, although its grammar is complex and poorly understood by modern linguists.

There seems to be no well-defined subject-verb-object word order in SSL. Verbs are made using one gesture, adding prefixes or suffixes as needed. FINGERSPELLING is rarely used and then only for proper names for when there is no gestural sign.

At present, the teaching of sign language in Spanish schools is under debate; some schools allow SSL and others do not. (See also SPAIN.

speech audiometry A measure of hearing spoken words presented at controlled intensity levels. (See also AUDIOMETRY.)

speech discrimination test A special speech/hearing test that tries to determine the ability to hear familiar words. (See also AUDIOMETRY.)

speech frequencies In audiometric testing, these are the pure-tone frequencies that can best predict the level at which speech can be understood (500, 1,000 and 2,000 Hz).

speech-language pathologist A specialist in human communication, its development and its disorders. Also known as a speech pathologist or speech therapist, the speech-language pathologist evaluates and treats persons with communication problems resulting from total or partial hearing loss, brain injury, cleft palate, voice pathology, emotional problems, foreign dialect, development delays, stroke, learning disabilities and so forth. They also provide clinical therapy to help those with speech and language disorders, and help them and their families understand the disorder and develop better communication skills.

In most settings, speech-language pathologists perform screening tests of auditory acuity and tympanometry (a measure of middle ear function). Only a speech-language pathologist is certified to make recommendations for the type of speech language treatment required. Treatment could include a specific program of exercises to improve language ability or speech together with support from the client's family and friends.

To practice speech-language pathology, states require a master's degree in speech-language pathology, more than 300 hours of supervised clinical experience and successful completion of a certifying exam.

speechreading The preferred term for lipreading, a way of recognizing spoken words by watching the speaker's lips, jaw and tongue movements. Speechreading is the least consistently visible of the communication choices available to deaf people; only about 30% of English sounds are visible on the lips, and half are homophonous (that is, they look like other words). For example, the words "kite," "height" and "night" look almost identical.

The ability to speechread is often contingent on the visibility, shape and configuration of the speaker's mouth. For example, it may be difficult to speechread someone who mumbles, who has a beard or who has no teeth.

Some deaf people become skilled speechreaders, especially if they can supplement what they see with some hearing. Many don't develop much skill at speechreading, but most do speechread to some extent. Because speechreading requires considerable guesswork, very few deaf people rely on speechreading alone when exchanging important information.

One system that has been designed to be used with speechreading is CUED SPEECH, developed by Dr. Orin Cornett of Gallaudet University. Cued speech is a method in which hand movements and location are used to make all of the sounds produced on the lips clear to the speechreader. (See also VISEME.)

speech reception threshold test A special speech hearing test that determines the softest speech a person can hear. (See also AUDIOMETRY.)

speech therapist See SPEECH-LANGUAGE PATHOLOGIST.

speech training Teaching speech to profoundly deaf individuals has been the center of a number of controversies in deaf education for hundreds of years. Today, controversy centers on how well deaf people can be taught to speak and the best methods to achieve that goal. Some still question the need to teach speech to deaf students at all.

The wide range of teaching methods vary according to the size of the speech unit taught and the number of senses the student uses in order to learn speech. Those methods that emphasize small units of speech (syllables and speech sounds) are called analytic; methods that teach units of speech no smaller than syllables and stress the importance of connected speech fall into the synthetic category.

speech training aids Devices that display speech electronically to teach those who cannot hear how to use their voice. One of the newest is the Matsushita speech system being evaluated jointly at the Lexington School for the Deaf in New York and the City University of New York.

With this speech system, which was developed in Japan, a speech therapist and client wear special sensors inside the mouth and on the nose that are linked to a computer. When the therapist pronounces a sound or a word, the computer generates an image on a video screen that illustrates the position of the tongue within the mouth, the vibration of the nose and the intensity of the voice. The student learns to pronounce the sound or word by trying to produce the same pattern on the screen.

According to Esther Lustig of the Lexington School, the device is still in the early stages of research but shows "great promise." Originally used in Japan, the school is testing it for use with American English-speaking students and are helping develop English language software for deaf individuals in the United States.

"It's a long-range project because you have to make sure the improvement you see is a result of the machine and not other factors," Lustig explained. "You need a sampling over a period of time." The school has been testing the system since February 1989. Although Lustig emphasized that the system is still in the experimental stages, she reports anecdotal improvement among students who use it.

Other devices have been developed including a computer-based system for children with displays that resemble video games and a laryngograph, which monitors the action of the larynx from two plates held against the throat, displaying voice pitch coordination with other movements and voice quality.

stapedectomy The purpose of this operation is to treat hearing loss caused by OTOSCLEROSIS, a familial form of deafness that is curable only by surgery. Otosclerosis causes the base of the stapes (stirrup), the innermost of the three bones in the middle ear, to become fixed to the opening of the inner ear by an overgrowth of spongy bone. This interferes with the stapes' ability to transmit sound to the inner ear.

While the patient is under a local or general anesthetic, a surgeon opens the ear canal and folds the eardrum forward. All (or most) of the stapes is removed, and a plastic or metal prosthesis is inserted into the entrance to the inner ear; the other end is attached to the incus. The eardrum is then repaired.

Antibiotics are usually used up to five days after surgery to prevent infection; packing and sutures are removed about a week after surgery. Hearing shows improvement within two weeks and continues to get better over the next three months.

Good candidates for a stapedectomy are patients who have fixed stapes from otosclerosis and a CONDUCTIVE HEARING LOSS of at least 20 dB with a speech discrimination score of at least 60%. Patients with a severe hearing loss might still profit from a stapedectomy, if only to bring their hearing up to a level where a hearing aid could be of help.

The operation improves hearing in more than 90% of cases, although about 1% of patients experience loss of hearing from damage to the COCHLEA. Because of this risk, a stapedectomy is normally done on one ear at a time, although otosclerosis usually affects both ears. It is almost never used on a patient with hearing in only one ear.

Other less common complications from the surgery include change in taste from damage to the chorda tympani nerve, perforated eardrum, vertigo and damage to the ossicular chain. Temporary Bell's palsy (facial nerve paralysis) can occur immediately after the operation. Occasionally, vertigo persists and may require surgery. (See also FENESTRATION; STAPES MOBILIZATION.)

stapedial footplate See FOOTPLATE.

stapedial muscle One of two intra-aural muscles in the middle ear, the stapedial muscle is attached to the top of the stapes and runs behind it.

stapedius A small muscle in the inner wall of the MIDDLE EAR that inserts into the neck of the STAPES and is responsible for retracting the stapes.

stapes Commonly called the stirrup, this is the smallest bone in the body and is one of the three tiny bones that make up the OSSICLES in the middle ear. The head of the stapes joins the middle ossicle (anvil). Its base fits into the oval window located in the wall of the inner ear and, as it vibrates, plunges in and out of the oval window.

The condition of OTOSCLEROSIS immobilizes the stapes in the entrance to the inner ear by an overgrowth of spongy bone, interfering with the ability of the stapes to move freely and transmit sound to the inner ear, thereby causing deafness. The condition can be helped by a hearing aid but is cured only by surgery (STAPEDECTOMY). Although the operation improves hearing in about 90% of patients, about 1% of patients actually experience a deterioration of hearing. This is why—although otosclerosis normally affects both ears—a stapedectomy is usually only done on one ear at a time.

stapes mobilization This operation for OTOSCLEROSIS was accidentally discovered during FENESTRATION (an operation creating a new oval window) when the stapes had been accidentally moved too much, loosening the otosclerosis and mobilizing the STAPES. After the operation, the patient had much better hearing than is normal after a simple fenestration.

But although this new type of operation seemed exciting at first, it was discovered that the otosclerosis continued to be active and would again fix the stapes to the OVAL WINDOW, losing all benefits of the mobilization. And for many patients, the otosclerosis had progressed too far and scarred or fixed their stapes too much to be helped with mobilization.

Mobilization today is used primarily for people who were born with problems of the stapes or oval window. In other patients, a STAPEDECTOMY is preferred to treat otosclerosis.

Stenger test A functional hearing impairment test in which both ears are stimulated by the same frequency but at different intensities. This test is used to assess a person's hearing loss in one ear. (See also AUDIOMETRY.)

stenosis A narrowing of the external ear canal as a result of various disease processes, including chronic OTITIS MEDIA (ear infection), inflammation, allergic reaction, injury or PERICHONDRITIS (an infection primarily of the cartilage covering the pinna).

stirrup See STAPES.

substance abuse The incidence of drug and alcohol abuse among deaf people is similar to the incidence among hearing people. However, deaf abusers historically have faced discrimination in treatment programs and services, with few professionals trained in chemical dependency and deafness, according to the National Information Center on Deafness.

There have been few studies of substance abuse in the deaf community, although it is generally believed that the problem is about the same as substance abuse in the hearing population: 1 in 10.

Deaf substance abusers generally have few ties with churches, organizations and clubs of the deaf community and live on the fringes of both the deaf and hearing societies. Substance abusers who are deaf high school students follow similar patterns.

Although treatment programs for substance abusers in the United States have proliferated since the 1930s, deaf people have found major barriers to existing treatment facilities. One of the biggest obstacles to treatment may be found in the deaf community itself, which has been reluctant in the past to admit that its members have a problem. Few referrals to substance abuse agencies come from the deaf community.

Further, deaf substance abusers find it difficult to admit to themselves that there is a problem, and self-referrals to treatment are lower in this population than in the general population.

A deaf person seeking treatment for a substance abuse problem, however, faces other hurdles: Most programs have been designed for hearing clients, and counselors lack an understanding of deafness, the deaf community and manual methods of communication. Agencies often can't afford to hire interpreters, and deafness experts aren't trained in substance abuse rehabilitation.

In 1973 the first treatment center for deaf alcoholics was established in St. Paul, Minneapolis, followed a year later by another in San Francisco.

In 1975, the first national conference on substance abuse in the deaf community was held in Cleveland, Ohio. During this time, inpatient treatment for deaf alcoholics, counseling programs and outreach projects were begun. In 1979 the quarterly *AID Bulletin* began to provide updated information to a national membership.

By 1985, alcohol treatment programs had begun in California, Illinois, New York, Ohio, Maryland, Minnesota and Massachusetts. These programs combine an outreach advocacy program run by specialists in substance abuse and deafness.

From the early 1970s on, programs for deaf alcoholics have featured outreach projects directed by substance abuse experts who understand the communication problems of deaf clients. When such treatment is therefore modified, deaf and hearing alcoholics recover at the same rate.

Sweden There are an estimated 208,000 deaf and hard-of-hearing people in Sweden. There are approximately 200 hard-of-hearing babies born each year and of these, about 50 are profoundly deaf. About 87 per 100,000 Swedes are deaf, according to 1930 statistics, one of the higher prevalence rates among developed countries (which range from 300 per 100,000 to 35 per 100,000).

The first school for deaf children in Sweden was opened in Stockholm in 1809, influenced by other European schools and relying on the oral approaches. But unlike many other schools in Europe, Sweden retained an interest in manual education and taught either method to children depending on individual preferences.

Today, deaf Swedes can attend either large state schools for deaf children or local community schools, where many children are mainstreamed.

More than 90% of Swedish children go on to a "gymnasium" (higher education) after completing the required nine years of school; although there are no special classes for hard-of-hearing students in these gymnasiums, there is a special gymnasium for deaf students in Orebro, where they may take vocational courses or pre-university studies.

Swedish Sign Language The language of more than 8,000 Swedish deaf citizens,

Swedish Sign Language is unrelated to any other sign language in the world and is not derived from any other sign system.

Still, it shares many characteristics of other sign languages, including a complex structure; signs are made with the hands, while facial expression, body movement and posture are used to indicate clause and sentence type. In addition, lip movements are always used with FINGERSPELLING and may also be used with signs. Sweden's manual alphabet was invented in the early 1800s by Swedish educator Per Aron Borg, who later took this alphabet to Portugal where he established schools for deaf students.

swimmer's ear Also known as external otitis or otitis externa, this ear problem is an infection of the ear canal that occurs after swimming in dirty or heavily chlorinated water. The risk of getting swimmer's ear increases with the frequency of swimming, the longer the person stays in the water and the more often the head is submerged.

Swimmer's ear usually results in redness and swelling of the ear canal, a discharge and sometimes excema around the ear opening. Itching may become painful and deafness can occur if pus blocks the ear.

It is treated with drying of the ear followed by antibiotic, antifungal or anti-inflammatory drugs.

For swimmers, this condition can be prevented by putting a few drops of rubbing alcohol in the ear after swimming. Because alcohol evaporates sooner than water, it helps draw water out of the ear. Physicians often recommend that sufferers limit time spent in the water to no longer than one hour with an hour or two wait between dips to allow the ear to dry out. Earplugs are not a good idea since they can irritate the skin of the canal.

Swimmer's ear can also be caused by excessive washing, perspiration, irritation of the ear canal after removal of foreign objects, allergies or a generalized skin disease such as atopic eczema or seborrheic dermatitis.

Swiss Sign Language Traditionally a country that favored the oral approach, sign language in SWITZERLAND today is slowly making a comeback in the deaf community.

In a country divided into three cultural sections (German, French and Italian), Swiss Sign Language varies widely from strictly sign language to mixtures of sign and spoken language.

Neither the German nor French areas of Switzerland have a manual alphabet. Because of this, the set of handshapes that make up the sign language is more restricted, and there is a tendency to mouth the equivalent word in the spoken language for those ideas that have no sign.

Research suggests that the various dialects of Swiss Sign Language have many similar characteristics in common with other sign languages, including the use of facial expressions, eye gaze and body posture.

In general, sign language is not widely used in the classroom, although both sign language and the pidgin forms of signing are used in the deaf community. There are still an insufficient number of sign language instructors and courses.

Switzerland Life in Switzerland for deaf citizens is a complicated affair since the decentralized country recognizes four languages (German, French, Italian and Romansh) with a bewildering number of dialects, particularly in German and Romansh. Prevalence of deafness is rather high (94 out of 100,000) when compared to other countries, but almost equal to the rate in the United States (100 out of 100,000).

Although education varies among the 23 different cantons (states), in general hard-of-hearing students who use amplification attend regular schools, and deaf students are taught to speechread and speak. Schools are open to deaf students between ages 6 and 16.

The manual approach is not widespread in Switzerland, but deaf students sign outside of class. Although there are differences among local sign languages, most deaf people can make each other understood across dialects.

sympathetic vibration A vibration in one object produced by vibrations of the same frequency in another object.

syntax The study of the rules of sentence formation. (See also LINGUISTICS.)

syphilis Whether contracted at birth or later in life, syphilis may cause an inner ear hearing loss. When a pregnant woman becomes infected with the disease, her unborn child usually also contracts the disease; 35% of these infants will eventually go on to experience some degree of hearing loss.

This eventual hearing loss from prenatal exposure to syphilis is hard to quantify since the deafness may show up suddenly later in childhood or even in adulthood.

Children tend to experience hearing loss in both ears suddenly, and if it appears before age 10, deafness is usually profound.

Hearing loss in adulthood from syphilis appears more gradually, as either a hearing loss or a fluctuation in intensity.

Treatment with penicillin and steroids is usually given for some months; if hearing improves, the steroids may be continued indefinitely to stave off a recurrent hearing loss. Although some syphilis-caused hearing loss responds immediately to treatment, other cases do not, in spite of continued treatment.

Because syphilis causes a SENSORINEURAL HEARING LOSS, sufferers have a poor understanding of speech even with the use of hearing aids. (See also PRENATAL CAUSES OF HEARING LOSS.)

syphilitic labyrinthitis See LABYRINTHITIS.

systemic infections and hearing loss Infections such as SCARLET FEVER, typhoid fever, MEASLES and tuberculosis can sometimes cause bilateral SENSORINEURAL HEARING loss.

In particular, scarlet fever can cause a moderate degree of sensorineural deafness with bilateral acute and, later, chronic OTITIS MEDIA.

T

tactile feedback device This device provides a substitute for sounds a deaf person cannot hear by converting sounds into a pattern of sensations on the skin. It is generally used in speech therapy, although it may also be used as an aid to speechreading.

One of the more recent devices, the Audiotact (produced by Sevrain-Tech of Madison, Wisconsin), uses 32 electrodes incorporated into a belt worn around the abdomen to stimulate the skin with electrical pulses that feel like finger taps, with different sounds producing different patterns of stimulation. By learning what these sounds ''feel'' like, a person can learn or pronounce them and eventually put these sounds together in words and sentences.

Unfortunately, it's hard to produce enough distinct patterns with 32 electrodes to represent the large variety of sounds in speech. As a result, the National Institute on Deafness and Other Communication Disorders is funding development of a device with 256 electrodes.

tangible reinforcement operant conditioning audiometry (TROCA) A type of hearing test used for preschool children, which rewards the young patient with positive reinforcement (candy, treats) for appropriate responses to sound (See also AUDIOMETRY.)

T-coil See TELECOIL.

TDD See TELECOMMUNICATIONS DEVICE FOR THE DEAF.

TDD distribution programs State programs—often established by legislative mandate—that provide eligible deaf and hard-of-hearing people access to telephone communication.

Usually, they are administered by the relevant state agency on deafness, which invites applications from residents who are deaf or hard-of-hearing, or have speech problems. Once applicants are screened for medical and financial eligibility, they may be given a TELECOMMUNICATIONS DEVICE FOR THE DEAF (TDD) at no charge or allowed to buy TDDs at substantially reduced rates.

tectorial membrane This fine, gelatinous membrane lies on top of the hair cells of the ORGAN OF CORTI, which in turn lies within the full length of the scala media.

When the ear transmits sound, high frequencies stimulate the hair cells at the lower end of the COCHLEA, and low frequencies stimulate hair cells toward the upper end. As the sound waves stimulate the hair cells, the nerves at the base of the cells gather the impulses and send them to the brain.

telecaption adapter See TELECAPTION DECODER.

TeleCaption decoder A device attached to a television set that interprets certain signals broadcast at the same time as the TV program, converting them to typed dialogue across the bottom of the TV screen. Manufactured and distributed by the NATIONAL CAPTIONING INSTITUTE, the devices are compatible with all TVs, video cassette recorders (VCRs) and cable hookups.

Since 1980, NCI has developed four generations of decoders. The current TeleCaption 4000 was introduced in 1989 and is less expensive than the first decoder available nine years earlier.

Together with ITT Corp., NCI is developing an integrated circuit chip that will allow TV manufacturers to provide built-in decoding capability in various sets. (See also CLOSED CAPTIONS; CAPTIONED FILMS/VIDEOS FOR THE DEAF; CAPTION CENTER.)

telecaptioning See CLOSED CAPTIONS.

telecoil The telecoil (also called the T-coil and the T-switch) is a tiny electrical component that can sense magnetic forces generated by another coil nearby, such as the speaker coil in a telephone or a loop or wire around the room or around a person's neck. The major use for a telecoil has been with the telephone, allowing clearer sound reception for the hard-of-hearing consumer.

When a hearing aid's control switch is set to the T-switch, the telecoil is connected and the hearing aid's microphone is disconnected. This allows the aid to receive magnetic signals instead of sound, enabling the wearer to hear only the "important" sound coming from the telecoil while screening out annoying background noise.

T-switches have become important with the advent of ASSISTIVE LISTENING DEVICES and assistive listening systems. More and more, public areas (churches, theaters, meeting rooms and so forth) have been fitted with assistive listening systems to help the hearing impaired. Where such an induction loop system is in place, the hearing aid wearer can turn on the T-mode to receive sound through the loop. Or, where certain public places feature FM or infrared systems, the wearer may use a special receiver to connect with the hearing aid in the T-mode.

In much the same way, assistive listening devices use the T-switch to improve hearing of TV and radio.

Not all HEARING AIDS have a telecoil, including most canal or in-the-ear aids. However, many behind-the-ear and all body aids have telecoils. Because there are no regulations or standards regarding telecoils, they can vary as much as 30 decibels in maximum sound output.

telecommunications device for the deaf Known as a TDD, this mechanical/electronic compensatory device allows people to type phone messages over the telephone network. The term TDD is generic and replaces the earlier term TTY, which refers specifically to teletypewriter machines.

Basically a visual typewriter, a TDD connects to a telephone line by a modular plug or acoustic modem. The conversation is displayed on a screen moving from right to left above the keyboard. Some TDDs have a printer, which provides a permanent record on special paper of all messages transmitted and received. A TDD is required at both ends of the phone line in order to communicate.

TDD keyboards follow the typical typewriter's layout, except that most TDDs have three-row keyboards on which the numerals 0 through 9 appear as upper case characters above the letters QWERTYUIOP. Some TDDs have four-row keyboards.

The TDD was invented in 1964 by ROBERT H. WEITBRECHT, a deaf physicist and licensed ham radio operator, together with James Marsters, a deaf orthodontist. The two wanted to investigate the possible ways a hard-of-hearing person might communicate by using a teletypewriter (TTY) with a radio or telephone. Working together in California, the two decided a telephone system would be more logical since many hard-of-hearing and deaf people already had telephones in their homes and a radio system would have required the deaf person to get a license from the Federal Communications Commission.

Weitbrecht developed an acoustic coupler that converted the electrical signals of the teletypewriter into audible tones that could be sent over the telephone network. A deaf person would place a telephone on Weitbrecht's special modem and a modified teleprinter machine. It took Weitbrecht several years to complete his "Weitbrecht Modem." At that same time, the telephone and telegraph companies were replacing their old teletypewriter equipment with newer devices.

Through an agreement between AT&T and the Alexander Graham Bell Association for the Deaf, surplus TTYs were obtained and equipped with acoustic couplers. These devices provided the first way for deaf people to communicate by telephone across the country. Both deaf organizations formed Teletypewriters for the Deaf Distribution Committee in Indianapolis, Indiana (now TELECOMMUNICATIONS FOR THE DEAF, INC.)

In some states, phone companies lend or sell TDDs at subsidized prices, and more and more public agencies are installing them. In addition, relay services are available to connect TDD and voice calls through an interpreter. By law, as of 1991 every state must have in place a TDD RELAY SERVICE.

New technology TDDs and computers use different codes for the letters of the alphabet and other characters, and therefore cannot normally communicate. However, it is possible to equip a personal computer with a special modem to make it function as a TDD. (A modem is a device that allows a computer to use a telephone line to transmit information to other computers with compatible modems).

Most TDDS with build-in modems can normally understand only transmissions in the BAUDOT CODE. Personal computers use the ASCII code, and modems designed for use with a computer accommodate only that code. However, there are four modems available that have the ability to communicate in both Baudot and ASCII codes.

Today there are a wide variety of other TDD products for deaf consumers. Some TDDs come in very small, lightweight, portable sizes. Others have built-in answering machines that respond only to TDD calls. For households that require it, there is an answering machine that responds to both voice and TDD calls.

Newest advances include a product that allows a deaf person to converse with anyone who owns a touchtone phone. The deaf person clamps the new device over the receiver, and the machine prints out a message on a tiny screen when the person on the other end taps out a special code on a touchtone phone.

In 1989, IBM introduced the Phone-Communicator, a system that allows a person with a TDD to communicate over phone lines with anyone owning an IBM-compatible personal computer. The Phone-Communicator includes an automatic answer mode capable of recording messages from touch-tone telephones and TDD callers.

Telecommunications for the Deaf, Inc. A consumer-oriented organization that sells caption decoders and a directory for deaf people. The group supports legislation and advocates the use of TELECOMMUNICATIONS DEVICES FOR THE DEAF, ASCII code, Emergency Access (911), telecaptioning and visual ALERTING DEVICES in the public, private and government sectors. Contact: Telecommunications for the Deaf, Inc., 814 Thayer Ave., Silver Spring, MD 20910; telephone: (voice) 301-589-3786, (TDD) 301-589-3006.

Telecommunications for the Disabled Act of 1982 See LEGAL RIGHTS.

Tele-Consumer Hotline Nonprofit, independent and impartial telephone consumer information service that provides free telephone assistance and publications on special telephone equipment, TDD directories, TDD/voice relay services, choosing a long distance company, selecting a phone, money saving tips and more. Contact: Tele-Consumer Hotline, 1910 K St., Suite 610, Washington, DC 20006; telephone: 800-332-1124 (outside D.C.) or (voice and TDD) 202-223-4371.

teletext A form of closed captioning that uses a different decoder than the LINE 21 system TELECAPTION DECODER. The teletext system uses several lines of the vertical blanking interval instead of just one line, as in the line 21 system.

Although similar in appearance to the line 21 system of closed captioning, teletext captioning may also include symbols, or icons, to indicate sound effects and may be quite elaborate. Teletext provides many "pages" of information that can be selected individually, and that don't move up on the screen.

The most well-known teletext system in the United States, the NORTH AMERICAN BASIC TELETEXT SPECIFICATION (NABTS) was adopted by CBS for text services and captioning, which is the only TV network to use the teletext system.

While NABTS decoders have been available since 1984, their use has not been widespread, in part because they require excellent television reception and cannot be used with video recorders. Since 1984 CBS has offered both teletext and line 21 closed captioning. (See also CAPTION CENTER, CLOSED CAPTIONS; NATIONAL CAPTIONING INSTITUTE; TELECAPTION DECODER.)

temporal bone fracture and hearing loss Head trauma with skull fracture involving the two temporal bones (which house the structures of the middle and inner ear) often involve the middle ear and causes a CONDUCTIVE HEARING LOSS. A transverse fracture of the temporal bone can also injure the inner ear or internal auditory meatus, causing SENSORINEURAL HEARING LOSS, VERTIGO, TINNITUS and facial nerve paralysis.

temporary hearing loss A nonpermanent hearing loss that often follows exposure to a loud, explosive noise such as a gunshot.

temporomandibular joint syndrome (TMJ) Severe pain in the jaw, face and head, especially around the ears, that researchers believe is caused by the improper function of the jaw (temporomandibular) joints and their muscles and ligaments.

Other symptoms of TMJ include jaw and ear clicking or popping, "locking" jaws and pain in opening the mouth, and hearing loss.

Clenching and grinding the teeth, which cause the muscles to go into spasm, is the most common cause of TMJ. An incorrect bite, excessive tension, head injury or, rarely, osteoarthritis can also lead to TMJ.

Treatment involves the application of moist heat to relieve the muscle spasm and the use of muscle relaxant medication and pain relievers. In severe cases, joint surgery may be required.

tensor tympani One of the two intra-aural muscles located in the middle ear. The tensor tympani is attached to the upper portion of the manubrium (the handle of the malleus) and crossed diagonally across the TYMPANUM into the tensor canal. It is supplied by a branch of the TRIGEMINAL NERVE.

threshold The softest sound or speech a person can hear. (See also AUDIOMETRY.)

tinnitus A ringing, buzzing, hissing or whistling noise heard inside the ear when the acoustic nerve transmits impulses to the brain impulses produced not from outside vibrations but as the result of stimuli produced inside the head. Actually, tinnitus is divided into two different types: tinnitus aurium (ringing in the ear) and tinnitus cerebri (ringing in the head).

Tinnitus is also classified as vibratory or nonvibratory. Vibratory tinnitus originates outside the inner ear and is caused by vibration from any of the middle ear hearing mechanisms, such as a dislocated ossicular chain or wax against the eardrum. It is possible for another person to hear vibratory tinnitus from as far away as several feet.

Nonvibratory tinnitus begins in either the inner ear or the auditory nervous system and is subjective, since only the patient can hear these sounds.

Tinnitus, which may affect as many as 40 million adults, usually involves almost continuous noise (although the affected person may only be aware of the noise occasionally). Tinnitus does not cause hearing disorders, but it may accompany decreased hearing and other ear symptoms, such as pressure or DIZZINESS, and may be psychologically uncomfortable as well.

Tinnitus often starts after an injury damages some of the sound-sensing hair cells of the inner ear, which lose their sensitivity to sound but still produce activity. Because these impulses travel along the hearing nerve, the brain interprets them as sound.

Causes

Noise Tinnitus can be produced by a wide variety of causes, but the most common is extensive exposure to very loud noise for long periods of time, which causes excessive wear of the inner ear. Although tinnitus can occur after a single loud noise, such as a gunshot, it is much more common after continuous noise overexposure, such as from industrial machinery, aircraft engines or loud music.

For example, a person who has worked for many years around mechanical equipment, uses a snowmobile frequently and who spends a lot of time cutting firewood with a power saw would be at much greater risk for developing tinnitus. Some people, however, appear to have a much higher tolerance for similar kinds of excessive noise and do not develop tinnitus under identical circumstances. Researchers as yet do not know why.

Head injury After excessive noise, head injury is the next most common cause of tinnitus. Because the delicate mechanisms involved in hearing are buried inside the skull, head injury of almost any kind can produce tinnitus. Even a slap—if it lands directly on the ear—can cause tinnitus, which may show up several days after the injury and then one day simply disappear.

Drugs Tinnitus can also be produced by OTOTOXIC DRUGS; aspirin is particularly well-known for a type of tinnitus that disappears after medication is stopped. On the other hand, quinine can produce a permanent tinnitus. Many of the aminoglycoside antibiotics may also produce tinnitus but only after longterm drug use and after extensive hearing loss has already occurred.

Diseases Diseases, such as MÉNIÈRE'S DISEASE, diabetes, thyroid problems, OTOSCLEROSIS, tumor on the hearing nerve, ear infections, or even excess wax against the eardrum, can cause tinnitus. Treatment of some diseases, such as otosclerosis, will also eliminate the tinnitus, but in others (notably, Meniere's disease), the tinnitus symptoms will be altered but not eliminated. Although the tinnitus that sometimes accompanies colds is temporary, people who travel in airplanes while nursing a cold may develop a severe and persistent form of tinnitus.

Physicians tend to consider tinnitus more of a nuisance than a medical condition; however, a person who has tinnitus in only one ear and who has not been exposed to excessive noise that might otherwise explain the tinnitus should immediately see an OTOLOGIST and an AUDIOLOGIST. Unilateral tinnitus can be a symptom of several serious ear diseases, including ACOUSTIC NEUROMA.

Treatment

Masking There is no cure for tinnitus, but there are ways to relieve the problem. Because the quieter the environment is, the worse tinnitus is, masking techniques that provide background noise will override the tinnitus impulses by keeping the ears busy with nerve signals from actual sounds to pass on to the brain. It takes advantage of a phenomenon called "residual inhibition," which means that following exposure to certain kinds of noise, there is a reduction in the level of tinnitus for a time.

However, not all tinnitus responds to masking; anyone considering buying a masker should first be tested to see if this treatment will bring relief. Playing a radio or tapes of natural sounds (waves or rain forest noises, for example) can often help.

Drug treatment Drug treatment may be effective in some cases, although there have been no definitive studies as yet. Studies have shown that the intravenous use of the local anesthetic lidocaine helps about 87% of tinnitus patients. But because the effects are only temporary, it is not practical as a permanent treatment.

The drug Tegretol is effective in about 62% of patients who had positive results from lidocaine, but its serious side effects make it a poor choice as a tinnitus treatment. In addition, vasodilators may help improve inner ear circulation and reduce tinnitus.

Stress reduction Because stress can make tinnitus worse, some people have been able to gain control of their tinnitus and suppress symptoms through the use of biofeedback. Biofeedback training helps individuals control some functions of their autonomic nervous system, such as heartbeat, blood pressure, sweating and temperature of hands and feet.

Electrical stimulation Scientists have found that a direct, positive electrical current can reduce or eliminate tinnitus for up to several weeks, although the time period varies from one person to the next. A transtympanic electrode is used to produce the current, which must be positive (a negative current produces pain or worsens the tinnitus). Although electrical currents can cause tissue damage, researchers hope to lessen the risk by designing stimulation that will lead to long-term suppression of tinnitus symptoms.

Support groups Because tinnitus can be psychologically crippling, help can be found through tinnitus support groups. Local hearing associations maintain listings for these groups. The AMERICAN TINNITUS ASSOCIATION sponsors such groups. Counseling may also be helpful in modifying the behavior of tinnitus patients, who sometimes allow their condition to dominate their lives.

Healthier lifestyle The American Academy of Otolaryngology/Head and Neck Surgery suggests that tinnitus patients avoid loud noises and stimulants such as caffeine and nicotine, monitor blood pressure, lower salt intake, exercise, get enough rest and reduce anxiety. It is also a good idea to use an aspirin substitute, such as acetaminophen, since aspirin may worsen tinnitus.

tinnitus masker There are three types of maskers available to relieve the problem of tinnitus (ringing and buzzing of the ears): simple maskers, HEARING AIDS and tinnitus instruments.

Simple Maskers Simple tinnitus maskers generally provide a high frequency band of noise designed to mask the frequency of the tinnitus.

Hearing Aids Although 90% of people with tinnitus also have a hearing problem, only a small percentage have ever used a hearing aid. If the pitch of the tinnitus is low, hearing aids usually help by raising the level of background noise and thereby masking the tinnitus. However, in cases of high-pitched tinnitus, even the highest-frequency hearing aids don't work very well as a masker since environmental noise is not high enough to mask the sound (environmental noise does not usually rise above 4,000 Hz).

Tinnitus Instrument This is a combination hearing aid and simple masker, used in cases of high-frequency tinnitus and high-frequency hearing loss. It is useful because a simple masker does not work in cases of high-frequency hearing loss since the person cannot hear the frequencies required to mask the tinnitus. There are behind-the-ear and in-the-ear models, and they have independent volume controls.

TMJ See TEMPOROMANDIBULAR JOINT SYNDROME.

tone control A special device on a hearing aid that changes the pitch of amplified sound. (See also HEARING AIDS.)

tone decay test A test that measures tone decay (auditory fatigue) that can be caused by pressure or damage to the AUDITORY (hearing, or eighth cranial) NERVE. In the test, constant tones are presented at the client's threshold. When it fades, the tone is increased 5 DECIBELS. The amount of decay is determined by subtracting the intensity of the initial signal from the intensity at the end of the test. Clients with a disorder of the auditory nerve will show a difference greater than 10 dB to 15 dB.

topophone A direction-finder for sound used in the 19th century, this device (worn over the shoulders) helped localize sound because its two ear trumpets were very widely spaced, and therefore one collected more sound than the other. Patented in 1880, it was originally designed for use by sea captains to determine the direction of a whistle in thick fog.

total communication This philosophy implies an acceptance, exposure and opportunity to use all possible methods of communication to help the deaf child learn to communicate. It is often confused with the SIMULTANEOUS COMMUNICATION (Sim-Com) method, which combines both speech and sign at the same time.

Total Communication provides exposure and opportunity to learn all modes of communication and allows the child to use whichever mode is easiest and with which he is best understood.

Rather than focus on one specific training method, parents and teachers who use a Total Communication approach try to decide which mode is best for a child in any one situation. Options can include SPEECHREADING, speech, SIGN LANGUAGE, auditory training and amplification, writing, audiovisual methods, FINGERSPELLING and graphics.

Total Communication was first described by a California teacher and parent of a deaf child, who combined signing and fingerspelling with speech and speechreading. In 1968, the idea was picked up and introduced by the supervisor of a program for deaf students in Santa Ana and then adopted at the Maryland School for the Deaf in the same year.

Within 10 years, two-thirds of schools for deaf students in the United States had begun to use a Total Communication approach to education. At the same time, the approach was gaining acceptance around the world, and by the 1980s it was widely used to describe a philosophical attitude toward education for deaf students.

Historically, the proponents of particular systems have often disagreed with each other. Total Communication has provided a compromise, adding to the increasing consensus that whatever system works best for the individual should be used to allow the hard-of-hearing or deaf person access to clear and understandable communication.

Still, schools that embrace Total Communication usually feature Simultaneous Communication, which combines the Manual and Oral Approaches at the same time. This combination remains controversial since some Oral Approach proponents claim Sim-Com doesn't produce good speech and Manual Approach supporters complain about the manual English systems used with Sim-Com. (See also MANUALLY CODED ENGLISH.)

toxoplasmosis A generalized protozoan infection that can be contracted by pregnant women who handle infected cats or their infected litter material. Toxoplasmosis can cause hearing loss in 17% of children infected while in the womb. (See also PRENATAL CAUSES OF HEARING LOSS.)

tragus A projecting bit of cartilage in the PINNA near the opening of the ear canal.

transliteration Technically, there are two separate terms for sign language interpretation. Transliteration refers to the interpretation process between a hearing person and a person using a manual code of a spoken language (such as SIGNED ENGLISH). Sign language interpretation refers only to the process of interpreting between speech and a true deaf sign language (such as AMERICAN SIGN LANGUAGE). (See also SIGN LANGUAGE INTERPRETERS.)

trigeminal nerve The fifth cranial nerve travels from the brain stem and divides into three branches, which supply sensation to the face, scalp, nose, teeth, lining of the mouth, upper eyelid, sinuses and front part of the tongue. The nerve also controls the production of saliva and tears and stimulates contraction of the jaw muscles responsible for chewing.

Abnormalities of the facial nerve branch are often associated with ear malformation. About 60% of the population do not have a completely-covered facial nerve canal in the middle ear cavity, which can result in a sensorineural hearing loss. On rare occasions, the facial nerve interrupts the OSSICULAR CHAIN and causes a conductive hearing loss.

TRIPOD This organization provides a national toll-free hotline for parents and individuals wanting information about raising and educating deaf children. TRIPOD operates a parent/infant/toddler program, a Montessori preschool and an elementary mainstream program for hard-of-hearing students. Contact: TRIPOD, 2901 N. Keystone St., Burbank, CA 91504; telephone: (nationwide) 800-352-8888, (California only) 800-346-8888 or (voice and TDD) 818-972-2080.

T-switch See TELECOIL.

TTY See TELECOMMUNICATIONS DEVICES FOR THE DEAF.

tumors of the middle ear These rare growths can remain undetected until they become quite large and invasive, when both malignant and benign tumors cause a CONDUCTIVE HEARING LOSS by blocking the middle ear and external auditory canal, destroying the ossicles and interfering with the eardrum's movement. Malignant tumors can also cause a SENSORINEURAL HEARING LOSS as the growth protrudes into the inner ear.

Symptoms of both types of tumor include DIZZINESS, bleeding from the ear, deep ear pain, drainage and paralysis of the facial nerve. Middle ear tumors include CHORISTOMA, congenital CHOLESTEATOMA, dermoid cysts, meningioma, facial nerve neuroma, ACOUSTIC NEUROMA, glomus tympanicum and glomus jugulare.

Generally, it is uncommon to find a malignant tumor in the middle ear, but the most common malignant tumor found here is a squamous cell carcinoma or glomus tumor.

Squamous cell carcinoma usually appears in the external ear canal and moves into the middle ear, interfering with sound transmission. It may appear after a chronic suppurative OTITIS MEDIA but can begin to grow for no apparent reason at any age, although it is most common in middle age. Symptoms include a conductive hearing loss, a bloody discharge from the ear and pain in the later stages. Survival rate of this lethal skin cancer, even after treatment with radiation and radical surgery, is only about 30%.

A glomus tumor is relatively slow-growing and develops from clusters of nerve cells that regulate body function. These cells are located in either the jugular vein or the back wall of the middle ear. Patients with this type of tumor experience a conductive hearing loss as the tumor grows, filling the middle ear and eroding into the inner ear. More common among women, the symptoms also include a pulselike TINNITUS, which may be followed by a sensorineural hearing loss, DIZZINESS and facial paralysis. Treatment includes radiation and surgery.

tuning forks An instrument developed in the 19th century and used today by a specialist to determine the presence of a hearing loss. Because it emits a remarkably pure tone as it vibrates, the tuning fork has been a basic tool for people trying to learn how the mind interprets sound. The standard frequencies of tuning forks include 128, 512, 1024 and 2048 Hertz. Four tuning fork tests used most often today are the WEBER, RINNE and SCHWABACH.

While the tuning fork has been replaced by electronic sound makers in some tests, forks are still used to support results of more formal audiological testing. Still, the usefulness of tuning forks is limited for a number of reasons: There is no way to accurately measure the intensity of tone; sound is distorted if the fork is struck too hard; there are problems in isolating response of the ear; and they are hard to use with young children. (See also AUDIOMETRY.)

tympanic cavity An air-filled space containing the OSSICULAR CHAIN this cavity is located in the temporal bone. It is linked to the nasopharynx via the eustachian tube.

tympanic membrane See EARDRUM.

tympanic plexus A group of nerves formed by branches of the facial and glossopharyngeal nerves and located on the mound between the round and oval windows. The tympanic plexus supplies sensation to the middle ear.

tympanogram The graphic representation of ACOUSTIC IMPEDANCE as a function of ear canal pressure. (See also AUDIOMETRY; TYMPANOMETRY.)

tympanometry The measure of ACOUSTIC-IMMITTANCE in the ear canal as a function of air pressure in the canal. The TYMPANOGRAM is the graphic representation of acoustic admittance or ACOUSTIC IMPEDANCE as a function of this air pressure.

In a person with normal hearing, the acoustic impedance (opposition to air flow) is least when the air pressure is close to 0 (atmospheric level). As the air pressure changes from this level, acoustic impedance increases and acoustic immittance decreases. The air pressure changes stiffen the eardrum and ossicles, reducing energy transfer through the middle ear.

In a patient with a middle ear disorder, acoustic-immittance measures are different and the specific disease can be diagnosed depending on the tympanogram configuration. For example, SEROUS OTITIS MEDIA with fluid results in a flat tympanogram; on the other hand, a disrupted ossicular chain will produce a tympanogram with an abnormally sharp peak. (See also AUDIOMETRY.)

tympanoplasty Surgery performed to repair the EARDRUM and/or OSSICLES (tiny bones in the middle ear). It is usually performed to treat CONDUCTIVE HEARING LOSS, provided that the COCHLEA and AUDITORY NERVE can benefit from the improved conductive function.

Normally, sound waves move from the eardrum to the inner ear by the three bones called the ossicles (hammer, stirrup and anvil). Chronic OTITIS MEDIA can erode or fuse these bones, causing some degree of conductive hearing loss. Tympanoplasty is the only way to restore some of the lost hearing.

One form of tympanoplasty (also called MYRINGOPLASTY) involves the repair of a perforated eardrum in order to prevent recurring infections and improve hearing. The hole is closed with a graft (usually taken from the patient's own body)—which is usually a piece of connective tissue from the surface of the temporalis muscle adjacent to the ear or the outer, thin covering of the cartilage from the tragus.

OSSICULOPLASTY is the surgical repair of a defect in the transmission of sound by the middle ear ossicles, usually as a result of chronic ear infection (otitis media), CHOLESTEATOMA or temporal bone fracture. Under general anesthesia, an incision is made next to the eardrum. Using a microscope, the surgeon repairs the ossicles by reshaping the bones or replacing them with either a plastic, cartilage or donor ossicle. The bones are reset, and the eardrum is repaired.

Although the operation often improves hearing, there is no guarantee of success, which depends on the complexity of the problem. If the malleus or stapes is missing, for example, the solution is less predictable.

tympanosclerosis A middle ear problem caused by a chronic middle ear infection. Often seen as a white area in the EARDRUM, it is caused when new bone is formed by calcification of the tissue in the lining of the middle ear. (See also OTITIS MEDIA.)

tympanum The main part of the middle ear cavity that lies between the tympanic membrane and the lateral bony wall of the internal ear.

typhoid fever An infectious disease contracted through food or water contaminated with the bacteria salmonella typhosa and sometimes resulting in hearing loss. The infection is found in the feces of an infected person and can be spread by drinking water contaminated by sewage, by flies carrying the bacteria from infected feces to food or by food handling by typhoid carriers.

The bacteria pass from the intestines into the blood, then to the spleen and liver, eventually accumulating in the gallbladder until they are released into the intestine. People who recover from typhoid fever can continue to have typhoid bacteria in the gallbladder, which can be released into the intestine for years.

Epidemics still occur in developing countries, and immunization against the disease is recommended for anyone traveling to these countries. The vaccine is given in two doses with a booster shot after two or three years. Even so, the vaccine does not provide complete protection, and tourists should drink only boiled water when traveling outside developed countries.

Typhoid fever symptoms can take up to two weeks to develop after infection, and the disease can vary from a mild infection to a life-threatening illness. Symptoms begin with a mild headache, fever, loss of appetite and malaise, often followed by delirium. Constipation gives way to diarrhea, and during the second week of the illness, a rash breaks out on the chest and abdomen. The illness usually resolves within one month, but if treatment is delayed, fatal complications can develop.

Treatment with antibiotics can usually control the disease in a few days, although very ill patients may also require corticosteroid drugs. People who recover from typhoid fever have permanent immunity, although failure to take antibiotics correctly can lead to relapses.

U

umbo The most inferior point where the MALLEUS is attached to the EARDRUM, the umbo is a prominent landmark for evaluating the normalcy of the eardrum during OTOSCOPY.

unisensory-auditory method See AUDITORY-ORAL METHOD.

United Kingdom The prevalance rate for profound prelingual deafness in the United Kingdom is estimated to be between .8 and 1.5 per 1,000 live births. About 62,000 people over age 16 have very severe hearing problems, and about 2.3 million have some degree of hearing difficulties. Approximately 30,000 people use BRITISH SIGN LANGUAGE as their main method of communication.

Early diagnosis (before age one) is emphasized in the United Kingdom; screening and subsequent diagnostic tests are free, as are HEARING AIDS, EARMOLDS, maintenance and batteries. Although only certain types of hearing aids are given to adults, children may be provided with any type of aid available. Once a child has been diagnosed, the family is placed in a home-based parent guidance program.

Education The Royal Commission of 1889 recommended that every child who is deaf should be educated with the oral approach; consequently, schools throughout the United Kingdom adopted this method. It was not until 1968 that, concerned about the results of the oral approach, the government decided that, while oralism was still desirable, research into the manual approach should be conducted.

In 1982, the British Association of Teachers of the Deaf issued a proclamation promoting the oral approach but recognized that some children might benefit from additional help in other types of communication.

There are both residential and day schools available in the United Kingdom, and since 1979 the trend has been leading away from residential schools and toward placing children in regular schools with special help.

Many special schools for deaf children arrange for their students to attend technical colleges or other types of further education, and some schools offer advanced education specifically for people who are hard-of-hearing. The National Study Group on Further and Higher Education for the Hearing Impaired in the United Kingdom publishes directories of available further education courses.

A few deaf students also go on to university or polytechnic schools, and specific facilities for deaf students are available at Sussex University and at the Colleges of St. Hilda and St. Bede of the University of Durham.

Continuing education for adult deaf people is also available through the Centre for the Deaf at the City Literary Institute in London.

Communication Services Telephone communications are available for deaf people in the United Kingdom through a portable keyboard telephone known as Vistel, replacing earlier teletypewriters. Vistel has an acoustic coupler to which any normal telephone handset may be attached. The message is typed on a conventional typewriter keyboard, displayed on a traveling display on the top of the equipment and sent over the phone lines to the receiver, who can read the same message on his or her own display.

In addition, deaf people in the United Kingdom can have access to Prestel, an interactive terminal with a large database of commercial and public service information. It provides thousands of pages of information with a TV, a Prestel decoder and a telephone.

Also available to deaf TV viewers is "teletext," a method of coding information in digital form in the unused lines of a TV picture. Teletext also offers the option to broadcast optional subtitles on ordinary TV programs at the press of a button.

In addition, special programs for deaf people are made available through the British Broadcasting system, called "SEE HEAR," a show including news and light entertainment in simultaneous speech, sign language and open subtitles. Other special BBC shows for deaf consumers include subtitles of daily news headlines, a news roundup and a series of educational programs in British Sign Language. In addition, some companies are producing special programs for deaf people in certain regional areas.

U.S. Deaf Skiers Association This group works with deaf members of U.S. ski teams involved in international competition and promotes recreational skiing for hard-of-hearing people. Contact: U.S. Deaf Skiers Association, Box USA, Gallaudet University, 800 Florida Ave. NE, Washington, DC; telephone (TDD): 202-651-5255.

Usher's syndrome type 2 A hereditary condition that begins with a profound congenital deafness, followed by a gradual loss of vision that often reaches complete blindness. Usher's syndrome is one form of retinitis pigmentosa, in which pigment is deposited in and damages the light-sensitive portion of the eye. Night blindness often begins during early teenage years, followed by a narrowing of the visual field. Originally described in 1959, Usher's syndrome may account for 10 percent of all cases of congenital deafness.

Usher's syndrome is one of the rarer autosomal recessive genetic conditions, in which both parents carry an abnormal gene at the same point on the chromosome. Both parents have normal hearing, however, because each also carries a normal dominant gene on the paired chromosome that counteracts the abnormal recessive one.

The effect of the abnormal gene is revealed when one-fourth of the children of a couple with this autosomal recessive condition inherit the abnormal gene from both parents. These children are then born with the paired abnormal genes and are profoundly deaf. There is no way of identifying which children carry two abnormal genes before birth.

Usher's syndrome accounts for about half of all deaf-blindness and affects from 3% to 6% of all congenitally deaf children.

Although there is no treatment, regular exams by an ophthalmologist are recommended for all deaf children, which can help identify Usher's syndrome early, usually before age six.

Most experts believe that telling a child of the impending blindness as soon as possible allows the child to take these conditions into consideration as they prepare for careers and family. The sooner education can be designed to help the student handle reduced input, the better. (See GENETIC MECHANISMS OF DEAFNESS; GENETICS AND HEARING LOSS.)

utricle A small sac in the VESTIBULE of the inner ear.

V

vertigo A feeling of dizziness together with a sensation of movement and—most important—a feeling of rotating in space. It is this sense of rotation (either of the individual or the surroundings) that is an essential ingredient of true vertigo and distinguishes it from simple dizziness.

Vertigo is caused by a disturbance of the SEMICIRCULAR CANALS in the inner ear or the nerve tracts leading from them. It can occur in anyone when sailing, or an amusement ride, while watching a movie, or simply by looking down from a height. It also may be set off by motion sickness, brain disease, drugs (such as streptomycin) or damage to the AUDITORY NERVE.

However, there are more severe forms of vertigo caused by disease: LABYRINTHITIS causes sudden vertigo accompanied by severe vomiting and unsteadiness in conjunction with an ear infection. MENIERE'S DISEASE is also characterized by vertigo, sometimes severe enough to cause collapse. Sudden attacks of vertigo are usually assumed to be associated with labyrinthitis and are treated with bed rest and antihistamine drugs.

vestibular Ménière's disease An atypical form of MÉNIÈRE'S DISEASE in which the sufferer experiences all the symptoms of classical Ménière's (VERTIGO, TINNITUS, nausea) except hearing loss. (See also COCHLEAR MÉNIÈRE'S DISEASE; VESTIBULAR SYSTEM.)

vestibular nerve section A surgical procedure that replaces LABYRINTHECTOMY (surgical excision of the entire inner ear) for incapacitating VERTIGO in patients with usable hearing in the diseased ear. The selective vestibular nerve section with preservation of hearing evolved from the earlier practice of severing the entire eighth cranial nerve.

vestibular system This system—with its primary receptors located in the inner ear (the cristae of the three semicircular canals and the maculae of the utricle and saccule)—is responsible for our sense of orientation in space, for maintaining an upright balance and posture and for the ability to keep moving objects in focus.

There are five separate vestibular detectors, whose connections in the central nervous system allow the brain to integrate information from a variety of receptors in the eyes, the skin, muscles and joints. The vestibular receptor organs deal with the forces associated with head accelerations and changes in head position. As a result, nerves send messages to the brain centers that use these signals to develop a sense of orientation and to activate muscles that control automatic movements of the eyes, movement and posture.

Many of the vestibular pathways in the central nervous system are organized into reflex pathways, called the vestibular reflex systems, that stabilize and coordinate movements of the eyes, head and body.

Vestibular Development Although the basic receptors and brain structures of the vestibular system are determined genetically, the development of vestibular function is a process that depends on use and interaction with the environment throughout life. These reflexes must be constantly adjusted in order to adapt to physical changes in the body's growing muscles and bones and to compensate for diseases or changes in the environment.

Research into the workings of the vestibular system is difficult because the fluid-filled receptor organs that detect motion and head position are encased in bone and therefore hard to study.

Vestibular Disorder Symptoms The vestibular system is complex and highly interactive, capable of continual adaptations to changes in the body and the environment. Because it has many different parts, there are many separate symptoms when things go wrong, ranging from mild discomfort to total incapacitation.

These symptoms may seem unrelated to the ears but result from the complex interactions of different sensory modes that contribute to vestibular function and balance. The symptoms of balance disorders also vary depending on cause, location (one or both ears), age of the patient and so forth. To make things more complicated, the type of symptom—DIZZINESS versus imbalance, for example—may depend on the type of movement the patient is making at the time.

Primary symptoms of a vestibular system gone awry include: VERTIGO, sensation of falling, imbalance, lightheadedness, disorientation, giddiness and visual blurring. Secondary symptoms include nausea and vomiting, faintness, drowsiness, fatigue and depression.

Vestibular Diseases Because vestibular signals interact with all of the major sensory systems and involve major brain centers, a large number of diseases can impair balance, especially among the elderly.

More than 90 million Americans have experienced dizziness or balance problems, and each year there are an estimated 97,000 new cases of MÉNIÈRE'S DISEASE, a disorder that affects the inner ear and causes episodes of vertigo, fluctuating hearing loss and TINNITUS.

There are many kinds of balance disorders, and motion sickness, with certain stimuli, can occur even in healthy people. Special environments (diving, high-speed flying and space travel) are situations for which humans are not genetically programmed, and therefore these reflexes must be overcome or reconditioned if humans are to be able to function in them.

vestibule A portion of the labyrinth of the inner ear located between the cochlea and the semicircular canals. (See also LABYRINTH; INNER EAR.)

viral labyrinthitis See LABYRINTHITIS.

viruses and hearing loss Viruses are common causes of high-frequency hearing loss. Among the viruses, herpes zoster (SHINGLES) has been known to cause a sudden severe deafness in one ear.

viseme A group of speech movements or shapes of the lips that are generally indistinguishable from one another. For example, one consonant category of visemes are the *p, b* and *m* sounds. These three consonants make up one viseme and are said to be homophonous.

However, researchers have not categorized vowels into visemes since no two vowels are produced with exactly the same movements. This does not mean, of course, that it is not possible to confuse the vowels when SPEECHREADING, as many do look similar.

visible speech A system of sound writing (or phonetic transcription) that describes oral sounds through written symbols. Developed by Alexander Melville Bell, it was the first attempt to systematize speech training. Although the system did seem to work for Bell and his sons, it was too intricate for other scientists and was not enthusiastically endorsed.

Bell's system included 29 symbols, with 52 consonants, 26 vowels and 12 diphthongs (a complex sound made by gliding from the position for one vowel to another; for example in ''boil'' or ''house'') that, Bell claimed, could be used to represent all of the distinctive sounds of speech (and therefore, all languages) by expressing the movements of the articulators for individual speech sounds.

The elder Bell considered his system to be a way to improve elocution and did not originally design the method to be used for teaching deaf students, although educator GARDINER GREENE HUBBARD saw the possibilities for use with deaf students and arranged lectures for Bell to discuss his system. But it was ALEXANDER GRAHAM BELL who first really developed the system as a way to teach deaf students.

Because his first experience in teaching deaf students with visible speech seemed promising, the younger Bell accepted an invitation to teach the method in Boston. In 1871, Bell introduced the system in the United States at the Horace Mann School in Boston and at the Clarke School for the Deaf in Northampton, Massachusetts, where it was taught for 10 years before it was discarded.

voice reflex test See LOMBARD TEST.

voice-to-sign interpreting Interpretation from a spoken language to a signed language. (See also SIGN LANGUAGE INTERPRETERS.)

Volta Bureau The headquarters of the ALEXANDER GRAHAM BELL ASSOCIATION FOR THE DEAF, this bureau houses the association's extensive library containing literature on deafness.

The bureau was created and endowed by ALEXANDER GRAHAM BELL from money he received from the Republic of France, which had awarded him its Volta Prize for his inventions. Bell envisioned the bureau as the best way to increase and publicize information about deafness and presented the bureau to the association in 1909.

Much of the archival collection belonging to the association is still housed at the Volta Bureau.

W

Waardenburg's syndrome About 50% of the people with this disorder may have nonprogressive SENSORINEURAL HEARING LOSS ranging from mild to severe in one or both ears, although only a slight few will be profoundly deaf in both ears.

Other symptoms include medial folds of the eyes associated with flattening of the root of the nose, a white forelock of hair and possibly two different colored eyes; about 15% of victims may undergo pigment changes.

The disorder, which is genetically transmitted to offspring in a dominant manner, carries a 50% risk that siblings may be born with a variation of the syndrome. Still, only a few people who have the abnormal form of the gene show all the features of the syndrome, and only a very small number have profound deafness in both ears. Researchers believe there may be some connection between the development of pigmentation, and hearing, during pregnancy. (See also GENETICS AND HEARING LOSS; GENETIC MECHANISMS OF DEAFNESS.)

wake-up alarms Audio alarms, such as ordinary clock radios or electronic alarms, that have been adapted to flash one or several lights or to turn on a small vibrator under the mattress or pillow. (See also ALERTING DEVICES; Appendix 3.)

Washoe See NONHUMAN SIGNING.

wavelength One of three measurements that describe a SOUND WAVE (the other two are amplitude and frequency). The wavelength is the longitudinal distance between the crests of two successive waves; the longer the wavelength of a sound, the lower its frequency.

Weber test This test determines which ear (if either) hears a tuning fork better by bone conduction. The base of the vibrating fork is held on the center of the forehead or upper front teeth, and the patient is asked in which ear the fork sounds louder. If hearing isn't the same in both ears, the fork's tone will be heard in only one ear, or appear to be displaced to one side of the head.

A patient complaining of hearing loss in one ear who can hear the fork in the good ear may have a sensorineural hearing loss. If the sound is lateralized to the poor ear, then a conductive loss is suspected.

A mixture of both types of hearing loss will not be accurately revealed by the Weber test.

Weitbrecht, Robert H. (1920–1983) The inventor of the teletypewriter (TTY) for deaf people, which is the forerunner of the present-day telecommunications device for the deaf (TDD).

Weitbrecht was a deaf physicist who adapted a teletype model so it could be used to communicate over a telephone line with another teletype machine. Weitbrecht's modification was also called a TTY.

Because Weitbrecht's teletype was a surplus machine contributed by AT&T and there were only a limited number of these extra machines, only 25 TTYs were in use by deaf people by 1968. In that year, however, AT&T decided to donate surplus TTYs to deaf people and within several years had distributed several thousand.

white noise A blend of audible frequencies over a wide range that can be used to convert disturbing silence into controlled quiet or to mask distracting noises. Often compared to the sound of escaping steam, white noise basically serves the same purpose as background music in restaurants. White noise has been used by dentists to mask the noise of the drill, which helps ease tension and pain. (See TINNITUS MASKER.)

Wing's symbols One of the first printed systems to help deaf children learn to speak, read and write syntactically correct sentences. Devised in 1883 by a deaf teacher named George Wing, it used numbers and letters to represent the different parts of speech in written language.

Specifically, Wing placed number and letter symbols over words, phrases or clauses. The symbols were grouped into the "essentials," "modifying forms," "correctives" and "special symbols." There were eight "essential" symbols: subject, transitive verb, intransitive verb, passive verb, object, adjective complement, noun and pronoun complement.

word deafness See AUDITORY AGNOSIA.

word recognition test Another name for speech discrimination test. (See also AUDIOMETRY.)

World Federation of the Deaf This organization, formed by conference members during the 1951 World Congress of the Deaf, provides international visibility for deaf people and serves as an information exchange for deaf experts from around the world. Its main function is to hold international conferences, to help attain full citizenship for deaf people in all countries. To that end, it has represented their interests before various international groups.

One of the interesting developments contributed by this group is the creation of the first international sign language. Born out of the problem of communication presented by members from 57 different nations with many different sign languages and dialects, the federation first adopted French and English as its official languages. Since 1959, members have been trying to develop a true international sign language that can be understandable by all.

Its efforts resulted in GESTUNO a sign language made up of 1,470 signs appropriated from existing sign languages that were the most easily-produced and the most natural referents.

The federation, which hopes to have gestuno accepted in other settings in addition to the annual congresses of the federation, now uses three sign languages at its plenary sessions: French and English sign language and gestuno. Contact: World Federation of the Deaf, Ilkantie 4, P.O. Box 65, SF-00401 Helsinki, Finland.

World Games for the Deaf The deaf athlete's Olympics, the World Summer and Winter Games for the Deaf, have been held every four years since they began in Paris in 1924. The games are administered by the COMITÉ INTERNATIONAL DES SPORTS DES SOURDS (CISS), a group recognized by the International Olympic Committee.

In 1924, Belgium, Czechoslovakia, France, Great Britain, the Netherlands and Poland met at Pershing Stadium in Paris for the first World Games, where deaf athletes competed in track, swimming, soccer, shooting and cycling. Since then, the World Games have grown in size and number of events.

Today, the summer games are held one year after the Olympic Games followed by the winter games two years later. Host countries are chosen by a majority vote at the Comité six years in advance.

To be eligible, athletes who wish to compete in the games must have an average hearing level for speech greater than 55 decibels in the better ear, documented by audiogram submitted in advance. In addition, an AUDIOLOGIST makes spot checks of competitors and retests all event winners. Hearing aids cannot be worn during competition.

Summer game competitions include badminton, basketball, cycling, shooting, soccer, swimming, table tennis, team handball, tennis, track, volleyball, water polo and wrestling. Both male and female athletes may compete, although women are barred from wrestling, cycling, soccer and water polo. Gold, silver and bronze medals are given to the first three winners, and diplomas are awarded to the next six finishers.

Winter games consist of alpine and nordic ski events and speed skating.

Competitions are conducted under the same rules as the Olympic Games, although some modifications are used to make auditory cues visible. The games are opened with a parade of athletes and raising of the CISS flag. Although the Olympic torch is not used, the International Olympic Committee allows the Olympic flag to be flown.

In 1966, the International Olympic Committee awarded its Olympic Cup in recognition of CISS' service to the cause of sports and the Olympic spirit.

World Recreation Association of the Deaf, Inc./USA This group promotes participation by hard-of-hearing people in a wide variety of recreational activities through its national and local chapters. Contact: World Recreation Association of the Deaf, Inc./USA, P.O. Box 321, Quartz Hill, CA 93586; telephone: (TDD) 805-943-8879 or (voice relay—California only) 800-342-5833.

Y

Y-cord A special cord found on a body-type hearing aid that carries amplified sound to two receivers.

APPENDIXES*

---

*Please note that Federal and State Resources were deleted from the Appendixes because all agencies are in the process of changing addresses.

APPENDIX 1: COMMUNITY PROGRAMS FOR DEAF PEOPLE

Listed below are community organizations offering services to deaf persons on a local or regional level. Included are state commissions or councils for deaf people.

ALABAMA

Deaf CONTACT
3224 Executive Park Circle
Mobile, AL 36606
205-342-3333
205-343-4555 (TDD)

E. H. Gentry Technical Facility
P.O. Box 698
Talladega, AL 35160
205-362-1050 (voice/TDD)

Janice Capilouto Center for the Deaf
1521 Mulberry St.
Montgomery, AL 36106
205-264-4533 (voice/TDD)

ALASKA

Louise Rude Center for Deaf Adults
1020 E. 4th Ave., Suite 2
Anchorage, AK 99501
907-276-3456 (voice/TDD)

ARIZONA

Community Outreach Program for the Deaf
268 W. Adams St.
Tucson, AZ 85705
602-792-1906 (voice/TDD)

Council for the Hearing Impaired
1300 W. Washington
Phoenix, AZ 85007
602-255-3323 (voice/TDD)

Good Samaritan Psychiatric Services for the Hearing Impaired
925 E. McDowell Road
Phoenix, AZ 85006
(voice) 602-239-5087
602-239-5085 (TDD)

Pima Community College
Disabled Student Resources
2202 W. Anklam Rd.
Tucson, AZ 85709
602-884-6688 (voice/TDD)

Signs of Communication
P.O. Box 44814
Phoenix, AZ 44814
602-956-2682 (voice/TDD)

Valley Center of the Deaf, Inc.
3130 E. Roosevelt
Phoenix, AZ 85008
602-267-1921 (voice/TDD)

ARKANSAS

Abilities Unlimited of Jonesboro
P.O. Box 5072
Jonesboro, AR 72401
501-932-1551

Crittendon County Sheltered Workshop
P.O. Box 1206
208 N. 4th St.
West Memphis, AR 72301
501-732-2750

Deaf Access
4601 W. Markham
Little Rock, AR 72205
501-371-6010 (voice)
501-371-6012 (TDD)

Deaf Outreach Center
4601 W. Markham
Little Rock, AR 72205
501-371-7647 (voice)
501-371-7647 (TDD)

Logan County Day Service Center
P.O. Box 454
Booneville, AR 72927
501-675-3770

Office for the Deaf and Hearing Impaired
1401 Brookwood Dr.
Box 3781
Little Rock, AR 72203
501-371-2502

Office for the Deaf and Hearing Impaired
4324 W. Markham
Little Rock, AR 72205
501-371-1922 (voice)
501-371-1924 (TDD)

Office of the Deaf and Hearing Impaired
P.O. Box 3800
Hwy. 25 N.
Batesville, AR 72503
501-793-4224

CALIFORNIA

Big Brothers/Big Sisters of San Francisco
Hearing Impaired Program
414 Mason St., Suite 500
San Francisco, CA 94102
415-434-4860 (voice)
415-434-4863 (TDD)

Deaf Community Services of San Diego, Inc.
3788 Park Blvd.
San Diego, CA 92103
619-692-0932 (voice/TDD)

Deaf CONTACT
1135 Carol Lane, #3
Lafayette, CA 94556
415-284-2002 (voice/TDD)

Deaf Counseling, Advocacy and Referral Agency (DCARA)
125 Parrot St.
San Leandro, CA 94577
415-895-2430 (voice)
415-895-2431 (TDD)

Deaf Self-Help, Inc.
2891 Bush St.
San Francisco, CA 94115
415-567-6360 (voice)
415-567-6361 (TDD)

GLAD—Kern County Outreach
122A Chester Ave.
Bakersfield, CA 93301
805-327-3781 (voice)
805-327-5652 (TDD)

GLAD San Gabriel Valley Outreach
536 E. Rowland Ave., Suite 102
Covina, CA 91723
818-967-3761

GLAD—San Fernando Valley Outreach
6851 Lennox Ave., Third Floor
Van Nuys, CA 91405
818-785-6583

Greater Los Angeles Council on Deafness, Inc. (GLAD)
616 S. Westmoreland Ave., Second Floor
Los Angeles, CA 90005
213-383-2220 (voice/TDD)

Greater LA Council on Deafness
536 E. Rowland Ave., #102
San Gabriel, CA 91723
818-967-3761 (voice/TDD)

HEAR Center
301 E. Del Mar Blvd.
Pasadena, CA 91101
213-681-4641

Hearing Society for the Bay Area, Inc.
1428 Bush St.
San Francisco, CA 94115
415-775-5700 (voice)
415-776-DEAF (TDD)

Independent Living Resource Center
423 W. Victoria
Santa Barbara, CA 93101
805-963-0595

Lanterman Developmental Center
P.O. Box 100
Pomona, CA 91769
714-595-1221

Napa State Hospital, Children's Program
2100 Napa Valley Hwy.
Napa, CA 94558
707-253-5571 (voice/TDD)

NorCal Center on Deafness
2400 Glendale Lane, Suite F
Sacramento, CA 95825
916-486-8570 (voice/TDD)

Orange County Deaf Equal Access Foundation
7700 Orangethorpe, Suite 6
Buena Park, CA 90621
714-523-7750 (voice/TDD)

Parker Hearing and Speech Institute
4201 Torrance Blvd., #140
Torrance, CA 90503
213-540-HEAR (voice/TDD)

Philadelphia Baptist Church and Deaf Center
823 W. Manchester Ave.
Los Angeles, CA 90044
213-231-0488

St. John's Mental Health Services for the Hearing Impaired
1328 22nd St.
Santa Monica, CA 90404
213-829-8536 (voice/TDD)

San Francisco Senior Center Deaf Seniors Program
890 Beach St.
San Francisco, CA 94109
415-775-1866 (voice)
415-771-2666 (TDD)

Speech, Hearing and Neurosensory Center
8001 Frost St.
San Diego, CA 92123
619-576-5838 (voice)
619-576-5831 (TDD)

TRIPOD Pre-School and Grapevine
955 N. Alfred St.
Los Angeles, CA 90069
213-656-4904 (voice/TDD)

UCSF Center on Deafness
1474 Fifth Ave.
San Francisco, CA 94143
415-731-9150 (voice)
415-731-7123 (TDD)

University of California/Irvine Deafness Center
101 City Drive S. Bldg. 53
Orange, CA 92668
714-634-6021

Valley Advocacy and Communication Center for the Deaf
441 W. Olive St., Suite 3
Fresno, CA 93728
209-486-8222

Valley Advocacy and Communication Center for the Deaf
1900 N. Dinuba Blvd., Suite H
Visalia, CA 93291
209-738-1001 (voice/TDD)

COLORADO

Pikes Peak Center on Deafness
11322 N. Academy Blvd., Suite 104
Colorado Springs, CO 80909
303-591-2777 (voice)
303-591-2333 (TDD)

Pikes Peak Mental Health Center, Inc.
Hearing Impaired Services
3090 N. Academy Blvd.
Colorado Springs, CO 80907
303-591-0300

CONNECTICUT

Connecticut Commission on the Deaf and Hearing Impaired
40 Woodland St.

Hartford, CT 06105
203-566-7414 (voice/TDD)

Contact of Southeastern Connecticut
P.O. Box 249
West Mystic, 06388
203-572-8143

Hearing Improvement Center
10 N. Main St.
West Hartford, CT 06107
203-232-5947 (voice)
203-236-5948 (TDD)

Newington Children's Hospital, Speech Pathology & Audiology
181 E. Cedar St.
Newington, CT 06111
203-667-5320

DISTRICT OF COLUMBIA

Deafpride, Inc.
1350 Potomac Ave. SE
Washington, DC 20003
202-675-6700 (voice/TDD)

Deaf REACH
3521 12th St. NE
Washington, DC 20017
202-832-6681 (voice/TDD)

National Health Care Foundation for the Deaf
3521 12th St. NE
Washington, DC 20017
202-832-6681 (voice/TDD)

Quota International
SHATTER SILENCE Program
1420 21st St. NW
Washington, DC 20036
202-331-9694 (voice/TDD)

FLORIDA

CONTACT Help Line
900 NE. 132 St.
N. Miami, 33161
305-751-9066 (voice/TDD)

CONTACT Tampa Help Line
P.O. Box 10117
Tampa, FL 33606
813-253-4040 (voice)
813-253-2020 (TDD)

Deaf Service Center
4000 W. Buffalo Ave., Suite 186
Tampa, FL 33614
813-272-3370 (voice)
813-876-3215 (TDD)

Deaf Services Bureau, Inc.
4800 W. Flagler St., Suite 213
Miami, FL 33134
305-444-2266 (voice)
305-444-2211 (TDD)

GEORGIA

Atlanta Center for Independent Living
1201 Glenwood Ave. SE
Atlanta, GA 30035
404-656-2952 (voice)
404-656-5911 (TDD)

CONTACT-Hall County
Box 1616
Gainesville, GA 30503
404-534-0617

Georgia Center for the Multi-Handicapped
1815 Ponce de Leon NE
Atlanta, GA 30307
404-378-5433

ILLINOIS

Center for Deafness
10100 Dee Rd.
Des Plaines, IL 60070
312-297-1022

Chicago Hearing Society
10 W. Jackson St., 4th Floor
Chicago, IL 60604
312-939-6888 (voice)
312-427-2166 (TDD)

CONTACT Rockford
Box 1976
Rockford, IL 61110

815-962-3323 (voice)
815-965-3277 (TDD)

Deaf CONTACT Chicago
505 N. Lake Shore Dr.
Chicago, IL 60601
312-644-4900 (voice)
312-644-5510 (TDD)

Kennedy Job Training Center
123rd & Wolf Rd.
Palos Park, IL 60464
312-448-4818 (voice/TDD)

Lutheran Child & Family Services,
Hearing Impaired Program
333 W. Lake St.
Addison, IL 60101
312-628-6488 (voice)
312-782-6555 (TDD)

Northwestern University Hearing Clinics
303 E. Chicago Ave.
Chicago, IL 60611
312-908-8107

Resurrection Hospital
7435 W. Talcott
Chicago, IL 60611
312-794-6058 (voice)
312-774-8170 (TDD)

Siegel Institute-Michael Reese Hospital
3033 S. Cottage Grove Ave.
Chicago, IL 60610
312-791-2900 (voice)
312-791-3449 (TDD)

Skills, Inc.
1122 5th Ave.
Moline, IL 61265
309-797-3586 (voice/TDD)

INDIANA

Community Services for the Deaf
445 N. Pennsylvania St., Suite 811
Indianapolis, IN 46204
317-637-3947 (voice/TDD)

Community Services with Adult Deaf
711 E. Colfax Ave.
South Bend, IN 46617
219-234-3136 (voice)
219-234-3130 (TDD)

CONTACT Cares, Inc., of NW Indiana
P.O. Box 10247
Merrillville, IN 46411
219-769-3141, 219-374-7660

Crossroads Rehabilitation Center/Speech
Pathology & Audiology
3242 Sutherland Ave.
Indianapolis, IN 46205
317-924-3251 (voice)
317-927-5469 (TDD)

Deaf Services, Inc.
7101 Broadway, Suite #3
Merrillville, IN 46410
219-769-6506 (voice/TDD)

Deaf Social Service Agency for the
Tri-State, Inc.
901 W. Virginia St.
Evansville, IN 47710
812-425-2726 (voice)
812-425-2841 (TDD)

The Rehabilitation Center, Inc.
3701 Bellemeade Ave.
Evansville, IN 47715
812-479-1411

IOWA

Arrowhead Area Educational Agency
1235 5th Ave. S
Box 1399
Fort Dodge, IA 50501
515-576-7434

Deaf Family Counseling Program
Family Counseling Center, Suite 401
507 10th St.
Des Moines, IA 50309
515-288-9023 (voice/TDD)

Deaf Services of Iowa
Iowa State Dept. of Health
Lucas State Office Building
Des Moines, IA 50319
515-281-3164 (voice/TDD)

KANSAS

Institute of Logopedics
2400 Jardine Dr.
Wichita, KS 67219
(316) 262-8271

Kansas Commission for the Deaf and
Hearing Impaired
2700 W. 6th St.
Biddle Building First Floor
Topeka, KS 66606
913-296-2874 (voice/TDD)

Kansas Vocational Rehabilitation Center
3140 Centennial Rd.
Salina, KS 67456
913-827-9356 (voice/TDD)

KENTUCKY

Kentucky Association of the Deaf
400 Brookview Place
Danville, KY 40422
606-236-5132

LOUISIANA

Deaf Resource and Communication Center
721 S. Ferdinand St.
New Orleans, LA 70117
504-949-4413 (voice/TDD)

MAINE

Maine Association of the Deaf, Inc.
P.O. Box 1014
Portland, ME 04104
207-787-2602 (voice/TDD)

MARYLAND

Deaf Referral Services, Inc.
3700 Greenspring Ave.
Baltimore, MD 21211
301-225-3323 (voice/TDD)

Family Service Foundation Institute on
Deafness
7580 Annapolis Rd.
Lanham, MD 20706
301-459-2121 (voice)
301-731-6141 (TDD)

Self Help for Hard of Hearing People, Inc.
7800 Wisconsin Ave.
Bethesda, MD 20814
301-657-2248 (voice)
301-657-2249 (TDD)

MASSACHUSETTS

CONTACT-Boston
P.O. Box 287
Newtonville, MA 02160
617-244-4353 (voice)
617-332-9416 (TDD)

D.E.A.F., Inc.
215 Brighton Ave.
Watertown, MA 02134
617-254-4041 (voice/TDD)

Deaf Community Center
75 Bethany Road
Framingham, MA 01701
617-875-3617 (voice)
617-875-0354 (TDD)

Hahnemann Rehabilitation Center
535 Lincoln St.
Worcester, MA 01605
617-792-8500 (voice)
617-792-8507 (TDD)

Massachusetts Commission for the Deaf
and Hard of Hearing
600 Washington St.
Boston, MA 02111
617-727-5106 (voice)
800-882-1155 (TDD)

Massachusetts Office of Deafness
20 Park Plaza, Suite 328
Boston, MA 02116
617-727-5236 (voice/TDD)

Stephen Miller House Project for the Deaf
P.O. Box 719
Falmouth, MA 02574
617-540-5052 (voice/TDD)

MICHIGAN

Community Services for the Hearing Impaired
50 Wayne St.
Pontiac, MI 48058
313-332-3323 (voice/TDD)

Hawthorn Center
18471 Haggerty Road
Northville, MI 48167
313-349-3000

Michigan Department of Labor
Division of Deaf and Deafened
309 N. Washington Square
Box 30015
Lansing, MI 48909
517-373-0378 (voice/TDD)

Social Services for the Hearing Impaired
302 E. Court St.
Flint, MI 48502
313-239-3112 (voice/TDD)

Valley Organization for Improved Communications and Equality
721 S. Washington St.
Saginaw, MI 48605
517-753-7111 (voice/TDD)

MINNESOTA

Ability Building Center, Inc.
1911 14th St. NW
Box 6938
Rochester, MN 55903
507-289-1891 (voice/TDD)

Central Area Regional Center
2015 S. First St.
Willmar, MN 56201
612-231-5175 (voice/TDD)

Central Area Regional Service Center
54 28th Ave. N
St. Cloud, MN 56374
612-255-2224 (voice/TDD)

Deafness Education and Advocacy Foundation
108 E. 7th St.
St. Paul, MN 55101
612-224-2515 (voice/TDD)

Deaf Services Division
Department of Human Services
Centennial Building, Fourth Floor
658 Cedar St.
St. Paul, MN 55155
612-296-3980 (voice/TDD)

First Call for Help
83 S. 12th St.
Minneapolis, MN 55403
612-340-7440 (voice/TDD)

Hearing Impaired Health and Wellness Services
640 Jackson St.
St. Paul, MN 55101
612-221-2719 (voice)
612-221-3761 (TDD)

Metro Area Regional Services Center
311 2nd Ave. S
Minneapolis, MN 55401
612-341-7100 (voice/TDD)

Minnesota Foundation for Better Hearing and Speech
508 Bremer Bldg.
7th and Robert Streets
St. Paul, MN 55101
612-223-5310 (voice/TDD)

Northeast Area Regional Service Center
505 W. 12th Ave.
Virginia, MN 55792
218-741-5855 (voice/TDD)

Northwest Area Regional Services Center
Government Services Building
320 W. 2nd St., Suite 611
Duluth, MN 55802
218-723-4962 (voice)
218-723-4961 (TDD)

Northwest Area Regional Services Center
125 W. Lincoln Ave., Suite 7
Fergus Falls, MN 56537
218-739-7589 (voice/TDD)

Northwest Area Regional Services Center
Hillview Offices

Highway 75 South & Minnesota St.
Crookston, MN 56716
218-281-1946 (voice/TDD)

Range Center, Inc.
P.O. Box 629
1001 NW 8th Ave.
Chisholm, MN 55719
218-254-3347 (voice)
218-254-4813 (TDD)

St. Paul Rehabilitation Center
319 Eagle St.
St. Paul, MN 55102
612-227-8471 (voice)
612-227-3779 (TDD)

Southern Area Regional Service Center
1200 S. Broadway, Suite 142
Rochester, MN 55901
507-285-7295 (voice/TDD)

Southwest Regional Services Center for Hearing Impaired People
709 ½ S. Front St.
Mankato, MN 45662
507-389-6517 (voice/TDD)

MISSISSIPPI

Golden Triangle-CONTACT
P.O. Box 1304
Columbus, MS 39703
601-328-0200

MISSOURI

Cochlear Implant Program
2940 Baltimore
Kansas City, MO 64108
816-531-0003 (voice/TDD)

CONTACT-St. Louis
P.O. Box 160070
St. Louis, MO 63116
314-771-8181

NEBRASKA

Commission for the Hearing Impaired
4600 Valley Road
Lincoln, NE 68510
402-471-3593 (voice/TDD)

NEVADA

University of Nevada Dept. of Speech Pathology & Audiology
108 Mackay Science Bldg.
Reno, NE 89557
702-784-4887

NEW HAMPSHIRE

Crotched Mountain Rehabilitation Center
Gilbert Verney Dr.
Greenfield, NH 03047
603-547-3311

New Hampshire Educational Services for the Hearing Impaired
17 S. Fruit St.
Concord, NH 03301
603-225-7073 (voice/TDD)

NEW JERSEY

CONTACT Atlantic
P.O. Box 181
Linwood, NJ 08221
609-646-6616 (voice)
609-645-1668

CONTACT of Burlington County
P.O. Box 333
Moorestown, NJ 08057
609-234-2223

Deaf CONTACT
c/o Katzenbach School for the Deaf
320 Sullivan Way
West Trenton, NJ 08628
609-587-3050 (voice)
609-452-1919 (TDD)

Deaf CONTACT Center
Box 75
Succasunna, NJ 07876
201-927-9333 (voice)
201-927-9334 (TDD)

Deaf CONTACT "609"
1050 N. Kings Hwy.

Cherry Hill, NJ 08034
609-667-3000, 609-428-2900 (both voice/TDD)

Deaf CONTACT "201"
P.O. Box 37
Westfield, NJ 07090
201-232-3333 (voice/TDD)

Jewish Deaf and Hearing Impaired Council
199 Scoles Ave.
Clifton, NJ 07012
201-779-2980 (voice)
201-779-2984 (TDD)

Jewish Deaf and Hearing Impaired Council
45 Blake Ave.
Cranford, NJ 07016
201-276-0201

New Jersey Association of the Deaf
3608 Park Ave.
Edison, NJ 08820
201-549-0621 (voice/TDD)

New Jersey Division of the Deaf
Labor and Industry Bldg.
Trenton, NJ 07920
609-984-7281 (voice/TDD)

Plainfield Hearing Society
518 Watchung Ave.
YMCA Building
Plainfield, NJ 07060
201-756-6060 (voice/TDD)

NEW YORK

Allegheny Rehabilitation Associates—Clinical Services Program
RD #1, Box 309
Allegheny, NY 14706
716-375-4740

Catholic Charities Bi-County Center Services for the Deaf
143 Schleigel Blvd.
Amityville, NY 11701
516-842-1400 (voice)
516-842-1540 (TDD)

Central New York Association for the Hearing Impaired
616 S. Salina St.
Syracuse, NY 13202
315-422-2321 (voice)
315-422-9746 (TDD)

CHEAR (Children's Hearing Education and Research)
928 McLean Ave.
Yonkers, NY 10704
914-237-2676

Deaf CONTACT
Div. of Help Line Telephone Services
3 W. 29th St., 10th Floor
New York, NY 10001
212-532-0994 (voice)
212-532-0942 (TDD)

Deafness Services, Catholic Charities
191 Joralemon St.
Brooklyn, NY 11201
718-598-5500, ext. 352 (voice)
718-596-0303 (TDD)

Educational Resource Center on Deafness
New York School for the Deaf
555 Knollwood Road
White Plains, NY 10603
914-949-7310, ext. 268

Lexington Hearing and Speech Center, Inc.
74-20 25th Ave.
Jackson Heights, NY 11370
718-899-8800, ext. 280 (voice)
718-898-5926 (TDD)

New York Catholic Deaf Center
1011 First Ave.
New York, NY 10012
212-988-8563 (voice)
212-988-1903 (TDD)

New York League for the Hard of Hearing
71 W. 23rd St.
New York, NY 10010
212-741-7650 (voice)
212-255-1932 (TDD)

New York Society for the Deaf
344 E. 14th St.
New York, NY 10003

212-673-6500 (voice)
212-673-6974 (TDD)

Prevention Services for Deaf Youths and Families
New York Foundling Hospital
1175 Third Ave.
New York, NY 10021
212-472-2233 (voice)
212-879-2059 (TDD)

Rochester Rehabilitation Center
1000 Elmwood Ave.
Rochester, NY 14620
716-271-2520 (voice)
716-271-2233 (TDD)

Rockland County Center for the Physically Handicapped
260 Little Tor Road N
New City, NY 10956
914-634-4648 (voice/TDD)

Southern Tier Independence Center
232 Clinton St.
Binghamton, NY 13905
607-797-1110

Speech & Hearing Center
Westchester County Medical Center
Grasslands Road
Valhalla, NY 10595
914-285-7294 (voice/TDD)

The Workshop, Inc.
339 Broadway
Menands, NY 12204
518-465-5201 (voice)
518-463-8597 (TDD)

NORTH CAROLINA

Asheville Community Service Center for the Hearing Impaired
518 Kenilworth Road, Suite C
Asheville, NC 28805
704-258-6190

Beginnings for Parents of Hearing Impaired Children
P.O. Box 10565
Raleigh, NC 27605
919-821-5479 (voice/TDD)

Charlotte Community Service Center for the Hearing Impaired
1926 E. Independence Blvd.
Charlotte, NC 28205
704-334-3481

CONTACT Winston-Salem
1111 W. First St.
Winston-Salem, NC 27101
919-723-4338 (voice)
919-724-1373 (TDD)

Greenville Community Service Center for the Hearing Impaired
226-A Commerce St.
P.O. Box 8166
Greenville, NC 27834
919-756-5737 (voice/TDD)

Guilford County Communications Center for the Deaf
1601 Walker Ave.
Greensboro, NC 27403
919-274-1461 (voice)
919-275-8878 (TDD)

Morganton Community Service Center for the Hearing Impaired
325 Enola Road
P.O. Box 2551
Morganton, NC 28655
704-433-2647 (voice/TDD)

North Carolina Council for the Hearing Impaired
620 N. West St.
P.O. Box 26053
Raleigh, NC 27611
919-733-3364 (voice)
919-733-5930 (TDD)

Raleigh Regional Community Service Center for the Hearing Impaired
436 N. Harrington St.
Raleigh, NC 27603
919-733-6714 (voice)
919-733-6715 (TDD)

Wilmington Regional Community Service Center for the Hearing Impaired
201-B Wallace Ave.
Wilmington, NC 28403
919-799-1490 (voice)
919-799-9564 (TDD)

Winston-Salem Deafness Center
2701 N. Cherry St.
Winston-Salem, NC 27105
919-724-3621 (voice)
919-724-7805 (TDD)

NORTH DAKOTA

Medical Center Rehabilitation Hospital
1300 S. Columbia Rd.
Grand Forks, ND 58201
701-780-2447

OHIO

AIM for the Handicapped, Inc.
945 Danbury Rd.
Dayton, OH 45420
513-294-4611

Cincinnati Speech & Hearing Center
3021 Vernon Place
Cincinnati, OH 45219
513-221-0527 (voice)
513-221-3300 (TDD)

Community Center for the Deaf
854 W. Town St.
Columbus, OH 43222
614-228-3323 (voice/TDD)

Community Services for the Deaf
212 E. Exchange St.
Akron, OH 44313
216-376-9494 (voice)
216-376-9351 (TDD)

Community Services for the Deaf
184 Salem Ave.
Dayton, OH 45406
513-222-9481

Comprehensive Program for the Deaf
4110 N. High St.
Columbus, OH 43214
614-263-5151 (voice/TDD)

CONTACT Community Connection
P.O. Box 1403
Warren, OH 44482
216-393-1565 (voice/TDD)

CONTACT-Queen City
P.O. Box 42071
Cincinnati, OH 45224
513-791-HOPE (voice)
513-891-1889 (TDD)

Hearing Impaired Services of Northwestern Ohio
One Stranahan Square, Suite 342
Toledo, OH 43612
419-255-1018 (voice/TDD)

Rehabilitation Services of North Central Ohio
Community Center for the Deaf
270 Sterkel Blvd.
Mansfield, OH 44907
419-756-1133 (voice/TDD)

Youngstown Hearing & Speech Center
6505 Market St.
Youngstown, OH 44512
216-726-8855 (voice)
216-726-8391 (TDD)

OKLAHOMA

Oklahoma Commission on the Deaf and Hearing Impaired
4901 N. Lincoln Blvd.
Oklahoma City, OK 73105
405-521-2754 (voice/TDD)

Tulsa Speech and Hearing Association
10301-E E. 51st St.
Tulsa, OK 74146
918-663-9920 (voice/TDD)

OREGON

Regional Resource Center on Deafness
Western Oregon State College
345 N. Monmouth Ave.
Monmouth, OR 97361

503-838-1220 (voice)
503-838-5151 (TDD)

PENNSYLVANIA

Berks County Association for the Hearing Impaired
223 N. 6th St.
Reading, PA 19601
215-373-6992 (voice)
215-374-7300 (TDD)

Center on Deafness
300 E. Swissvale Ave.
Pittsburgh, PA 15218
412-371-7000

CONTACT Altoona
P.O. Box 11
Altoona, PA 16603
814-946-9050 (voice)
814-946-1933 (TDD)

CONTACT E.A.R.S.
P.O. Box 7804
New Castle, PA 16107
412-658-5529

CONTACT Philadelphia
4360 Monument Road
Philadelphia, PA 19131
215-877-9099

CONTACT York
145 S. Duke St.
York, PA 17403
717-845-3656 (voice/TDD)

Deaf CONTACT
447 E. King St.
Lancaster, PA 17602
717-299-7184 (voice/TDD)

Deaf CONTACT
P.O. Box 376
Newton, PA 18940
215-860-1800 (voice)
215-860-1802 (TDD)

Deaf CONTACT Harrisburg
P.O. Box 2328
Harrisburg, PA 17105
717-652-4987 (voice)
717-652-5555 (TDD)

Easter Seal Society of York County
2201 S. Queen St.
York, PA 17404
717-741-3891 (voice/TDD)

Elwyn-Nevil Center for Deaf & Hearing Impaired
4031 Ludlow St.
Philadelphia, PA 19104
215-895-5509 (voice)
215-895-5695 (TDD)

Harmarville Rehabilitation Center, Inc.
Communication Skills Dept.
P.O. Box 11460
Guys Run Rd.
Pittsburgh, PA 15238
412-781-5700

Jewish Family & Children's Agency
8900 Roosevelt Blvd.
Philadelphia, PA 19115
215-673-0100 (voice)
215-552-9525 (TDD)

Lutheran Social Services, Deaf Services Program
144 S. 8th St.
Chambersburg, PA 17201
717-264-8178 (voice/TDD)

Pittsburgh Hearing, Speech & Deaf Services
1945 Fifth Ave.
Pittsburgh, PA 15219
412-281-1375 (voice/TDD)

Vocational Rehabilitation Center
1323 Forbes Ave.
Pittsburgh, PA 15219
412-471-2600

Westmoreland County Deaf Services
110 E. Otterman St.
Greensburg, PA 15601
412-832-7600 (voice/TDD)

SOUTH CAROLINA

HELPLINE of the Midlands, Inc.
P.O. Box 6336

Columbia, SC 29260
803-771-4357 (voice/TDD)

SOUTH DAKOTA

Communication Services for the Deaf
421 N. Lewis
Sioux Falls, SD 57103
605-339-6718 (voice/TDD)

TENNESSEE

CONTACT Ministries, Inc.
P.O. Box 1403
Johnson City, TN 37605
615-926-0144

CONTACT of Chattanooga
1202 Duncan Ave.
Chattanooga, TN 37404
615-266-8228 (voice/TDD)

CONTACT Teleministries of Knoxville
P.O. Box 11234
Knoxville, TN 37939
615-523-9108 (voice)
615-523-9125

Daniel Arthur Rehabilitation Center
728 Emory Valley Road
Oak Ridge, TN 37830
615-482-4081

Interpreting Service for the Deaf
YMCA
3548 Walker
Memphis, TN 38111
901-324-8270 (voice)
901-327-4233 (TDD)

Knoxville Area Community Center for the Deaf
134 Maryville Pike, Suite B
Knoxville, TN 37920
615-577-3559 (voice)
615-577-4419 (TDD)

League for the Hearing Impaired, Inc.
1810 Edgehill Ave.
Nashville, TN 37212
615-320-7347 (voice)
615-329-9271 (TDD)

Library Service for the Hearing Impaired
700 Second Ave. S, Room 211
Nashville, TN 37210
615-259-5410 (voice/TDD)

Services for the Deaf
317 Oak St., Suite 316
Chattanooga, TN 37412
615-755-2850 (voice/TDD)

TEXAS

Bay Area Deaf Services
701 W. Sterling
Baytown, TX 77520
713-428-2121

Corpus Christi Area Council for the Deaf
5115 McArdle
Corpus Christi, TX 78411
512-993-1154 (voice/TDD)

Deaf Council of Greater Houston
6910 Fannin St., Suite 204
Houston, TX 77030
713-796-0520 (voice)
713-796-2416 (TDD)

East Texas Deaf and Hearing Association
215 W. Bow
Tyler, TX 75702
214-593-3355 (voice/TDD)

El Paso Center of the Deaf, Inc.
1005 E. Yandell
El Paso, TX 79902
915-544-6032 (voice/TDD)

Goodrich Center of the Deaf
2500 Lipscomb St.
Fort Worth, TX 76110
817-926-5305 (voice)
817-926-4101 (TDD)

Goodwill Industries of South Texas, Inc.
2961 S. Poret
Corpus Christi, TX 78405
512-884-4068

Lubbock County Services for the Deaf
4324 22nd Place

Lubbock, TX 79410
806-795-2345 (voice/TDD)

San Antonio Council for the Deaf
2803 E. Commerce
San Antonio, TX 78203
512-223-9200 (voice/TDD)

Southeast Texas Council for the Hearing Impaired
P.O. Box 1748
Beaumont, TX 77704
409-833-6679 (voice)
409-833-6689 (TDD)

Southwest Center for the Hearing Impaired
6487 Whitby Road
San Antonio, TX 78240
512-699-3311 (voice/TDD)

Texas Commission for the Deaf
510 S. Congress
Austin, TX 78704
512-469-9891 (voice/TDD)

Texoma Council for the Deaf
800 N. Travis
Sherman, TX 75090
214-892-6531 (voice/TDD)

Travis County Services for the Deaf
2201 Post Rd., Room 100
Austin, TX 78704
512-448-7597 (voice)
512-444-4181 (TDD)

Vaughn House, Inc.
P.O. Box 3178
Austin, TX 78764
512-444-9763 (voice/TDD)

West Texas Service for the Deaf
1600 Campus Ct.
ACU Box 8107
Abilene, TX 79699
915-674-2425 (voice/TDD)

VIRGINIA

CONTACT Tidewater, Inc.
P.O. Box 23
Virginia Beach, VA 23458
807-428-2211 (voice)
807-422-5740 (TDD)

Deaf Project
Woodrow Wilson Rehabilitation Center
Fishersville, VA 22939
703-332-7327 (voice)
703-885-9775 (TDD)

Virginia Department for the Deaf and Hard of Hearing
James Monroe Bldg., 7th Floor
101 N. 14th St.
Richmond, VA 23219
804-225-2570 (voice/TDD)
In Virginia, 800-552-7917 (voice/TDD)

WASHINGTON

Deaf CONTACT
P.O. Box 684
Richland, WA 99352
509-946-5911 (voice/TDD)

Hearing, Speech & Deafness Center
1620 18th Ave.
Seattle, WA 98122
206-323-5770

Lighthouse for the Blind, Inc.
Deaf-Blind Program
2501 S. Plum St.
Seattle, WA 98114
206-322-4200 (voice/TDD)

WEST VIRGINIA

Deaf CONTACT
Quarrier & Morris Sts.
Charleston, WV 25301
304-346-0826 (voice)/TDD)

Deaf CONTACT
520 11th St.
Huntington, WV 25701
304-523-3447 (voice)
304-523-0060 (TDD)

West Virginia Rehabilitation Center
Barron Dr., P.O. Box 1004
Institute, WV 25112
304-766-4797 (voice/TDD)

WISCONSIN

Department of Health and Social Services
819 N. 6th St., Sixth Floor
Milwaukee, WI 53203
414-224-4504 (voice/TDD)

Goodwill Industries of South Central Wisconsin, Inc.
1302 Mendota St.
Madison, WI 53714
608-246-3140 (voice/TDD)

Office for the Hearing Impaired
718 W. Clairemont Ave.
Eau Claire, WI 54701
713-836-2062 (voice/TDD)

Office for the Hearing Impaired
One W. Wilson St., Room 412
P.O. Box 7851
Madison, WI 53707
608-266-8081 (voice)
608-266-8083 (TDD)

S.E. Wisconsin Center for Independent Living
3680 S. Layton Blvd.
Milwaukee, WI 53215
414-643-0910 (voice)
414-643-5807 (TDD)

APPENDIX 2: GENERAL ORGANIZATIONS AND RESOURCES FOR DEAF PEOPLE

Alexander Graham Bell Association for the Deaf
3417 Volta Place NW
Washington, DC 20007
202-337-5220 (voice/TDD)

American Academy of Otolaryngology—Head and Neck Surgery
One Prince St.
Alexandria, VA 22316
703-836-4444 (voice)

American Association of the Deaf-Blind
814 Thayer Ave., Third Floor
Silver Spring, MD 20910
301-588-6545

American Athletic Association of the Deaf, Inc.
1052 Darling St.
Ogden, UT 84403

American Deafness and Rehabilitation Association
P.O. Box 55369
Little Rock, AR 72225
501-663-7074 (voice/TDD)

American Hearing Research Foundation
55 E. Washington St., Suite 2022
Chicago, IL 60602
312-726-9670 (voice)

American Medical Assn., Section
Council on Otorhinolaryngology
Department of Otolaryngology
University of Texas Health Science Center
5323 Harry Hines Blvd.
Dallas, TX 75235

American Society for Deaf Children
814 Thayer Ave.
Silver Spring, MD 20910
301-585-5400 (voice/TDD)

American Speech-Language-Hearing Association
10801 Rockville Pike
Rockville, MD 20852
301-897-5700 (voice/TDD)
800-897-8682 (helpline)

American Tinnitus Association
P.O. Box 5
Portland, OR 97207
503-248-9985 (voice)

Association of Late-Deafened Adults
1027 Oakton
Evanston, IL 60202

Better Hearing Institute
P.O. Box 1840
Washington, DC 20013
800-EAR-WELL (voice)
703-642-0580 (voice)

The Caption Center
125 Western Ave.
Boston, MA 02134
617-492-9225 (voice/TDD)

Captioned Films for the Deaf
5000 Park St. N

St. Petersburg, FL 33709
800-237-6213 (voice/TDD)

Center for Bicultural Studies, Inc.
5506 Kenilworth Ave., Suite 105
Riverdale, MD 20737
301-277-3945

Children of Deaf Adults
c/o Texas School for the Deaf
P.O. Box 3538
Austin, TX 78764
512-440-5300

Cochlear Implant Club International
P.O. Box 464
Buffalo, NY 14223
716-838-4662 (voice/TDD)

Cochlear Implant Information Center
800-458-4999 (voice/TDD) (except Colorado)
303-790-9010 (in Colorado, voice/TDD)

Conference of Educational Administrators Serving the Deaf
American School for the Deaf
139 N. Main St.
West Hartford, CT 06107
203-727-1304 (voice/TDD)

Convention of American Instructors of the Deaf
P.O. Box 2025
Austin, TX 78768
512-441-2225 (voice/TDD)

D.E.A.F., INC.
215 Brighton Ave.
Allston, MA 02134
617-254-4041 (voice/TDD)

Deaf Artists of America
87 N. Clinton Ave., Suite 408
Rochester, NY 14604
716-325-2400 (voice/TDD)

Deafness Research Foundation
9 E. 38th St.
New York, NY 10016
212-684-6556 (voice)
212-684-6559 (TDD)
800-535-DEAF

DEAFPRIDE, Inc.
1350 Potomac Ave. SE
Washington, DC 20003
202-675-6700 (voice/TDD)

Deaf Women United
215 Brighton Ave.
Allston, MA 02134
617-254-4041 (voice/TDD)

The Ear Foundation
(The Ménière's Network)
2000 Church St.
Box 111
Nashville, TN 37326
800-545-HEAR (voice/TDD)

Gallaudet Research Institute
800 Florida Ave. NE
Washington, DC 20002
202-651-5400
800-451-8834

Genetic Services Center
Gallaudet Research Institute
Gallaudet University
800 Florida Ave. NE
Washington, DC 20002
202-651-5258 (voice/TDD)
800-672-6720, ext. 5258 (voice/TDD)

Hearing Industries' Association
1800 M St. NW
Washington, DC 20036
202-833-1411

Hear Now
4001 S. Magnolia Way, Suite 100
Denver, CO 80237
800-648-HEAR (voice/TDD)
financial assistance

Helen Keller National Center for Deaf-Blind Youths and Adults
111 Middle Neck Road
Sands Point, NY 11050
516-944-8900 (voice/TDD)

House Ear Institute
256 S. Lake
Los Angeles, CA 90057

213-483-4431 (voice)
213-484-2642 (TDD)

International Association of Parents of the Deaf
814 Thayer Ave.
Silver Spring, MD 20910

International Foundation for Children's Hearing, Education and Research
871 McLean Ave.
Yonkers, NY 10704

Junior National Association of the Deaf Youth Programs
445 N. Pennsylvania St., Suite 804
Indianapolis, IN 46204
301-587-1788 (voice/TDD)

National Association for Hearing and Speech Action
Rockville, MD
800-638-TALK (voice/TDD)

National Association of the Deaf (NAD)
814 Thayer Ave.
Silver Spring, MD 20910
301-587-1788 (voice/TDD)

National Black Deaf Advocates, Inc.
P.O. Box 91166
Washington, DC 20066
301-559-5398 (TDD)

National Captioning Institute, Inc.
5203 Leesburg Pike
Falls Church, VA 22041
703-998-2400 (voice/TDD)

National Center for Law and the Deaf
Gallaudet University
800 Florida Ave. NE
Washington, DC 20002
202-651-5373 (voice/TDD)

National Crisis Center for the Deaf
University of Virginia Medical Center
P.O. Box 484
Charlottesville, VA 22908
800-446-9876 (outside Virginia, voice/TDD)
800-552-3723 (inside Virginia, voice/TDD)

National Cued Speech Association
P.O. Box 31345
Raleigh, NC 27622
919-828-1218 (voice/TDD)

National Foundation for Children's Hearing Education and Research
928 McLean Ave.
Yonders, NY 10704
914-237-2676

National Fraternal Society of the Deaf
1300 W. Northwest Hwy.
Mt. Prospect, IL 60056
312-392-9282 (voice)
312-392-1409 (TDD)
800-876-NFSD (voice/TDD)

National Hearing Aid Society
20361 Middlebelt
Livonia, MI 48152
313-478-2610 (voice)
800-521-5247 (helpline)

National Hearing Association
1010 Jorie Blvd., Suite 308
Oak Brook, IL 60521
312-323-7200

National Information Center for Children and Youth with Handicaps
P.O. Box 1492
Washington, DC 20013
703-893-6061 (voice/TDD)
800-999-5599

National Information Center on Deafness
Gallaudet College
800 Florida Ave. NE
Washington, DC 20002
202-651-5051 (voice)
202-651-5052 (TDD)

National Rehabilitation Information Center
8455 Colesville Road, Sutie 935
Silver Spring, MD 20910
301-588-9284 (voice/TDD)
800-34-NARIC

National Research Register for Heredity Hearing Loss
Boys Town National Research Hospital

555 30th St.
Omaha, NE 68154
402-498-6631 (voice/TDD)

The National Theatre of the Deaf
P.O. Box 659
Chester, CT 06412
203-526-4971 (voice)
203-526-4974 (TDD)

Parmly Hearing Institute
Loyola University of Chicago
6525 N. Sheridan Rd.
Chicago, IL 60626
312-508-2710

Project ALAS
c/o D.E.A.F., Inc.
215 Brighton Ave.
Allston, MA 02134
617-254-4041 (voice/TDD)

Quota International, Inc.
1420 21st St. NW
Washington, DC 20036
202-331-9694 (voice/TDD)

Rainbow Alliance of the Deaf
P.O. Box 14182
Washington, DC 20044
202-779-6459 (TDD)

Registry of Interpreters for the Deaf, Inc.
511 Monroe St., Suite 1107
Rockville, MD 20850
301-779-0555 (voice/TDD)

The See Center for the Advancement of Deaf Children
P.O. Box 1181
Los Alamitos, CA 90720

Self Help for Hard of Hearing People, Inc.
7800 Wisconsin Ave.
Bethesda, MD 20814
301-657-2248 (voice)
TTY-657-2249 (TDD)

Sign Instructors Guidance Network (SIGN)
814 Thayer Ave.
Silver Spring, MD 20910
301-587-1788

Telecommunications for the Deaf, Inc.
814 Thayer Ave.
Silver Spring, MD 20910
301-589-3786 (voice)
301-589-3006 (TDD)

Tele-Consumer Hotline
1910 K St. NW, Suite 610
Washington, DC 20006
202-223-4371 (voice/TDD)
800-332-1124 (voice/TDD) (outside D.C.)

TRIPOD
2901 N. Keystone St.
Burbank, CA 91504
800-352-8888
800-346-8888 (California only)
818-972-2080 (voice/TDD)

U.S. Deaf Skiers Association
Box USA
Gallaudet University
800 Florida Ave. NE
Washington, DC 20002
202-651-5255 (TDD)

Vestibular Disorders Association of America
1015 NW 22nd Avenue, D230
Portland OR 97120
503-229-7705 (voice)

World Federation of the Deaf
Ilkantie 4, P.O. Box 65
SF-00401 Helsinki, Finland

World Recreation Association of the Deaf, Inc./USA
P.O. Box 321
Quartz Hill, CA 93586
800-342-5833 (voice relay; California only)
805-943-8879 (TDD)

APPENDIX 3: DEVICES FOR PEOPLE WITH HEARING LOSS*

ASSISTIVE LISTENING DEVICES

AT&T National Special Needs Center
2001 Rte. 46, #310
Parsippany, NJ 07054
800-233-1222 (voice)
800-833-3232 (TDD)

Hear You Are, Inc.
4 Musconetcong Ave.
Stanhope, NJ 07874
201-347-7662

Potomac Technology, Inc.
1010 Rockville Pike
Rockville, MD 20852
301-762-4005

Radio Shack stores
Circulation Dept.
300 One Tandy Center
Fort Worth, TX 76102
components/catalogs
817-390-3011

Sound Resources, Inc.
201-E. Ogden
Hinsdale, IL 60521
708-325-6133

Tele-Consumer Hotline
1910 K St. NW, Suite 610
Washington, DC 20006
202-223-4371 (voice/TDD)
800-332-1244

(*Note: Inclusion does not indicate endorsement; exclusion does not indicate disapproval.)

HEARING AID INFORMATION

Consumer Reports
P.O. Box 1949
Marion, OH 43305
How To Buy a Hearing Aid (reprint)

Council of Better Business Bureaus, Inc.
1515 Wilson Blvd.
Arlington, VA 22209
Facts About Hearing and Hearing Aids
15-page pamphlet, one copy free

FDA—Office of Consumer Communication
5600 Fishers Lane
Rockville, MD 29857
Tuning In on Hearing Aids
(one copy free)

Superintendent of Documents
U.S. Government Printing Office
Washington, DC 20402
Facts About Hearing and Hearing Aids
31-page pamphlet;
order #SN 003-003-02024-9
Hearing Aids
order #SN 003-003-00751-0

SIGNALING DEVICES

Nationwide Flashing Signal Systems
8120 Fenton St.
Silver Spring, MD 20910
301-589-6670 (TDD)
301-589-6671 (voice)
301-589-5153 (FAX)
Burglar alarms, baby criers, doorbell signalers, fire/smoke alarms, answering

machines, pagers, phone signalers, telecaption decoders, bed vibrators, wake up alarms

American Communications Corp.
180 Roberts St.
East Hartford, CT 06108
203-289-3491 (voice/TDD)
baby criers, doorbell and phone signalers

AT&T National Special Needs Center
2001 Rte. 46, #310
Parsippany, NJ 07054
800-233-1222 (voice)
800-833-3232 (TDD)
phone amplifiers, doorbell and phone signalers, answering machines, telecaption decoders

Audex
713 N. 4th St.
Longview, TX 75601
800-237-0716 (voice/TDD)
phone amplifiers

G. N. Danavox, Inc.
6400 Flying Cloud Dr.
Eden Prairie, MN 55344
612-941-0690 (voice)
800-247-5343 (voice in Minnesota)
800-328-6297 (TDD)
phone amplifiers

Eye Festival, Inc.
1530 N. Gower St., Suite 201
Hollywood, CA 90028
213-873-3325 (voice)
800-873-3327 (TDD)
bed vibrators; wake-up alarms

Hal-Hen Co.
35–53 24th St.
Long Island, NY 11106
718-392-6020
phone amplifiers; baby criers; doorbell, phone, fire, smoke signalers; bed vibrators; wake-up alarms

Julian McDermott Corp.
1639 Stephen St.
Ridgewood, NY 11385
718-456-3606 (voice)
burglar alarms; doorbell, fire, smoke signalers, wake-up alarms

Phone-TTY, Inc.
202 Lexington Ave.
Hackensack, NJ 07601
201-489-7889 (voice)
201-489-7890 (TDD)
baby criers; doorbell, fire, smoke, phone signalers; bed vibrators; wake-up alarms

Precision Controls, Inc.
14 Doty Rd.
Haskell, NJ 07420
201-835-5000 (voice/TDD)
baby criers; doorbell, fire, smoke, phone signalers; bed vibrators; wake-up alarms

Silent Call Corp
P.O. Box 16348
Clarkston, MI 48016
313-391-1710
baby criers; doorbell, fire, smoke, phone signalers

Sonic Alert, Inc.
1750 W. Hamlin
Rochester, MI 48309
313-656-3110 (voice/TDD)
baby crier; doorbell, fire, smoke, phone signalers; bed vibrators; wake-up alarms

Ultratec, Inc.
6442 Normandy Lane
Madison, WI 53719
608-273-0707
baby crier; doorbell, fire, smoke, phone signalers; wake-up alarms

TELECAPTION DECODERS

National Captioning Institute
5203 Leesburg Pike
Falls Church, VA 22041
800-845-1992 (voice)
800-321-8337 (TDD)

AT&T National Special Needs Center
2001 Rte. 46, #310
Parsippany, NJ 07054

800-233-1222 (voice)
800-833-3232 (TDD)

TELECOMMUNICATIONS DEVICES FOR THE DEAF (TDD)

General Information

AT&T National Special Needs Center
2001 Rte. 46, #310
Parsippany, NJ 07054
800-233-1222 (voice)
800-833-3232 (TDD)

National Center for Law and the Deaf
Gallaudet University
800 Florida Ave. NE
Washington, DC 20002
202-651-5373 (voice/TDD)
information on mandated state and federal relay systems

National Information Center on Deafness
Gallaudet University
800 Florida Ave. NE
Washington, DC 20002
202-651-5109 (voice)
202-651-5976 (TDD)

NTID
Department of Public Affairs
One Lomb Memorial Dr.
Rochester, NY 14623
What You Should know About TDDs

Self Help for Hard Of Hearing People, Inc.
7800 Wisconsin Ave.
Bethesda, MD 20814
301-657-2248 (voice)
301-657-2249 (TDD)
Beyond the Hearing Aid with Assistive Devices
SHHH Information Series #251

Telecommunications for the Deaf, Inc.
814 Thayer Ave.
Silver Spring, MD 20910
301-589-3786 (voice)
301-589-3006 (TDD)
International Telephone Directory of the Deaf

Tele-Consumer Hotline
1910 K St. NW, Suite 610
Washington, DC 20006
800-332-1124 (voice/TDD)
202-223-4371 (voice/TDD)
TDD Relay Center comparison chart

TDD/voice answering machine distributors

Deaf Communications of Cincinnati
550 Palmerston Dr.
Cincinnati, OH 45231
513-451-3722 (voice/TDD)
Brand: Mirac

Guardian Communications Corp., Inc.
105 E. Annadale Road, Suite 200
Falls Church, VA 22046
703-241-5805 (voice)
Brand: Takachiho

Nationwide Flashing Signal Systems, Inc.
8120 Fenton St.
Silver Sping, MD 20910
301-589-6671 (voice)
301-589-6670 (TDD)
Brand: Panasonic

TDD and TDD/computer manufacturers

American Communication Corp.
180 Roberts St.
East Hartford, CT 06108
203-289-3491 (voice/TDD)

AT&T Information Products and Systems
60 Columbia Turnpike, Room A-A210
Morristown NJ 07960
800-233-1222 (voice)
800-833-3232 (TDD)

Cascade Medical, Inc.
10180 Viking Dr.
Eden Prarie, MN 55344
612-941-7345

Hearing Impaired Technology
Gallaudet University
P.O. Box 1742
800 Florida Ave. NE
Washington, DC 20002

IBM
National Support Center for Persons with Disabilities

P.O. Box 2150
Altanta, GA 30055
800-426-2133 (voice)
800-284-9482 (TDD)

Integrated Microcomputer Systems, Inc.
2 Research Place
Rockville, MD 20850
301-948-4790 (voice)
301-869-6391 (TDD/ASCII 300)

Krown Research, Inc.
10371 W. Jefferson Blvd.
Culver City, CA 90232
800-833-4968 (outside CA only)
213-839-0181 (voice/TDD)

Phone-TTY, Inc.
202 Lexington Ave.
Hackensack, NJ 07061
201-489-7889 (voice)
201-489-7890 (TDD)

Specialized Systems, Inc.
2525 Pioneer Ave., Suite 3
Vista, CA 92083
800-854-1559 (voice/TDD outside CA)
619-598-7337 (voice/TDD)

Ultratec, Inc.
6442 Normandy Lane
Madison, WI 53719
800-482-2424 (voice/TDD outside WI)
608-272-0707 (voice/TDD)

Zicom Technologies, Inc.
2485-A Coral St.
Vista, CA 92083
800-748-5633 (voice/TDD)
619-727-7110 (voice/TDD)

APPENDIX 4: GENETICS AND DEAFNESS INFORMATION

In addition, many large universities and hospitals have clinical genetic services. Ask your doctor or local health department for a list of genetic service providers.

American Society of Human Genetics
American Board of Medical Genetics
9650 Rockville Pike
Bethesda, MD 20814
301-571-1825

Genetic Services Center
Gallaudet University
800 Florida Ave. NE
Washington, DC 20002
202-651-5258 (voice/TDD)
800-451-8834, ext. 5258 (voice/TDD)

March of Dimes Birth Defects Foundation
Professional Education
1275 Mamaroneck Ave.
White Plains, NY 10605

National Society of Genetic Counselors
233 Canterbury Dr.
Wallingford, PA 19086
215-872-7608

APPENDIX 5: HOMES AND HOUSING FOR AGED DEAF PERSONS

ARIZONA

Good Shepherd
2701 Aldersgate
Little Rock, AR 72205
501-224-7200 (voice)

CALIFORNIA

California Home for the Aged Deaf
529 Las Tunas Dr.
Arcadia, CA 91006
818-445-2259 (voice)
818-445-0875 (TDD)

Pilgrim Tower
1207 S. Vermont Ave.
Los Angeles, CA 90006
213-387-6541 (voice/TDD)

GEORGIA

Crussell-Freeman Center of the Deaf
740 Erin Ave. SW
Atlanta, GA 30310
404-758-8254 (voice/TDD)

INDIANA

Archibald Memorial Home for the Deaf
RR 2
Brookston, IN 47923
317-563-3582 (voice/TDD)

IOWA

Park Place
615 Park St.
Des Moines, IA 50309
515-284-5900 (voice)

LOUISIANA

Village DuLac
1404 Carmel Ave.
Lafayette, LA 70501
318-234-5106 (voice)
318-232-3463 (TDD)

MASSACHUSETTS

New England Home for the Deaf
154 Water St.
Danvers, MA 09123
508-774-0445 (voice/TDD)

MINNESOTA

Ebenezer Park Apartments
2700 Park Ave.
Minneapolis, MN 55407
612-879-2233 (voice/TDD)

NEW YORK

Tanya Towers
c/o New York Society for the Deaf
620 E. 13th St.
New York, NY 10009
212-777-3840 (voice/TDD)
212-777-2804 (voice/TDD)

OHIO

Columbus Colony, Inc.
1150 Colony Dr.

Westerville, OH 43081
614-891-5055 (voice/TDD)

Columbus Colony Housing, Inc.
1165 Colony Dr.
Westerville, OH 43081
614-890-6152 (voice/TDD)

PENNSYLVANIA

The George W. Nevil Home
Elwyn Institute
111 Elwyn Rd.
Elwyn, PA 19063
215-891-2000 (voice)
215-891-2359 (TDD)

SOUTH DAKOTA

Maple Creek
2815 E. 11th St., #100
Sioux Falls, SD 57103
605-339-6718 (voice)
605-339-3748 (TDD)

VIRGINIA

George Washington Home for Adults
P.O. Box 280
Winchester, VA 22601
703-667-3000 (voice)

The Meadows
5800 Meadow Dr.
Crozet, VA 22932
804-823-4683 (voice)

APPENDIX 6: HOUSING FOR DEAF ADULTS WITH SPECIAL NEEDS

The following is a list of group homes or supervised living arrangements for deaf adults, designed primarily for people with additional handicaps. Several programs offer vocational training in or near the home.

ARIZONA

Community Outreach Program for the Deaf
268 W. Adams
Tucson, AZ 85705
602-792-1906 (voice/TDD)

CALIFORNIA

Concord House
2301 Mt. Diablo St.
Concord, CA 94520
415-825-4423 (voice)

Deafness Counseling, Advocacy
and Referral Agency
125 Parrot St.
San Leandro, CA 94577
415-895-2430 (voice/TDD)
referrals in the San Francisco Bay area

Hampshire House
3556 N. Vineland Ave.
Baldwin Park, CA 91706
818-962-3458 (voice/TDD)

Harmony House
19169 Lowell Ave.
Hayward, CA 94541
415-276-3480 (voice/TDD)

Independent Living Resource Center, Inc.
423 W. Victoria St.
Santa Barbara, CA 93101
805-963-0595 (voice/TDD)

San Gabriel/Pomona Regional Center
P.O. Box 2280
West Covina, CA 91793
818-814-8811 (voice)
818-960-3609 (TDD)

Self Actualization Institution for the Deaf,
Inc. (SAID)
6253 Hollywood Blvd., Suite 422
Hollywood, CA 90028
213-462-7243 (voice/TDD)

CONNECTICUT

Connecticut Valley Hospital
Leak Hall
Middletown, CT 06457
203-344-2434 (voice)
203-347-9301 (TDD)

Robinson House
South Quaker Lane
West Hartford, CA 06119
203-232-0818 (voice/TDD)

Robinson House
c/o Mental Health Association of
Connecticut
20–30 Beaver Road
Wethersfield, CT 06109

203-529-1970 (voice)
203-529-6833 (TDD)

DISTRICT OF COLUMBIA

Aspen House
6809 9th St. NW
Washington, DC 20012
202-722-2318 (voice/TDD)

CHHI (Key) House
1203½ Otis St. NE
Washington, DC 20017
202-832-6681 (voice/TDD)

Gallatin House
1501 Gallatin St. NE
Washington, DC 20017
202-722-2318 (voice/TDD)

Otis House
1203 Otis St. NE
Washington, DC 20017
202-832-2660 (voice/TDD)

GEORGIA

Crussel Freeman Watchful Care Home
740 Erin St. SW
Atlanta, GA 30321
404-758-8254 (voice/TDD)

IDAHO

The Center of Resources for Independent People
P.O. Box 4185
707 N. 7th Ave.
Pocatello, ID 83201
208-232-2747 (voice/TDD)

ILLINOIS

Center on Deafness
10100 Dee Road
Des Plaines, IL 60016
312-297-1022 (voice/TDD)

McLean House
2335 W. McLean St.
Chicago, IL 60647
312-772-2322 (voice/TDD)

Thresholds Bridge for the Hearing Impaired
4814 N. California
Chicago, IL 60625
312-989-8568 (voice)
312-989-8547 (TDD)

INDIANA

Tri-County Center, Inc.
8945 N. Meridian
Indianapolis, IN 46260
317-574-0055 (voice)

Tri-County Mental Health Group Home for the Hearing Impaired
6825 Township Line Road
Indianapolis, IN 46260
317-257-5134 (voice/TDD)

MAINE

Caron Street
26 Caron St.
Portland, ME 04103
207-797-8046 (voice/TDD)

Deaf Services Coordinator's Office
Bureau of Mental Health
State House, Station #40
Augusta, ME 04333
207-289-2000 (voice/TDD)

MARYLAND

Deaf Independent Living Association, Inc.
Alternate Living Clinic
106 Plaza West, Suite 402
Salisbury, MD 21801
301-742-5052 (voice/TDD)

Family Services Foundation, Inc.
7580 Annapolis Road
Lanham, MD 20706
301-731-6141 (voice/TDD)

People Encouraging People
4201 Primrose Ave.
Baltimore, MD 21215
301-764-8560 (voice)
301-764-7016 (TDD)

MASSACHUSETTS

Bay House
5 Lincoln St.
Winthrop, MA 02152
617-846-8690 (voice/TDD)

Bedford House
87 Bedford Ave.
Lowell, MA 01854
508-452-3002 (voice/TDD)

The Cape Cod Avenue Program
96 Cape Cod Ave.
Plymouth, MA 02360
508-224-6774

The Charles Street Program
40 Charles St.
Weymouth, MA 02189
617-335-7222 (voice/TDD)

Deaf Community Center
75 Bethany Hill Road
Framingham, MA 01701
508-875-3617

Deaf Developmentally Disabled Staffed Apartment Program
229 School St.
Waltham, MA 02154
617-899-9422 (voice/TDD)

Deaf MR Residence
23 Winter St.
Amesbury, MA 01913
508-388-1177 (voice/TDD)

F.F.S., Inc.
40 Pond St.
Worcester, MA 01604
508-753-0734

Lynn Deaf Program
24 Wave St.
Lynn, MA 01905
617-595-4923 (voice/TDD)

Mayo House
46 Gordon St.
Framingham, MA 01701
508-620-0481 (voice/TDD)

New England Residential Services
P.O. Box 3822
Plymouth Center, MA 02361
508-747-5090 (voice)

North Shore Association for Retarded Citizens
184 Lafayette St.
Salem, MA 01970
508-744-1225 (voice/TDD)

On Our Way, Inc. (office)
227 Dedham St.
Norfolk, MA 02056
508-384-2517 (voice)

On Our Way, Inc.
31 Wollaston Ave.
Quincy, MA 02170
617-479-9515 (TDD)

Swampscott Deaf Apartment Program
12 Ryan Place
Swampscott, MA 01907
617-599-9249 (voice/TDD)
617-599-9273 (voice/TDD)

Turning Point, Inc.
Box 6127
Newburyport, MA 01950
508-462-8251 (voice/TDD)

Waltham Committee, Inc.
564 Main St.
Waltham, MA 02154
617-899-8220 (voice/TDD)

MICHIGAN

Genessee County Community Mental Health Deaf Services
1102 Mackin Road
Flint, MI 48503
313-257-3676 (voice)
313-767-7736 (TDD)

Mid-Michigan Youth and Family Development, Inc.
2306 Miller Road
Flint, MI 48503
313-290-2524 (voice)
612-290-9062 (TDD)

MINNESOTA

Journey House of People, Inc.
18135 13th Ave. N
Plymouth, MN 55447
612-476-6410 (voice)
612-476-6412 (TDD)

Petra Howard House
700 E. 8th St.
St. Paul, MN 55106
612-771-5575 (voice)
612-771-5576 (TDD)

MISSOURI

Woodhaven Learning Center
P.O. Box 1796
Columbia, MO 65205
314-875-6181 (voice)
314-876-7310 (TDD)

NEW YORK

Cardinal Cooks
2465 Bathgate Ave.
Brooklyn, NY 10458
212-354-3581 (voice)

Cribben House
218–20 104 Ave.
Queens Village, NY 11429
718-776-4190 (voice/TDD)

New York Society for the Deaf
817 Broadway, 7th Floor
New York, NY 10003
212-777-3900 (voice/TDD)

Rockland Psychiatric Center
Deafness Unit, Bldg. #36
Orangeburg, NY 10962
914-359-1000 ext. 3628 (voice)
914-359-8039 (TDD)

Supervised Apartment Program
500 South Ave.
Rochester, NY 14620
716-325-4304 (voice/TDD)

NORTH CAROLINA

Goodwill Program for the Hearing Impaired
P.O. Box 668768
Charlotte, NC 28266
704-372-3434 (voice/TDD)
for referrals in North Carolina

Pioneer House
2115 The Plaza
Charlotte, NC 28205
704-376-8113 (TDD)

Starens Pioneer House
Goodwill Industries of South Piedmont
P.O. Box 668768
Charlotte, NC 28266
704-392-2039 (voice/TDD)

PENNSYLVANIA

InterCommunity Action, Inc.
6012 Ridge Ave.
Philadelphia, PA 19128
215-487-1982 (voice)
215-543-3065 (TDD, relay service)
referrals in the Philadelphia area

Pittsburgh Hearing, Speech and Deaf Services
1945 5th Ave.
Pittsburgh, PA 15219
412-281-1375 (voice/TDD)
referrals in the Pittsburgh area

RHODE ISLAND

Corliss Institute/Corliss Cooperative Center
292 Main St.
Warren, RI 20885
401-245-3609 (voice)
401-245-2223 (TDD)

SOUTH DAKOTA

Evergreen Place
4909 W. 43rd St.
Sioux Falls, SD 57106
605-361-9976 (voice/TDD)

TEXAS

Southwest Center for the Hearing Impaired
6487 Whitby Road

San Antonio, TX 78240
512-699-3311 (voice/TDD)

Travis County Mental Health and
Retardation Center
708 Patterson Ave.
Austin, TX 78703
512-477-6975 (voice)
512-444-4181 (TDD)

Vaughn House, Inc.
P.O. Box 3178
Austin, TX 78764
512-444-9763 (voice/TDD)

VERMONT

Austine Transition House
112 Maple St.
Brattleboro, VT 05301
802-257-4510

VIRGINIA

Deaf Services Unit
P.O. Box 521
Fisherville, VA 22939
703-332-7239 (voice/TDD)

Supervised Apartment Program for Hearing
Impaired Persons
Riverside Hospital CMHC
500 J. Clyde Morris Blvd.
Newport News, VA 23601
804-599-2060 (voice/TDD)

WEST VIRGINIA

West Virginia Dept. of Health
Office of Behavioral Health
Capitol Complex
Bldg. 3, Rm. 451
Charleston, WV 25305
304-348-2276 (voice/TDD)
304-348-0627 (voice/TDD)

APPENDIX 7: PERFORMANCE GROUPS

The following list of performance groups of and for deaf people are both professional and amateur, some touring locally, some nationally.

Access Theatre
2428 Chapala St.
Santa Barbara, CA 93105
805-682-8184 (voice/TDD)

Callier Theatre of the Deaf
University of Texas
Dallas-Callier Center for Communication Disorders
1966 Inwood Road
Dallas, TX 75235
214-905-3049 (voice/TDD)

Chicagoland Advocates for Signed Theatre
67 E. Madison, Suite 2115
Chicago, IL 60603
312-346-5588 (voice)
312-346-5589 (TDD)

Expression
Southwest Collegiate Institute for the Deaf
Avenue C
Big Spring, TX 79720
915-264-3700 (voice/TDD)

Fairmount Theatre of the Deaf
8500 Euclid Ave.
Cleveland, OH 44106
216-229-2838

Fantasy
East Carolina University
A114 Brewster Bldg.
Greenville, NC 27834
919-757-6729 (voice/TDD)

Florissant Valley Theatre of the Deaf
St. Louis Community College
Florissant Valley
3400 Pershall Rd.
Ferguson, MO 63135
314-595-4477 (voice)
314-595-4488 (TDD)

Gallaudet University Theatre
800 Florida Ave. NE
Washington, DC 20002
202-651-5501 (voice)
202-651-5502 (TDD)

Gallaudet Dance Company
Physical Education Dept.
800 Florida Ave. NE
Washington, DC 20002
202-651-7572 (voice/TDD)

Hands in Harmony
P.O. Box 104
Cheyenne, WY 82003
307-638-9506 (voice)

Kinzie Dancers
5625 S. Mobile
Chicago, IL 60638
312-838-5352 (voice)

Lenoir-Rhyne Sign Troupe
Box 7483, Lenoir-Rhyne College
Hickory, NC 28603
704-328-7299 (voice)
704-328-7298 (TDD)

The National Theatre of the Deaf
5 W. Main St.
Chester, CT 06412
203-526-4971 (voice)
203-526-4974 (TDD)

NTID Music Program
NTID Performing Arts
Rochester Institute of Technology
P.O. Box 9887
Rochester, NY 14623
716-475-6796 (voice/TDD)

RIT Dance Company
NTID Theatre-NTID/RIT
One Lomb Memorial Dr.
Bldg. 60, Room 1828
Rochester, NY 14623
716-475-6252 (voice/TDD)

The Silent Sounds, Inc.
P.O. Box 8204
Chicago, IL 14623
312-829-7631 (voice)
312-381-1640 (TDD)

Stage Hands, Inc.
1020 DeKalb Ave., Suite 26
Atlanta, GA 30307
404-659-2684 (voice/TDD)

Starfire
Indiana School for the Deaf
1200 E. 42nd St.
Indianapolis, IN 46205
317-924-4347 (voice/TDD)
317-255-1997 (voice/TDD)

Sunshine, Too
NTID Performing Arts
Rochester Institute of Technology
P.O. Box 9887
Rochester, NY 14623
716-475-6251 (voice/TDD)

Theatre of Silence
Montana State University
Bozeman, MT 59717
406-994-3815 (voice)

APPENDIX 8: PERIODICALS OF INTEREST TO DEAF PEOPLE

AAAD Bulletin
American Athletic Association of the Deaf
1052 Darling St.
Ogden, UT 84403

ADARA Newsletter
P.O. Box 55369
Little Rock, AR 72225
(American Deafness and Rehabilitation Association)

ALDA News
Association of Late-Deafened Adults
1027 Oakton
Evanston, IL 60202

American Annals of the Deaf
Gallaudet University
800 Florida Ave. NE
Washington, DC 20002
(Scholarly journal of research related to deaf education; published 5 times a year; $40/year)

American Athletic Association of the Deaf Bulletin
134 Davenport Dr.
Burton, MI 48529
(Quarterly sports publication; $4/year)

ASHA
9030 Old Georgetown Road
Washington, DC 20014
(Monthly journal of the American Speech-Language-Hearing Association)

Audecibel
20361 Middlebelt
Livonia, MI 48152
(Quarterly journal of the National Hearing Aid Society)

The Broadcaster
193 Main St.
Lincoln Park, NJ 07035
(Published by the National Association of the Deaf)

The Bulletin
1 Prince St.
Alexandria, VA 22316
(Newsletter of the American Academy of Otolaryngology)

Communicator
P.O. Box 1840
Washington, DC 20013
(Better Hearing Institute)

Cued Speech Journal
P.O. Box 31345
Raleigh, NC 27622
(Journal of the National Cued Speech Association)

Cued Speech News
Dept. of Audiology and Speech-Language Pathology
Cued Speech Team/Mary Thornberry Bldg.
Gallaudet University
800 Florida Ave. NE
Washington, DC 20002
(Published quarterly; $6/year)

The Deaf American
445 N. Pennsylvania St., Suite 804
Indianapolis, IN 46204

(Published by the National Association of the Deaf; $20/year, free to members of NAD)

The Deaf Catholic
814 Thayer Ave.
Silver Spring, MD 20910
(International Catholic Deaf Assoc.)

The Deaf Episcopalian
1616 Calle Santiago
Pleasanton, CA 94566
(Episcopal Conference of the Deaf)

Deaf Life
c/o MSM Productions, Ltd.
Box 63083
Marketplace Mall
Rochester, NY 14623
(Published monthly; $30/year; Special interest stories in the deaf community)

The Deaf Lutheran
1333 S. Kirkwood Road
St. Louis, MO 63122

The Deafpride Advocate
1350 Potomac Ave. SE
Washington, DC 20003

Deaf USA
Eye Festival Communications, Inc.
1530 N. Gower St., Suite 201
Hollywood, CA 90028
(Published monthly; $16/year; general community news of interest to the deaf community)

The Endeavor
The American Society for Deaf Children
814 Thayer Ave.
Silver Spring, MD 20910
(Organization newsletter for parents of deaf children; published bimonthly; $25/year; fee includes membership)

The Exceptional Parent
264 Beacon St.
Boston, MA 02116
(Bimonthly consumer magazine dealing with all handicaps; $10/year)

The Frat
National Fraternal Society of the Deaf
1300 W. Northwest Hwy.
Mt. Prospect, IL 60056
(Published bimonthly; $5/year; insurance information and news about members)

Gallaudet Media Distribution Catalog
Gallaudet Media Distribution
Gallaudet University Library
Gallaudet University
800 Florida Ave. NE
Washington, DC 20002
(Published once every 18 months; deaf awareness and sign language instructional audiovisual resources available for free loan and for sale)

Gallaudet Research Institute Newsletter
Gallaudet Research Institute
Fay House
Gallaudet University
800 Florida Ave. NE
Washington, DC 20002
(Biannual; highlights work of the GRI.)

Gallaudet Today
The National Center for Law and the Deaf
Gallaudet University
800 Florida Ave. NE
Washington, DC 20002
(Published quarterly; $10/year. Special issues on deafness-related topics)

Gallaudet University Bookstore Catalog
Gallaudet University Bookstore
Gallaudet University
800 Florida Ave. NE
Washington, DC 20002
(Annual with periodic flyers; list of popular books on deafness and sign language, gift items and electronic devices for the deaf)

Gallaudet University Extension Catalog
Office of Extension and Summer Programs
College for Continuing Education
Gallaudet University
800 Florida Ave. NE
Washington, DC 20002

(Information on graduate credit courses, workshops and training sessions that can be offered throughout the country on request)

Gallaudet University Press Catalog
Gallaudet University Press
Gallaudet University
800 Florida Ave. NE
Washington, DC 20002
(Annual periodic flyers; catalog of books on deafness from scholarly works to children's materials)

GA-SK
Telecommunications for the Deaf, Inc.
814 Thayer Ave.
Silver Spring, MD 20910
(Published quarterly; $15/year; publication for telecommunication users)

Hearing Aid Journal
205 Benson Bldg.
Sioux City, IA 51101
(Monthly commercial trade magazine; $5/year)

Hearing Heart Magazine
The American Ministries to the Deaf
7564 Brown's Mill Road, Kaufman Station
Chambersburg, PA 17291

The Hearing Instrument
1 E. First St.
Duluth, MN 55802
(Monthly commercial trade magazine; $10/year)

International Perspectives
International Center on Deafness
Gallaudet University
800 Florida Ave. NE
Washington, DC 20002
(Three to five times yearly; highlights international activities relating to deafness and deaf education)

Journal of American Deafness and Rehabilitation Association
P.O. Box 55369
Little Rock, AR 72225
(Published four times yearly, newsletter every other month with membership; $36/year; for professionals working with deaf people)

Junior NAD Newsletter
Junior National Association of the Deaf
Branch Office
445 N. Pennsylvania St., Suite 804
Indianapolis, IN 46204
(Published nine times a year from September through May; $8/year; for young people who are members of Junior NAD)

Listening
The National Catholic Office of the Deaf
814 Thayer Ave.
Silver Spring, MD 20910

NAD Broadcaster
National Association of the Deaf
814 Thayer Ave.
Silver Spring, MD 20910
(Published 11 times a year; $10/year; free for NAD members; a deaf community national newspaper)

Nat-Cent News, The
The Helen Keller National Center for Deaf-Blind Youths and Adults
111 Middle Neck Road
Sands Point, NY 11050

Newsounds
Alexander Graham Bell Association for the Deaf, Inc.
3417 Volta Place NW
Washington, DC 20007
(See *Volta Review*)

NTID Focus
National Technical Institute for the Deaf
One Lomb Memorial Dr., Box 9887
Rochester, NY 14623
(Published quarterly; free; NTID technical and professional education programs)

On Cue
The National Cued Speech Assoc.

P.O. Box 31345
Raleigh, NC 27622

Otolaryngology—Head and Neck Surgery
1 Prince St.
Alexandria, VA 22316
(Journal of the American Academy of Otolaryngology—Head/Neck Surgery)

OTO Review
House Ear Institute
256 S. Lake
Los Angeles, CA 90057

Our Kids Magazine
Alexander Graham Bell Association for the Deaf
3417 Volta Place NW
Washington, DC 20007

Perspectives for Teachers of the Hearing Impaired
KDES, PAS 6
Gallaudet University
800 Florida Ave. NE
Washington, DC 20002
(Five times yearly, $15/year; magazine for teachers of hearing-impaired students with helpful information that can be used by parents at home)

The Quotarian
Quota International, Inc.
1420 21st St. NW
Washington, DC 20036

The Receiver
Deafness Research Foundation
9 E. 38th St.
New York, NY 10016

SHHH
Self Help for Hard of Hearing People, Inc.
7800 Wisconsin Ave.
Bethesda, MD 20814
(Published 6 times a year; $15/year; educational journal about hearing loss for hard-of-hearing people)

Silent News
Williamsville Branch
P.O. Box 23330
Rochester, NY 14692
(Published monthly; $15/year; newspaper devoted to current events in the deaf community)

Tattler
Rainbow Alliance of the Deaf
P.O. Box 14182
Washington, DC 20044

Tinnitus Today
American Tinnitus Assoc.
P.O. Box 5
Portland, OR 97207

Transaction
100 17th St. NW
Washington, DC 20036
(Bimonthly published by the American Academy of Ophthalmology and Otolaryngology)

The Voice
11931 N. Central Expressway, #11
Dallas, TX 75243
(Published nine times annually; $10/year; for deaf and hard-of-hearing people, health care professionals, libraries, agencies, schools and organizations)

Volta Review
Newsounds
Alexander Graham Bell Association for the Deaf
3417 Volta Place, NW
Washington, DC 20007
(Newsounds published 10 times, Volta Review 7 times yearly; $35/year membership includes both; promotes the association's goals of teaching speech and speechreading and the use of residual hearing)

Washington Sounds
National Association for Hearing and Speech Action
814 Thayer Ave.
Silver Spring, MD 20910

The World Around You
Gallaudet University
800 Florida Ave. NE
Washington, DC 20002

(Published nine times a year from September to May; $6.50/year; magazine for deaf and hard-of-hearing junior and senior high schoolers)

APPENDIX 9: RELIGIOUS MINISTRIES AND ORGANIZATIONS FOR DEAF PEOPLE

American Ministries to the Deaf
7564 Brown's Mill Road, Kaufman Station
Chambersburg, PA 17201
717-375-2610 (voice/TDD)

Baptist Sunday School Board Special Ministries
127 Ninth Ave. N
Nashville, TN 37234
615-251-2762 (voice)

Catholic Charities Office for Disabled Persons
Deafness Services
191 Joralmon St., 14th Floor
Brooklyn, NY 11201
718-596-5500 (voice)
718-596-0303 (TDD)

Catholic Deaf Apostolate
243 Steele Road
West Hartford, CT 06117
203-523-7530 (voice/TDD)

Cave Spring United Methodist Church
Ministries to Deaf Children
P.O. Box 305
Cave Spring, GA 30124
404-777-3582 (voice/TDD)

Central Bible College
3000 N. Grant St.
Springfield, MO 65803
417-833-2551 (voice)

Christian Record Services
Division for the Deaf
4444 S. 52nd St.
P.O. Box 6097
Lincoln, NE 68506
402-488-0981 (voice)
402-488-1902 (TDD)

Christian Reformed Church
Committee on Disability Concerns
2850 Kalamazoo Ave. SE
Grand Rapids, MI 49560
616-246-0837

Deaf International Bible College
808 Tenth St. E, Suite 5
Minneapolis, MN 55404
612-332-2081 (voice/TDD)

Deaf Missions
RR2, Box 26
Council Bluffs, IA 51503
712-322-5493 (voice/TDD)

Episcopal Conference of the Deaf
1616 Calle Santiago
Pleasanton, CA 94566

Evangelical Lutheran Church of America
Division of Social Ministry Organizations
8765 W. Higgins Rd.
Chicago, IL 60631
312-380-2690 (voice)
312-380-2685 (TDD)

General Council of the Assemblies of God
Division of Home Missions
Deaf Culture Ministries

1445 Boonville Ave.
Springfield, MO 65802
417-862-2781 ext. 3258 (voice)
417-862-1217 (TDD)

Gospel Ministries for the Deaf
P.O. Box 12
Oregon City, OR 97045
503-235-3551 (voice)

Home Mission Board, Southern Baptist Convention
Language, Church, Extension Division
1350 Spring St. NW
Atlanta, GA 30367
404-898-7000 (voice)

International Catholic Deaf Association
814 Thayer Ave.
Silver Spring, MD 20910
301-588-4009 (TDD)

International Lutheran Deaf Association
1333 S. Kirkwood Road
St. Louis, MO 63122
314-965-9000, ext. 315 (voice)
800-433-3954 (TDD)

Lutheran Church Missouri Synod
Mission to the Deaf and Blind
1333 S. Kirkwood Road
St. Louis, MO 63122
314-965-9917, ext. 321 (voice/TDD)

Mennonite Board of Missions
Office of Deaf Ministries
P.O. Box 370
Elkhart, IN 46515
219-294-7523, ext. 254 (voice/TDD)

Mill Neck Foundation
Lutheran Friends of the Deaf
P.O. Box 100
Mill Neck, NY 11765
516-922-4100 (voice/TDD)

National Catholic Office for the Deaf
814 Thayer Ave.
Silver Spring, MD 20910
301-587-7992 (voice)
301-585-5084 (TDD)

National Congress of Jewish Deaf
4960 Sabal Palm Blvd., Bldg. 7, Apt. 207
Tamarac, FL 33319

Presbyterian Church USA
Education and Congregational Nurture
100 Witherspoon, Room 5627
Louisville, KY 40202
502-569-5454 (voice)

United Methodist Church
Health and Welfare Ministries Program
475 Riverside Dr., Room 350
New York, NY 10115
212-870-3870 (voice)

APPENDIX 10: RESIDENTIAL PROGRAMS FOR DEAF/EMOTIONALLY DISTURBED CHILDREN

ALABAMA

The Learning Tree, Inc.
Box 9428
Mobile, AL 36609
205-649-4420 (voice/TDD)

CONNECTICUT

Paces Program
American School for the Deaf
139 N. Main St.
West Hartford, CT 06107
203-727-1300, 727-1496, 727-1421
(all voice/TDD)

MASSACHUSETTS

Adapt Unit
Beverly School for the Deaf
6 Echo Ave.
Beverly, MA 01915
508-927-7070 (voice/TDD)

Hayden Hearing Impaired Program
21 Queen St.
Dorchester, MA 02122
617-436-6866, 436-6867
(both voice/TDD)

MICHIGAN

Hawthorn Center
18471 Haggerty Rd.
Northville, MI 48167
313-349-3000 (voice)
313-349-8218 (TDD)

NEW YORK

The Lake Grove School
Open Gates Program for Hearing Impaired Adolescents with Adjustment Difficulties
P.O. Box L
Lake Grove, NY 11755
516-585-8776

Residential Treatment Facility for Emotionally Disturbed Hearing Impaired Children and Youth at Hillside Center
1183 Monroe Ave.
Rochester, NY 14620
716-473-5150 (voice)
716-473-7426 (TDD)

PENNSYLVANIA

Elwyn Institute
Program for Deaf and Hearing Impaired
111 Elwyn Rd.
Elwyn, PA 19063
215-891-2000 (voice)
800-345-8111 (voice)
215-891-2359 (TDD)

Friendship House Children's Center
Scranton State School for the Deaf
1615 E. Elm St.
Scranton, PA 18505
717-342-8305 (voice/TDD)

Mental Health Program
Western Pennsylvania School for the Deaf
300 Swissvale Ave.
Pittsburgh, PA 15218
412-371-7000 (voice)
412-371-2233 (TDD)

APPENDIX 11: SUMMER CAMPS FOR DEAF AND HARD-OF-HEARING CHILDREN

ALABAMA

Alabama Institute for Deaf and Blind
P.O. Box 698
Talladega, AL 35160
205-761-3650 (voice/TDD)

ARIZONA

Tucson Parks and Recreation Dept.
900 S. Randolph Way
Tucson, AZ 85716
602-791-4504

ARKANSAS

Arkansas School for the Deaf
2400 W. Markham
Little Rock, AR 72203
501-371-1555 (voice/TDD)

CALIFORNIA

California School for the Deaf—Riverside
Family Learning Vacation
3044 Horace St.
Riverside, CA 92506
714-782-6500 (voice/TDD)

Camp Scherman
Girl Scout Council of Orange County
P.O. Box 3739
Costa Mesa, CA 92628
714-979-7900 (voice)

Camp Signshine
Sky Mountain Christian Camp
P.O. Box 1488
Truckee, CA 95734
916-587-2801 (voice)

John Tracy Clinic
806 W. Adams Blvd.
Los Angeles, CA 90007
213-748-5481 (voice/TDD)
800-522-4582 (voice/TDD)

Leadership Training Program
Camp Signshine
P.O. Box 1488
Truckee, CA 95734
916-587-2801 (voice)

COLORADO

Aspen Camp School for the Deaf
Box 1494
Aspen, CO 81612
303-923-2511 (voice)
303-923-6609 (TDD)

Colorado Lions Camp
P.O. Box 9043
Woodland Park, CO 80866
719-687-2087

CONNECTICUT

Camp Isola Bella
American School for the Deaf
139 N. Main St.
West Hartford, CT 06107
203-727-1304 (voice/TDD)

DISTRICT OF COLUMBIA

Cued Speech Family Program
Gallaudet University/Cued Speech Dept.
800 Florida Ave. NE
Washington, DC 20002
202-651-5330 (voice/TDD)

Family Learning Vacation
Gallaudet University
National Academy
Family Life Program
800 Florida Ave. NE
Washington, DC 20002
202-651-5096 (voice/TDD)

ILLINOIS

Camp Lions Adventure Wilderness School
(by invitation only)
Lions of Illinois Foundation
1701 S. 1st. Ave.
Maywood, IL 60153
708-681-8800 (voice)
800-955-5466 (voice)

Camp Lions "Little Giant"
Lions of Illinois Foundation
1701 S. 1st Ave.
Maywood, IL 60153
708-681-8800 (voice)
800-955-5466 (voice)

Camp Lions "Ravenswood"
Lions of Illinois Foundation
1701 S. 1st. Ave.
Maywood, IL 60153
708-681-8800 (voice)
800-955-5466 (voice)

Institute for Parents of Hearing Impaired
Children
Illinois School for the Deaf
125 Webster Ave.
Jacksonville, IL 62650
217-245-5141, ext. 255 (voice/TDD)

Summer Vocational Program for Hearing
Impaired Adolescents
Admissions and Records
Illinois School for the Deaf
125 Webster Ave.
Jacksonville, IL 62650
217-245-5141 (voice/TDD)

INDIANA

Camp Adventure Deaf Camp
7484 N. Park Ave.
Indianapolis, IN 46240
317-251-3732 (voice)

KANSAS

Institute of Logopedics Summer Program
Institute of Logopedics
2400 Jardine Dr.
Wichita, KS 67219
316-262-8271 (voice/TDD)
800-835-1043 (voice/TDD)

KENTUCKY

Camp Piomingo
Deaf Community Center
P.O. Box 5455
Louisville, KY 40205
502-452-2053 (voice/TDD)

MARYLAND

Camp for the Deaf, Inc.
7202 Buchanan St.
Landover Hills, MD 20784
301-577-8057 (voice/TDD)

MASSACHUSETTS

Clarke School for the Deaf Summer
Program
Round Hill Road
Northampton, MA 01060
413-584-3450 (voice/TDD)

New England Deaf Camp
15 Ledgewood Rd.
Wakefield, MA 01880
617-245-9369 (voice/TDD)

MICHIGAN

Summer Remedial Clinics
Central Michigan University

Moore Hall, Room 441
Mt. Pleasant, MI 48859
517-774-3472 (voice)

MINNESOTA

Courage Center
3915 Golden Valley Dr.
Golden Valley, MN 55422
612-520-0520 (voice/TDD)

MISSISSIPPI

Mississippi School for the Deaf
1253 Eastover Dr.
Jackson, MS 39211
601-987-3936 (voice/TDD)

NEBRASKA

Christian Record Services
Division for the Deaf
4444 S. 52nd St.
Lincoln, NE 68506
402-488-0981 (voice)
402-488-1902 (TDD)

NEW YORK

Children's Aid Society
Wagon Road Camp
431 Quaker Road
P.O. Box 47
Chappaqua, NY 10514
914-238-4761 (voice)

Empire State Speech and Hearing Clinic, Inc.
P.O. Box 261
Elmira, NY 14902
607-732-7069 (voice/TDD)

Explore Your Future Camp
National Technical Institute for the Deaf
One Lomb Memorial Dr.
P.O. Box 9887
Rochester, NY 14623
716-475-6705 (voice/TDD)

Mid-Hudson Valley
St. Frances DeSalles School for the Deaf
260 Eastern Pkwy.
Brooklyn, NY 11225
718-636-4573 (voice)
718-636-1190 (TDD)

NYFRS Mitzvah Corps Chevrah
New York Federation of Reform Synagogues
838 Fifth Ave.
New York, NY 10021
212-249-0100, ext. 552 (voice)

NORTH DAKOTA

North Dakota School for the Deaf Summer Camp
14th St. and College Dr.
Devils Lake, ND 58301
701-662-5082 (voice/TDD)

PENNSYLVANIA

Beacon Lodge Camp
P.O. Box 428
Lewistown, PA 17044
717-242-1113 (voice)

TENNESSEE

Bill Rice Ranch
627 Bill Rice Ranch Road
Murfreesboro, TN 37129
615-893-2767 (voice/TDD)

TEXAS

Camp Sign
Texas Commission for the Deaf
P.O. Box 12904, Capitol Station
Austin, TX 78711
512-469-9891 (voice/TDD)

WASHINGTON

Camp Sealth
8511 15th Ave. NE
Seattle, WA 98115
206-524-8550 (voice)

Camp DonBosco
CYO Outdoor Ministries
Archdiocese of Seattle
910 Marion St.
Seattle, WA 98104
206-382-4851 (voice)

WISCONSIN

Wisconsin Lions Camp
46 County Road A
Rosholt, WI 54473
715-677-4761 (voice/TDD)

APPENDIX 12: TRAINING CENTERS FOR HEARING EAR DOGS

NATIONAL PROGRAMS

American Humane Association
P.O. Box 1266
Denver, CO 80201
303-695-0811 (voice)
303-695-4531 (TDD)

Canine Companions for Independence
Executive Office
P.O. Box 446
Santa Rosa, CA 95402
707-528-0830

Canine Helpers for the Handicapped, Inc.
5705 Ridge Road
Lockport, NY 14094
716-433-4035 (voice/TDD)

Center for Hearing Ear Dogs
9725 E. Hampden Ave.
Denver, CO 80231
303-695-0811 (voice)
303-695-4531 (TDD)

Dogs for the Deaf, Inc.
110175 Wheeler Road
Central Point, OR 97502
503-899-7177 (voice)
503-846-6783 (TDD)

Hearing Ear Dog Program
Executive Office
P.O. Box 213
West Boylston, MA 01583
508-835-3304 (voice/TDD)

International Hearing Dogs, Inc.
5901 E. 89th Ave.
Henderson, CO 80640
303-287-3277 (voice/TDD)

National Hearing Dog Center
1116 S. Main
Athol, MA 01331
508-249-9264 (voice)

Red Acre Farm Hearing Dog Center
109 Red Acre Road
P.O. Box 278
Stow, MA 01775
508-897-5370 (voice)
508-897-8343 (TDD)

REGIONAL PROGRAMS

California
Companion Animal Program for the Deaf
Riverside Humane Society
5791 Fremont St.
Riverside, CA 92504
714-688-4382 (voice)
714-688-8612 (TDD)

San Francisco SPCA
Hearing Dog Program
2500 16th St.
San Francisco, CA 94103
415-554-3020 (voice)
415-554-3022 (TDD)

Maryland, Virginia, Washington, D.C.
Canine Companions
14238 Briarwood Terrace
Rockville, MD 20853
301-460-3040 (voice/TDD)

North Carolina, South Carolina, Georgia
Southeastern Assistance Dogs (SEAD)
Speech, Hearing and Learning Center
811 Pendleton St.
9–11 Medical Court
Greenville, SC 29601
803-235-6065 (voice/TDD)

Connecticut
Connecticut Hearing Dog Program
239 Maple Hill Ave.
Newington, CT 06111
203-666-4646 (voice)
203-666-4648 (TDD)

Minnesota, Indiana, Ohio, Illinois
Ears for the Deaf, Inc.
1235 100th St. SE
Byron Center, MI 49302
616-698-0688 (voice/TDD)

Hearing Dogs of Columbus, Inc.
290 N. Hamilton Rd.
Gahanna, OH 43230
614-471-7397 (voice/TDD)
(serves Ohio)

Hearing Dog Program of Minnesota
4229 30th Ave. S
Minneapolis, MN 55406
612-722-2093 (voice/TDD)
(serves Minnesota)

APPENDIX 13: WHERE TO LEARN COMMUNICATION SKILLS

AUDITORY TRAINING CLASSES

Auditory training classes and instruction in listening skills help hard-of-hearing people learn to use their remaining hearing. For more information, call:

American Speech-Language-Hearing Association Helpline
800-638-8255 (voice/TDD)

CUED SPEECH

National Cued Speech Association
Cued Speech Center, Inc.
P.O. Box 31345
Raleigh, NC 27622
919-828-1218

Cued Speech—Dept. of Audiology
Gallaudet University, MTB 217
800 Florida Ave. NE
Washington, DC 20002
202-651-5330

North Coast Cued Speech Services
23970 Hermitage Road
Cleveland, OH 44122
216-292-6213

West Coast Cued Speech Programs
348 Cernon St.
Vacaville, CA 95688
707-448-4060

SIGN LANGUAGE

The best way to learn sign is with a teacher in a class. Contact the following:

- local school system, community college or university extension program
- state or county department of public instruction, education or special education
- county vocational rehabilitation services (many states have a coordinator of services for the deaf)
- United Way
- recreation and community centers (YWCA, YMCA)
- adult education/continuing education centers
- religious organizations
- libraries
- deafness-related organizations or groups (see Appendixes A and C)
- state school for the deaf
- state office/commission or state association for the deaf (see Appendixes A and B)

In addition, each April the *American Annals of the Deaf* includes a comprehensive list of services, schools and classes for deaf students. These would be good contacts for information on the availability of sign language.

If there are no classes available, text and tape materials are available. Check your local library.

SPEECHREADING

For more information, contact:

American Speech-Language-Hearing Association Helpline
800-638-8255 (voice/TDD)

Alexander Graham Bell Association for the Deaf
202-337-5220 (voice/TDD)

BIBLIOGRAPHY

Abercrombie, D. *Elements of General Phonetics.* Chicago: Aldine, 1967.

Aiello, B. *The Hearing-Impaired Child in the Regular Class.* Washington, DC: The AFT Teachers' Network for Education of the Handicapped, 1981.

Akens, David. *Loss of Hearing and You.* Huntsville, AL: Strode, 1970.

Albertini, J., B. Meath-Lang and Caccamise, F. "Sign Language Use: Development of English and Communication Skills." *Audiology* 9 (1984): 111–126.

Allen, J. C., and M. L. Allen. "Discovering and Accepting Hearing Impairment." *Volta Review* 81, no. 5 (1979): 279–285.

Allen, T. E., and T. I. Osborn. "Academic Integration of Hearing-Impaired Students: Demographic, Handicapping and Achievement Factors." *American Annals of the Deaf* 129, no. 2 (1984): 100–113.

———, C. S. White, and M. A. Karchmer. "Issues in the Development of a Special Edition for Hearing-Impaired Students of the Seventh Edition of the Stanford Achievement Test." *American Annals of the Deaf* 128, no. 1 (1983): 34–39.

Altshuler, K. A. "Psychiatric Considerations in the Adult Deaf." *American Annals of the Deaf* 107, no. 5 (1962): 560–561.

———. "The Social and Psychological Development of the Deaf Child: Problems, Their Treatment and Prevention." *American Annals of the Deaf* 119, no. 4 (1974): 365–376.

———, W. E. Deming, and J. Vollenweider. "Impulsivity and Profound Early Deafness." *American Annals of the Deaf* 121, (3) (1976): 331–345.

———, and J. Rainer, eds. *Mental Health and the Deaf: Approach and Prospects.* Washington, DC: U.S. Department of Health, Education and Welfare, Social and Rehabilitation Services, 1968.

American Society for Deaf Children. *Position Statements on Education, Educational Options, Parental Involvement in Education, Communication, Total Communication.* Silver Spring, MD: American Society for Deaf Children, 1983.

Angus, Jean Rich. *Watch My Words: An Open Letter to Parents of Young Deaf Children.* Cincinnati, OH: Forward Movement Publications, 1974.

Anthony, D., W. Dekkers, and C. Erikson. *Seeing Essential English: Code-breaker.* Boulder, CO: Pruett, 1978.

Baker, C., and R. Battison. *Sign Language and the Deaf Community.* Silver Spring, MD: National Association of the Deaf, 1980.

———, and D. Cokely. *American Sign Language: A Teacher's Resource Text on Grammar and Culture.* Silver Spring, MD: T. J. Publishers, 1980.

Bale, J. F., J. A. Blackman, J. Murph and R. D. Anderson. "Congenital Cytomegalovirus Infection: Information for Educational Personnel." *American Journal of Diseases of Children* 140 (1986): 128–131.

Battison, Robbin. *Lexical Borrowing in American Sign Language.* Silver Spring, MD: Linstok Press, 1978.

Beck, B. "Self-assessment of selected interpersonal abilities in hard of hearing and deaf adolescents," *International Journal of Rehabilitation Research* 11, no. 4 (1988): 343–9.

Becker, G. *Growing Old in Silence.* Berkeley: University of California Press, 1980.

Bekesy, G. *Experiments in Hearing.* New York: McGraw-Hill, 1960.

Bellugi, Ursula, and D. Newkirk. "Formal Devices for Creating New Signs in American Sign Language." *Sign Language Studies* 30 (1981): 1–35.

———, H. Poizner and E. Klima. "Brain Organization for Language: Clues from Sign Aphasia." *Human Neurobiology* 2 (1983): 155–170.

Bender, R. *The Conquest of Deafness.* Cleveland, OH: Case Western Reserve, 1970.

Bennett, W., and D. Ling. "Teaching a Complex Verbal Response to a Hearing-Impaired Girl." *Journal of Applied Behavioral Analysis* 5 (1972): 321–327.

Berendt, R. D., E. Corliss and M. Ojalvo. *Quieting: A Practical Guide to Noise Control.* U.S. Dept. of Commerce, National Bureau of Standards, Washington, DC, 1976.

Berg, F. S. *Educational Audiology: Hearing and Speech Management.* New York: Grune & Stratton, 1976.

Berger, Kenneth W. *Hearing Aids.* Detroit: National Hearing Aid Society, 1974.

———, E. Hagberg and R. Rane. *Prescription of Hearing Aids: Rationale, Procedure, and Results.* Kent, OH: Herald Publishing House, 1979.

Bergman, M. *Aging and the Perception of Speech.* Baltimore, MD: University Park Press, 1980.

Bergstrom, L. "Causes of Severe Hearing Loss in Early Childhood." Pediatric Annals 9 (1980): 23–30.

Bess, F. *Childhood Deafness: Causation, Assessment and Management.* New York: Grune & Stratton, 1977.

———, B. A. Freeman and J. S. Sinclair, eds. *Amplification in Education.* Washington, DC: Alexander Graham Bell Association for the Deaf, 1981.

Birch, J. *Hearing-Impaired Pupils in the Mainstream of Education.* Reston, VA: Council for Exceptional Children, 1974.

Blackwell, P. *Teaching Hearing Impaired Children in Regular Classrooms.* Washington, DC: Center for Applied Linguistics, 1983.

Block, M., and M. Okrand. "Real-time Closed Captioned Television as an Educational Tool." *American Annals of the Deaf* 128, no. 5 (1983): 636–641.

Bodner-Johnson, B. A. "The Family Environment and Achievement of Deaf Students." *Exceptional Children* 52 (1986): 443–449.

Bolinger, D. *Aspects of Language.* New York: Harcourt Brace Jovanovich, 1968.

Bonnickson, K. "A Functional Language Program That Works." *Volta Review* 87, no. 2 (1985): 67–76.

Boothroyd, A. H. *Hearing Impairments in Young Children.* Englewood Cliffs, NJ: Prentice-Hall, 1982.

Bornstein, Harry. "A Description of Some Current Systems Designed to Represent English." *American Annals of the Deaf* 118 (1973): 454–464.

———. "Towards a Theory of Use for Signed English: From Birth Through Adulthood." *American Annals of the Deaf* 127, no. 1 (1982): 26–31.

———, and Karen Saulnier. *The Signed English School Book.* Washington, DC: Kendall Green Publications, Gallaudet University Press, 1987.

———, K. Saulnier and Lillian Hamilton, eds. *The Comprehensive Signed English Dictionary.* Washington, DC: Gallaudet University Press, 1983.

Boughman, J. A., and K. A. Shaver. "Genetic Aspects of Deafness: Understanding the Counseling Process." *American Annals of the Deaf* 127, no. 4 (1982): 393–400.

Braddy, N. *Anne Sullivan Macy: The Story Behind Helen Keller.* New York: Doubleday, 1933.

Bradford, L. and W. Hardy, eds. *Hearing and Hearing Impairment.* New York: Grune & Stratton, 1979.

Brasel, K., and S. P. Quigley. "Influence of Certain Language and Communication Environments in Early Childhood on the Development of Language in Deaf Individuals." *Journal of Speech and Hearing Research* 20 (1977): 95–107.

Brill, Richard G. *Administrative and Professional Developments in the Education of the Deaf.* Washington, DC: Gallaudet University Press, 1971.

———. *Mainstreaming the Prelingually Deaf Child.* Washington, DC: Gallaudet University Press, 1978.

Bruce, Robert. *Alexander Graham Bell and the Conquest of Solitude.* Boston: Little, Brown, 1973.

Caccamise, F., ed. "Sign Language and Simultaneous Communication: Linguistic, Psychological and Instructional Ramifications." *American Annals of the Deaf,* November 1978.

———, et al., eds. *Introduction to Interpreting for Interpreters/Transliterators, Hearing-Impaired Consumers, Hearing Consumers.* Silver Spring, MD: Registry of Interpreters for the Deaf, 1980.

———, and D. Hicks, eds. *American Sign Language in a Bilingual Bicultural Context.* Silver Spring, MD: National Association of the Deaf, 1980.

———, and W. Newell. "A Review of Current Terminology in Deaf Education and Signing." *Journal of the Academy of Rehabilitative Audiology* 17 (1984).

Caldwell, D. "Closed Captioned Television and the Hearing Impaired." *Volta Review* 83, no. 5 (1981): 285–289.

Calvert, D. *A Parent's Guide to Speech and Deafness.* Washington, DC: Alexander Graham Bell Association for the Deaf, 1984.

———, and S. R. Silverman. *Speech and Deafness.* Washington, DC: Alexander Graham Bell Association for the Deaf, 1983.

Carmen, Richard. *Our Endangered Hearing: Understanding and Coping With Hearing Loss.* Emmaus, PA: Rodale Press, 1977.

Catford, J. *Fundamental Problems in Phonetics.* Bloomington: University of Indiana Press, 1966.

Chess, S., and P. Fernandez. "Impulsivity in Rubella Deaf Children: A Longitudinal Study." *American Annals of the Deaf* 125, no. 40 (1980): 505–9.

Chomsky, N. *Language and Mind.* New York: Harcourt Brace Jovanovich, 1968.

Chouard, D., B. Meyer and D. Maridat. "Transcutaneous Electrotherapy for Severe Tinnitus." *Acta Otolaryngology* 91 (1981): 415–422.

Chough, S. K. "Speech is Not Equivalent to Personality Development." *Social Work* 22, no. 4 (1977): 310–312.

———. "Social Services for Deaf Citizens: Some Proposals of Effectiveness." In *Deafness,* vol. 3. Silver Spring, MD: Professional Rehabilitation Workers with the Adult Deaf, 1973.

Christiansen, J. B., and D. P. Polakoff. "Characteristics of Social Workers and Social Work Programs at Residential and Day Schools for the Deaf." *American Annals for the Deaf,* June 125(4), 1980: 482–7.

Clarke, B. R., and D. Ling. "The Effects of Using Cued Speech." *Volta Review* 78 (1976): 23–34.

Cokely, D. "When Is a Pidgin Not a Pidgin? An Alternate Analysis of the ASL-English Contact Situation." *Sign Language Studies* 38 (1983): 1–24.

———, and R. Gawlik. "A Position Paper on the Relationship between Manual English and Sign." *Deaf American,* May 7–11, 1973.

Cole, E., and H. Gregory, eds. *Auditory Learning.* Washington, DC: Alexander Graham Bell Association for the Deaf, 1986.

Combs, Alec. *Hearing Loss Help.* Santa Maria, CA: Alpenglow Press, 1986.

Compton, Cynthia, and Fred Brandt. *Assistive Listening Devices.* Washington, DC: National Information Center on Deafness.

Connor, L., ed. *Speech for the Deaf Child: Knowledge and Use.* Washington, DC: Alexander Graham Bell Association for the Deaf, 1971.

Conrad, R. *The Deaf School Child.* London: Harper & Row, 1979.

Corbett, E. E., Jr. and C. J. Jensema. *Teachers of the Deaf: Descriptive Profiles.* Washington, DC: Gallaudet University Press, 1981.

Corliss, Edith L. *Hearing Aids.* Washington, DC: U.S. Department of Commerce, 1970.

Craig, H. B. "Parent-Infant Education in Schools for Deaf Children." *American Annals of the Deaf* 128, no. 21 (1983): 82–98.

Craig, W. "Effects of Pre-School Training on the Development of Reading and Lipreading Skills of Deaf Children." *American Annals of the Deaf* 109, no. 3 (1964): 280–296.

Crammatte, A. B. *Deaf Persons in Professional Employment.* Springfield, IL: Thomas, 1968.

———. *Meeting the Challenge: Hearing Impaired Professionals in the Workplace.* Washington, DC: Gallaudet University Press, 1987.

———. *Questions and Answers About Employment of Deaf People.* Washington, DC: National Information Center on Deafness, 1988.

Crandall, K. E., and N. A. Orlando. "The Use and Learning of Spoken Language Systems." *American Annals of the Deaf* 125, no. 3 (1980): 335–448.

———. "A Comparison of Signs Used By Mothers and Deaf Children During Early Childhood." In *Proceedings of the Convention of American Instructors of the Deaf, 1975.*

Dale, D. M. *Individualized Integration: Studies of Deaf and Partially-Hearing Children and Students in Ordinary Schools and Colleges.* Springfield, IL: Thomas, 1984.

Daniloff, R., G. Schuckers and L. Feth. *The Physiology of Speech and Hearing: An Introduction.* Englewood Cliffs, NJ: Prentice-Hall, 1980.

Davis, Hallowell, and S. Richard Silverman, eds. *Hearing and Deafness.* New York: Holt, Rinehart and Winston, 1978.

Davis, Julia, and Edward Hardick. *Rehabilitative Audiology for Children and Adults.* New York: Macmillan, 1986.

Day, P. S. "Deaf Children's Expression of Communication Intentions." *Journal of Communication Disorders* 19, no. 5 (1986): 376–386.

DiPietro, L. *A Look at Fingerspelling.* Washington, DC: The National Academy, Gallaudet University, 1976.

Dobie, R., and C. Berlin. "Binaural interaction in brainstem-evoked responses." *Ann. Otol. Rhinol. Laryngol,* Archives of Otolaryngology 105 (7): 391–8 July 1979.

DuBow, S. "Courts Interpret Mainstreaming: How Residential Schools Can Adapt." *American Annals of the Deaf* 129, no. 2 (1984): 92–94.

Dunan, J. G. "Recent Legislation Affecting Hearing-Impaired Persons." *American Annals of the Deaf* 129, no. 2 (1984): 83–91.

Eisenberg, R. "The Development of Hearing in Man: An Assessment of Current Status." *ASHA* 12 (1970): 119–123.

Erber, N. P. *Auditory Training.* Washington, DC: Alexander Graham Bell Association for the Deaf, 1972.

Erting, C., and R. Meiesegeier, eds. *Social Aspects of Deafness.* Washington, DC: Gallaudet University Press, 1982.

Evans, L. *Total Communication: Structure and Strategy.* Washington, DC: Gallaudet University Press, 1982.

Farrugia, D., and G. F. Austin. "A Study of Social-Emotional Adjustment Patterns of Hearing-Impaired Students in Different Educational Settings." *American Annals of the Deaf* 125, no. 5 (1980): 535–541.

Fasold, R. *The Sociolinguistics of Society.* Oxford, England: Blackwell, 1984.

Fellendorf, G. *Current Developments in Assistive Devices for Hearing-Impaired Persons.* Washington, DC: Gallaudet Research Institute, 1982.

Ferris, C. *A Hug Isn't Enough.* Washington, DC: Gallaudet College Press, 1980.

Fine, P. J., ed. *Deafness in Infancy and Early Childhood.* New York: Medcom Press, 1974.

Flexer, C. "Audiological rehabilitation in the schools," *ASHA* 32, no. 4 (April 1990): 44–5.

Fraser, G. *The Causes of Profound Deafness in Childhood.* Baltimore: Johns Hopkins University Press, 1976.

Frederickson, J. *Life After Deaf.* Silver Spring, MD: National Association of the Deaf, 1985.

Freeman, Roger D., Clifton F. Carbin and Robert J. Boese. *Can't Your Child Hear?* Baltimore: University Park Press, 1981.

Freese, Arthur S. *You and Your Hearing: How To Protect It, Preserve It and Restore It.* New York: Scribner, 1979.

Frishberg, N. "Arbitrariness and Iconicity: Historical Change in American Sign Language." *Language* 51, no. 3 (1975): 696–719.

———. *Interpreting: An Introduction.* Silver Spring, MD: RID Publications, 1985.

Froehlinger, V. *Today's Hearing Impaired Child: Into the Mainstream of Education.* Washington, DC: Alexander Graham Bell Association for the Deaf, 1981.

Funk, B. "Being Ignored Can Be Bliss—How To Use a Sign Language Interpreter." Deaf American, 34, no. 6 (1982).

Furth, Hans G. *Thinking Without Language: Psychological Implications of Deafness.* New York: Free Press, 1966.

Galenson, E., and R. Miller, E. Kaplan, A. Rothstein et al. "Assessment of Development in the Deaf Child." *Journal of the American Academy of Child Psychiatry* 18, no. 1 (1979): 128–42.

Gannon, J. *Deaf Heritage: A Narrative History of Deaf Americans.* Silver Spring, MD: National Association of the Deaf, 1981.

Garcia, W. J., ed. *Medical Sign Language.* Springfield, IL: Thomas, 1983.

Garrity, J. H., and H. Mengle. "Early Identification of Hearing Loss: Practices and Procedures." *American Annals of the Deaf* 128, no. 2 (1983): 99–106.

Gelfland, S. *Hearing: An Introduction to Psychological and Physiological Acoustics.* New York: Dekker, 1981.

Gerber, S. E., ed. *Audiometry in Infancy.* New York: Grune & Stratton, 1977.

Gerkin, K. P. "The High-Risk Register for Deafness." ASHA 26, no. 3 (1984): 17–23.

Gibbs, K. W. "Individual differences in cognitive skills related to reading ability in the deaf." *American Annals of the Deaf* 134, no. 3 (July 1989): 214–8.

Gilbert, L., ed. "Deafness and Aging in the USA." *Gallaudet Today* 12, no. 2 (Winter 1982).

Glick, F. P., and D. Pellman. *Breaking Silence.* Scottsdale, AZ: Herald Press, 1982.

Goldstein, M. H., Jr. and A. Proctor. "Tactile Aids for Profoundly Deaf Children." *Journal of the Acoustical Society of America* 77, no. 11 (1985): 258–265.

Graff, Stewart and Polly Anne. *Helen Keller: Toward the Light.* New York: Dell, 1971.

Graham, J. M., and J. Hazell. "Electrical Stimulation of the Human Cochlea Using a Transtympanic Electrode." *Brit. J. Audio.* 11 (1977): 59–62.

Greenberg, M. T. "Family Stress and Child Competence: The Effects of Early Intervention for Families with Deaf Infants." *American Annals of the Deaf* 128, no. 4 (1980): 407–417.

———, and R. Calderon. "Early Intervention for Deaf Children: Outcomes and Issues." *Topics in Early Childhood Special Education* 4 (1984): 1–9.

Gregory, S. *The Deaf Child and His Family.* New York: Wiley, 1976.

Groce, N. *Everyone Here Spoke Sign Language.* Cambridge, MA: Harvard University Press, 1985.

Grosjean, F. *Life With Two Languages: An Introduction to Bilingualism.* Cambridge, MA: Harvard University Press, 1982.

Gustason, G., E. Pfetzing and E. Zawolkow. *Signing Exact English.* Silver Spring, MD: National Association of the Deaf, 1980.

Hagborg, W. J. "A sociometric investigation of sex and race peer preferences among deaf adolescents," *American Annals of the Deaf* 134, no. 4 (Oct. 1989): 265–7.

Hairston, E., and L. Smith. *Black and Deaf in America: Are We That Different?* Silver Spring, MD: T. J. Publishers, 1983.

Hardy, R., and J. Cull, eds. *Educational and Psycho-Social Aspects of Deafness.* Springfield, IL: Thomas, 1974.

Haring, Norris, ed. *Exceptional Children and Youth.* Columbus, OH: Merrill, 1981.

Harris, G. *Broken Ears, Wounded Hearts.* Washington, DC: Gallaudet University Press, 1983.

Harris, S., M. Casselbrant, A. Ivarsson, O. Tjernström. "Hearing Threshold Measurement in Menieres Disease" *Audiology* 1984 23(1): 46–52.

Heffner, R. *General Phonetics.* Madison: University of Wisconsin Press, 1960.

Helleberg, Marilyn M. *Your Hearing Loss: How To Break The Sound Barrier.* Chicago: Nelson-Hall, 1979.

Henggeler, S. W., and P. F. Cooper. "Deaf Child-Hearing Mother Interaction." *Journal of Pediatric Psychology* 8 (1983): 83–95.

Higgins, P. *Outsiders in a Hearing World: A Sociology of Deafness.* Beverly Hills, CA: Sage Publications, 1980.

Hochberg, I., H. Levitt and M. J. Osberger, eds. *Speech of the Hearing Impaired: Research, Training and Personnel Preparation.* Baltimore, MD: University Park Press, 1983.

Holborow, C. "Deafness as a World Problem." *Advances in Oto-Rhino-Laryngology* 29 (1983): 174–182.

Holm, V. and L. Kunze. "Effect of Chronic Otitis Media on Language and Speech Development." *Pediatrics* 43 (1969): 833–9.

Hopkinson, N. ed. "Speech Reception Threshold." In *Handbook of Clinical Audiology.* Baltimore, MD: Williams and Wilkins, 1978.

House, W. F. "Cochlear Implants." *Annals of Otolaryngology, Rhinology, Laryngology* 85, suppl. 27 (1976): 1–93.

House, J., L. Miller and P. House. "Severe Tinnitus: Treatment with Biofeedback Training, Results in 41 Cases." *Trans. American Academy of Opthalmology and Otolaryngology* 84 (1976): 697–703.

Hughes, Gordon B., M. D., and Lawrence Koegel, M.D. "Ototoxicity." In *Textbook of Clinical Otology.* New York: Thieme-Stratton, 1985.

Hull, R., and K. Dilka, eds. *The Hearing Impaired Child In School.* Orlando, FL: Grune & Stratton, 1984.

Jacobs, L. *A Deaf Adult Speaks Out.* Washington, DC: Gallaudet University Press, 1980.

———. "The Community of the Adult Deaf." *American Annals of the Deaf* 119, no. 11 (1974): 41–46.

Jamison, S. L., ed. *Signs for Commuting Terminology.* Silver Spring, MD: National Association of the Deaf, 1983.

Jeffers, J., and M. Barley. *Speechreading (Lipreading).* Springfield, IL: Thomas, 1971.

Jensema, C., and J. Mullins. "Onset, Cause, and Additional Handicaps in Hearing-Impaired Children." *American Annals of the Deaf* 119, no. 6 (1974): 701–705.

Kampfe, C. M. "Parental reaction to a child's hearing impairment," *American Annals of the Deaf* 134, no. 4 (Oct. 1989): 255–9.

Kannapell, B., Lillian Hamilton and H. Bornstein. *Signs for Instructional Purposes.* Washington, DC: Gallaudet University Press, 1969.

Kaplan, H. *Anatomy and Physiology of Speech.* New York: McGraw-Hill, 1971.

Katsuki, J., et al. "Application of Theory of Signal Detection to Dichotic Listening." *Journal of Speech and Hearing Research* 27 (1984): 444–448.

Katz, J. *Handbook of Clinical Audiology.* 3d ed. Baltimore, MD: Williams and Wilkins, 1985.

Katz, L., S. Mathis and E. C. Merrill Jr. *The Deaf Child in the Public Schools: A Handbook for Parents of Deaf Children.* Danville, IL: Interstate Printers and Publishers, 1978.

Kettrick, Catherine. *American Sign Language: A Beginning Course.* Silver Spring, MD.: National Association of the Deaf, 1984.

King, S. "Comparing two causal models of career maturity for hearing-impaired adolescents," *American Annals of the Deaf* 135, no. 1 (Spring 1990): 43–9.

Klima, E., and U. Bellugi. *The Signs of Language.* Cambridge, MA: Harvard University Press, 1979.

Kluwin, T. N. "The Grammaticality of Manual Representations of English in Classroom Settings." *American Annals of the Deaf* 126 (4) (June 1981): 417–421.

———. "A Rationale for Modifying Classroom Signing Systems." *Sign Language Studies* 23 (1979): 99–136.

Konigsmark, B. W., and R. Gorlin. *Genetic and Metabolic Deafness.* Philadelphia: Saunders, 1976.

Kothman, V. "Classroom Auditory Trainers." *Hearing Aid Journal* Dec. 1981, 8–9, 41–43.

Kretschmer, R., and L. Kretschmer. *Language Development and Intervention with the Hearing Impaired.* Baltimore MD: University Park Press, 1978.

Ladefoged, P. *A Course in Phonetics.* New York: Harcourt Brace Jovanovich, 1975.

Lash, J. *Helen and Teacher: The Story of Helen Keller and Anne Sullivan Macy.* New York: American Foundation for the Blind, 1980.

Lass, N. *Speech and Language: Advances in Basic Research and Practice.* Vol. 8. New York: Academic Press, 1982.

———, *Speech, Language and Hearing.* Philadelphia: Saunders, 1982.

Levine, E. *The Ecology of Early Deafness: Guide to Fashioning Environments and Psychological Assessments.* New York: Columbia University Press, 1981.

———. "Psychological Tests and Practices with the Deaf: A Survey of the State of the Art." *Volta Review* 76, no. 5 (1974): 298–319.

———. *The Psychology of Deafness: Techniques of Appraisal for Rehabilitation.* New York: Columbia University Press, 1960.

———, and E. Wagner. "Personality of Deaf Persons." *Perceptual and Motor Skills* 39 (1974): 1167–1236.

Levine, S. C. "A complex case of cochlear implant electrode placement," *American Journal of Otolaryngology* 10, no. 6 (November 1989): 477–80.

Levitt, H. "Hearing Impairment and Sensory Aids." *Journal of Rehabilitation Research and Development* 23, no. 1 (1986): xiii–xviii.

Locke, J. *Phonological Acquisition and Change.* New York: Academic Press, 1984.

Libbey, S. S., and W. Pronovost. "Communication Practices of Mainstreamed Hearing-Impaired Adolescents." *Volta Review* 82, no. 4 (1980): 197–213.

Liben, L. S., ed. *Deaf Children: Developmental Perspectives.* New York: Academic Press, 1978.

Ling, D. *Early Intervention for Hearing-Impaired Children: Oral Options.* San Diego, CA: College-Hill Press, 1984.

———. *Early Intervention for Hearing-Impaired Children: Total Communication Options.* San Diego, CA: College-Hill Press, 1984.

———. *Speech and the Hearing Impaired Child.* Washington, DC: Alexander Graham Bell Association for the Deaf, 1976.

Liston, S. L. "Beethoven's deafness." *Laryngoscope* 99, no. 12 (Dec. 1989): 1301–4.

Lubinski, R. B. "A Review of Recent Research on Verbal Communication Among the Elderly." *International Journal of Aging and Human Development* 9 (1978–79): 237–245.

Luey, H. S., and M. Per-Lee. *What Should I do Now: Problems and Adaptations of the Deafened Adult.* Washington, DC: Gallaudet University Press, 1983.

Luterman, D. M., ed. *Deafness in Perspective.* San Diego, CA: College-Hill Press, 1986.

———. *Counseling Parents of Hearing Impaired Children.* Boston: Little, Brown, 1979.

———. *Deafness in the Family.* Boston: Little, Brown, 1987.

Markowicz, H. "American Sign Language: Fact and Fancy." Washington, DC: The National Academy, Gallaudet University, 1977.

Marshall, L. "Auditory Processing in Aging Listeners." *Journal of Speech and Hearing Disorders* 46, no. 3 (August 1981).

Martin, F. N. *Introduction to Audiology.* Englewood Cliffs, NJ: Prentice-Hall, 1981.

McArthur, Shirley H. *Raising Your Hearing-Impaired Child: A Guideline for Parents.* Washington, DC: Alexander Graham Bell Association for the Deaf, 1982.

McCrone, W. P. "Learned Helplessness and Level of Underachievement Among Deaf Adolescents." *Psychology in the Schools* 16, no. 3 (1979): 298–319.

McFarland, W., and B. P. Cox. *Aging and Hearing Loss.* Washington, DC: National Information Center on Deafness/American Speech-Language-Hearing Association, 1987.

Meadow, K. P. *Deafness and Child Development.* Berkeley, CA: University of California Press, 1980.

———. Greenberg, M. T., and C. Erting. "Attachment Behavior of Deaf Children with Deaf Parents." *Journal of the American Academy of Child Psychiatry* 22 (1983): 23–28.

———, M. T. Greenberg, C. Erting, H. Carmichael. "Interactions of Deaf Mothers and Deaf Preschool Children: Comparisons with Three Other Groups of Deaf and Hearing Dyads." *American Annals of the Deaf* 126, no. 4 (1981): 454–468.

Mendel, M. "Infant Responses to Recorded Sounds." *Journal of Speech and Hearing Research* 11 (1968): 811–816.

Mendelsohn, J. Z., and B. Fairchild. *Years of Challenge, A Guide for Parents of Hearing-Impaired Adolescents*. Silver Spring, MD: National Association of the Deaf, 1982.

Miller, Alfred, Barbara Farrel Rohman and Frances Vena Thompson. *Your Child's Hearing and Speech*. Springfield, IL: Thomas, 1974.

Mills, J. H., and J. A. Going. "Review of Environmental Factors Affecting Hearing." *Environmental Health Perspectives* 44 (1982): 119–127.

Mindel, E. D. "A Child Psychiatrist Looks at Deafness." *The Deaf American* 20 (1968): 15–19.

———, & Vernon McCay. *They Grow in Silence: Understanding Deaf Children and Adults*. 2d ed. Silver Spring, MD: National Association of the Deaf, 1987.

Moeller, M. P. "Parents' use of Signing Exact English: a descriptive analysis," *Journal of Speech and Hearing Disorders* 55, no. 2 (May 1990): 327–37.

Moore, B. *An Introduction to the Psychology of Hearing*. 2d ed. New York: Academic Press, 1982.

Moores, D. *Educating the Deaf: Psychology, Principles, and Practices*. 3d ed. Boston: Houghton Mifflin, 1987.

Moses, K. "Parenting a Hearing-Impaired Child." *Volta Review* 81, no. 2 (1979): 73–80.

Murphy, A. T., ed. "The Families of Hearing-Impaired Children." *Volta Review* 81, no. 5 (1979).

Myklebust, H. *The Psychology of Deafness*. New York: Grune & Stratton, 1960.

Naiman, D., and J. Schein. *For Parents of Deaf Children*. Silver Spring, MD: National Association of the Deaf, 1978.

Nash, J., and A. Nash. *Deafness in Society*. Lexington, MA: Heath, 1981.

National Center for Law and the Deaf. *Legal Rights of Hearing-Impaired People*. Washington, DC: Gallaudet University Press, 1986.

National Information Center on Deafness. *Communicating with Deaf People*. Washington, DC: Gallaudet University Press, 1987.

———. *Learning Sign Language: Audio Visual/Computer Programs*. Washington, DC: National Information Center on Deafness, 1989.

———. *Growing Together: Information for Parents of Hearing Impaired Children*. Washington, DC: National Information Center on Deafness and the Center for Curriculum Development Training and Outreach, Gallaudet University Press, 1987.

Neisser, A. *The Other Side of Silence: Sign Language and the Deaf Community in America*. New York: Knopf, 1983.

Newby, Hayes A. *Audiology*. New York: Appleton-Century-Crofts, 1972.

Nix, G. W. "The Right To Be Heard." *Volta Review* 83, no. 4 (1981): 199–205.

———. *Mainstream Education for Hearing Impaired Children and Youth*. New York: Grune & Stratton, 1976.

Northcott, W. H. *The Hearing Impaired Child in a Regular Classroom.* Washington, DC: Alexander Graham Bell Association, 1973.

Northern, J. L., and M. P. Downs. *Hearing in Children.* Baltimore, MD: Williams & Wilkins, 1974.

Ogden, P., and S. Lipsett. *The Silent Garden: Understanding the Hearing Impaired Child.* New York: St. Martin's Press, 1982.

Olsen, W., and N. Matkin. "Speech Audiometry." In *Hearing Assessment,* edited by W. Rintelmann. Baltimore, MD: University Park Press, 1979.

Orlans, H. *Adjustment to Adult Hearing Loss.* San Diego, CA: College-Hill Press, 1985.

O'Neil, J., and H. Oyer. *Visual Communication for the Hard of Hearing.* Englewood Cliffs, NJ: Prentice-Hall, 1961.

Osberger, M. J. "Audiological rehabilitation with cochlear implants and tactile aids." *ASHA* 32, no. 4 (April 1990): 38–43.

Ozdamor, O., N. Kraus and L. Stein. "Auditory Brainstem Responses in Infants Recovering from Bacterial Meningitis." *Archives of Otolaryngology* 109 (January 1983): 13–18.

Panara, R. F. "Cultural Arts Among the Deaf." *The Deaf American* 32, no 9 (1980): 9–11.

———, and J. Panara. *Great Deaf Americans.* Silver Spring, MD: T. J. Publishers, 1983.

Panjvani, Z., and J. Hanshaw. "Cytomegalovirus in the Perinatal Period." *American Journal of the Disabled Child* 135 (January 1981): 56–60.

Parasnis, I. "Visual Perceptual Skills and Deafness." *Journal of the Academy of Rehabilitative Audiology* 16 (1983): 148–160.

Pickett, J. "Speech Technology and Communication for the Hearing Impaired." In *Learning Technology and the Hearing Impaired,* edited by F. Withrow. *Volta Review* 83, no. 5 (1981): 301–309.

———. *The Sounds of Speech Communication.* Baltimore, MD: University Park Press, 1980.

———, and W. F. McFarland. "Auditory Implants and Tactile Aids for the Profoundly Deaf." *Journal of Speech and Hearing Research* 28 (1985): 134–150.

Pimental A. T. "A Barrier-Free Environment for Deaf People." *The Deaf American* 32, no. 5 (1980): 7–9.

Plomp, R. *Aspects of Tone Sensation.* New York: Academic Press, 1976.

Poizner, H. "Visual and Phonetic Coding of Movement: Evidence from American Sign Language." *Science* 212 (1981): 691–693.

Polack, D. *Educational Audiology for the Limited-Hearing Infant.* Springfield, IL: Thomas, 1970.

Pollack, M., ed. *Amplification for the Hearing Impaired.* New York: Grune & Stratton, 1980.

Potter, R., G. Kopp and H. Kopp. *Visible Speech.* New York: Van Nostrand, 1947.

Punch, J. "The Prevalence of Hearing Impairment." *ASHA* 25, no. 4 (1983): 27.

Quigley, S. P., and R. E. Kretshmer. *The Eduation of Deaf Children: Issues, Theory and Practice.* Baltimore, MD: University Park Press, 1982.

Rainer, J. D., K. Z. Altshuler and F. J. Kallmann, eds. *Family and Mental Health Problems in a Deaf Population.* Springfield, IL: Thomas, 1969.

Ramsdell, D. A. "The Psychology of the Hard of Hearing and Deafened Adult." In *Hearing and Deafness,* 499–510. New York: Rinehart & Winston, 1978.

Reardon, W. "Sex-linked deafness," *Journal of Medical Genetics* 27, no. 6 (June 1990): 376–9.

Riccardi, V. M. "A Geneticist's Approach to Deafness." *Volta Review* 81, no. 1 (1979): 9–14.

Riekehof, Lottie L. *The Joy of Signing.* Springfield, MO: Gospel Publishing House, 1987.

Roeser, Ross, and Marion Downs. *Auditory Disorders in School Children: The Law—Identification—Remediation.* New York: Thieme-Stratton, 1981.

Ross, M., and T. Giolas. *Auditory Management of Hearing-Impaired Children.* Baltimore, MD: University Park Press, 1978.

———, and L. Nober, eds. *Educating Hard of Hearing Children.* Washington, DC: Alexander Graham Bell Association for the Deaf, 1981.

Rupp, R. "The Roles of the Audiologist." *Journal of the Academy of Rehabilitation Audiology* 10, no. 1 (1977): 10–17.

Rutman, D. "The impact and experience of adventitious deafness," *American Annals of the Deaf* 134, no. 5 (Dec. 1989): 305–11.

Rybak, L. P. "Drug Ototoxicity." *Annual Review of Pharmacology and Toxiology* 26 (1986): 79–99.

Sanders, D. *Aural Rehabilitation: A Management Approach.* Englewood Cliffs, NJ: Prentice-Hall, 1982.

Sataloff, Joseph, M.D., and Paul L. Michael, Ph.D. *Hearing Conservation.* Springfield, IL: Thomas, 1973.

Sattler, J. *Assessment of Children's Intelligence and Special Abilities.* 2d ed. Boston: Allyn and Bacon, 1982.

Schaeffer, Benson, Arlene Musil and George Kollinzas. *Total Communication: A Signed Speech Program for Nonverbal Children.* Springfield, IL: Research Press, 1980.

Schein, J., and M. T. Delk. *Deaf Population of the United States.* Silver Spring, MD: National Association of the Deaf, 1974.

———. *The Deaf Community.* Washington, DC: Gallaudet College Press, 1968.

———, "Survey of Health Care for Deaf People." *The Deaf American* 32, no. 5 (1980): 5–6, 17.

Schlesinger, H., and K. Meadow. *Sound and Sign: Childhood Deafness and Mental Health.* Berkeley, University of California, 1974.

———. "Language Acquisition in Four Deaf Children." *Hearing and Speech News* 40 (1972): 4–7, 22–29.

———. "The Effects of Deafness on Childhood Development." In *Deaf Children, Developmental Perspectives,* edited by L. Liben. New York: Academic Press, 1978.

Schildroth, A. N., and M. A. Karchmer, eds. *Deaf Children in America.* San Diego, CA: College-Hill Press, 1986.

Schleuning, A., R. M. Johson and J. A. Vernon. "Masking and Tinnitus." *Ear and Hearing* 6 March–April (2): 71–4 1980.

Schowe, B. *Identity Crisis in Deafness.* Tempe, AZ: Scholars Press, 1979.

Schwartz, Sue. *Choices in Deafness: A Parents' Guide.* Kensington, MD: Woodbine House, 1987.

Scouten, E. L. *Turning Points in the Eduation of Deaf People*. Danville, IL: Interstate, 1984.

Schow, R. L., and M. A. Nerbonne. "Hearing Levels Among Elderly Nursing Home Residents." *Journal of Speech and Hearing Disorders* 45, no 1 (1980): 124.

Schroedel, J. G., and W. Schiff. "Attitudes Towards Deafness Among Several Deaf and Hearing Populations." *Rehabilitative Psychology* 19 (1972): 59–70.

Shambaugh, G. "Diplacusis: A Localizing Symptom of Disease of the Organ of Corti." *Archives of Otolaryngology* 31 (1940): 160.

Sherrick, C. "Basic and Applied Research on Tactile Aids for Deaf People." *Journal of the Acoustical Society of America* 75 (1984) 1325–1342.

Shulman, Joel B. "Ototoxicity." *Ear Diseases, Deafness and Dizziness*. Hagerstown, MD: Harper and Row, 1979.

Solow, S. *Sign Language Interpreting: A Basic Resource Book*. Silver Spring, MD: National Association of the Deaf, 1981.

Spradley, Thomas S., and James P. Spradley. *Deaf Like Me*. Washington, DC: Gallaudet University Press, 1978.

Spellman, E. D. "Community Services for the Deaf." In *Deafness Annual*. Vol. IV, 91–95. Silver Spring, MD: Professional Rehabilitation Workers With the Adult Deaf, 1974.

Stern, V. W., and M. R. Redden. *Selected Telecommunication Devices for Hearing-Impaired Persons*. Washington, DC: Congress of the United States, Office of Technology Assessment, 1982.

Sternberg, M., C. Tipton and J. Schein. *Curriculum Guide for Interpreter Training*. New York: New York University, 1973.

Stone, H. "Hearing Loss and Mental Health." *Shhh* 3, no. 6 (November/December 1982).

Sullivan, P., and M. Vernon. "Psychological Assessment of Hearing-Impaired Children." *School Psychology Review* 8, no. 3 (1979): 271–290.

Switzer, M. E., and B. R. Williams. "Life Problems of Deaf People: Prevention and Treatment." *Archives of Environmental Health* 15 (1967): 249–256.

Taylor, D., and G. Mencher. "Neonate Response: The Effect of Infant State and Auditory Stimuli." *Archives of Otolaryngology* 95 (1972): 120–124.

Travis, Lee Edward. *Handbook of Speech Pathology and Audiology*. New York: Appleton-Century-Crofts, 1971.

Van Cleve, J. V., ed. *Gallaudet Encyclopedia of Deaf People and Deafness*. New York: McGraw-Hill, 1987.

Van Itallie, Philip. *How to Live With a Hearing Handicap*. New York: Eriksson, 1963.

Vernon, M. "Sociological and Psychological Factors Associated with Hearing Loss." *Journal of Speech and Hearing Research* 12 (1969): 541–563.

———. "Current Etiological Factors in Deafness." *American Annals of the Deaf* 113, no. 2 (1968): 106–115.

———. "Prematurity and Deafness." *Exceptional Children* 33, no. 5 (1967): 289–298.

———. "Tinnitus." *Hearing Aid Journal* 13 (1975): 82–83.

———. "The Employment Picture: Deafness and Mental Health," *Rehabilitation Lit.* 38 (6–7): 188–92 June–July 1977.

———. "Fifty Years of Research on the Intelligence of the Deaf and Hard-of-Hearing." *Journal of Rehabilitation of the Deaf* 1 (1968) 1–12.

Walker, C. H. "Neonatology—then and now. Deafness in children of very low birth weight," *Archives of the Disabled Child* November 64(11), 1989: 1646.

Wallenfels, Herman. *Hearing Aids for Nerve Deafness.* Springfield, IL: Thomas, 1971.

Wax, Teena, and Loraine DiPietro. *Managing Hearing Loss Later in Life.* Washington, DC: National Information Center on Deafness/American Speech-Language-Hearing Association, 1987.

Webster, D., and M. Webster. "Neonatal Sound Deprivation Affects Brainstem Auditory Nuclei." *Archives of Otolaryngology* 103 (1977): 392–6.

Wightman, F., and D. Green. "The Perception of Pitch." *American Scientist* 62 (1974): 208–215.

Wilbur, R. *American Sign Language and Sign Systems.* Baltimore, MD: University Park Press, 1979.

Williamson, W. D., M. M. Desmond, N. LaFevers, L. H. Taber, F. I. Catlin, and T. G. Weaver. "Symptomatic Congenital Cytomegalovirus: Disorders of Language, Learning and Hearing." *American Journal of Diseases of Children* 136 (1982): 902–905.

Williams, Peggy and Linda Jacobs-Condit. *Hearing Aids: What Are They?* Washington, DC: National Information Center on Deafness/American Speech-Language-Hearing Association, 1987.

Woodward, J. "Historical Bases of American Sign Language." In *Understanding Language Through Sign Language Research,* edited by R. Siple. New York: Academic Press, 1978.

Yoken, C., ed. *Interpreter Training: The State of the Art.* Washington, DC: The National Academy of Gallaudet College, 1980.

Yost, William, and D. Nielsen. *Fundamentals of Hearing: An Introduction.* New York: Holt, Rinehart and Winston, 1972.

Youniss, J. *Parents and Peers in Social Development.* Chicago: University of Chicago Press, 1980.

Zieziula, F., ed. *Assessment of Hearing Impaired People: A Guide for Selecting Psychological, Educational and Vocational Tests.* Washington, DC: Gallaudet College Press, 1982.

SUGGESTED READINGS FOR CHILDREN AND PARENTS

For Children:

Arthur, Catherine. *My Sister's Silent World.* Chicago: Children's Press, 1979.

Blatchford, Claire. *Yes, I Wear A Hearing Aid.* New York: Lexington School for the Deaf, 1976.

Glazzard, Margaret H. *Meet Camille & Danielle: They Are Special Persons.* Lawrence, KS: H&H Enterprises, 1978.

Hlibok, Bruce. *Silent Dancer.* New York: Messner, 1981.

LaMore, Gregory S. *Now I Understand.* Washington, DC: Gallaudet University Press.

Peter, Diana. *Claire and Emma.* New York: John Day, 1976.

Peterson, Jeanne W. *I Have A Sister, My Sister Is Deaf.* New York: Harper and Row, 1977.

Rosenberg, Maxine. *My Friend Leslie: The Story of a Handicapped Child.* New York: Lothrop, Lee & Shepard, 1983.

Scott, Virginia. *Belonging.* Washington, DC: Gallaudet University Press, 1986.

Sullivan, Mary Beth, Alan Brightman, Joseph Blatt, Margaret Roberts, JoAnn W. Fiske. *Feeling Free.* Reading, MA: Addison-Wesley, 1979.

Walker, Lou Ann. *Amy, the Story of a Deaf Child.* New York: Lodestar Books/Dutton, 1985.

Wolf, Bernard. *Anna's Silent World.* New York: Lippincott, 1977.

For Parents:

Angus, Jean R. *Watch My Words: An Open Letter to Parents of Young Deaf Children.* Cincinnati, OH: Forward Movement Publications, 1974.

Benderly, Beryl L. *Dancing Without Music: Deafness in America.* New York: Anchor Press/Doubleday, 1980.

Featherstone, Helen. *A Difference In The Family, Living With a Disabled Child.* New York: Penguin Books, 1981.

Ferris, Caren. *A Hug Just Isn't Enough.* Washington, DC: Gallaudet University Press, 1980.

Forecki, Marcia C. *Speak to Me.* Washington, DC: Gallaudet University Press, 1985.

Frederickson, Jeannette. *Life After Deaf.* Silver Spring, MD: National Association of the Deaf, 1985.

Glick, Ferne P., and D. Pellman. *Breaking Silence: A Family Grows With Deafness.* Scotsdale, PA: Herald Press, 1982.

Harris, George. *Broken Ears, Wounded Hearts.* Washington, DC: Gallaudet University Press, 1983.

Katz, Lee, Steve Mathis and Edward Merrill. *The Deaf Child in the Public Schools: A Handbook for Parents.* Danville, IL: Interstate Printers and Publishers, 1978.

Ling, Daniel, ed. *Early Intervention for Hearing-Impaired Children: Oral Options.* San Diego, CA: College Hill Press, 1984.

Luterman, David. *Deafness in the Family.* Boston, MA: Little, Brown, 1987.

McArthur, Shirley. *Raising Your Hearing-Impaired Child: A Guideline for Parents.* Washington, DC: Alexander Graham Bell Association for the Deaf, 1982.

Meadow, Kathryn P. *Deafness and Child Development.* Berkeley, CA: University of California Press, 1980.

Mendelsohn, Jacqueline Z., and Bonnie Fairchild. *Years of Challenge, A Guide For Parents of Hearing Impaired Adolescents.* Silver Spring, MD: National Association of the Deaf, 1982.

Ogden, Paul, and Suzanne Lipsett. *The Silent Garden: Understanding The Hearing Impaired Child.* New York: St. Martin's Press, 1982.

Schein, Jerome, and D. Naiman. *For Parents of Deaf Children.* Silver Spring, MD: National Association of the Deaf, 1978.

Schwartz, Sue, ed. *Choices in Deafness: A Parents' Guide.* Kensington, MD: Woodbine House, 1987.

Spradley, Thomas S., and James P. Spradley. *Deaf Like Me.* Washington, DC: Gallaudet University Press, 1985.

Tweedie, David, and Edgar Shroyer, eds. *The Multihandicapped Hearing Impaired: Identification and Instruction.* Washington, DC: Gallaudet University Press, 1982.

INDEX

C

D

E

F

G